Donated To: Cardiology Library
St. Luke's Episcopal Hospital

Date: April 10, 1989

By: C.M.E. Associates
1022 Main Street
Dunedin, Florida 34698

1988
YEAR BOOK OF
CARDIOLOGY®

The 1988 Year Book® Series

Year Book of Anesthesia®: Drs. Miller, Kirby, Ostheimer, Roizen, and Stoelting

Year Book of Cancer®: Drs. Hickey and Saunders

Year Book of Cardiology®: Drs. Schlant, Collins, Engle, Frye, Kaplan, and O'Rourke

Year Book of Critical Care Medicine®: Drs. Rogers, Allo, Dean, McPherson, Michael, Miller, Traystman, and Wetzel

Year Book of Dentistry®: Drs. Cohen, Hendler, Johnson, Jordan, Moyers, Robinson, and Silverman

Year Book of Dermatology®: Drs. Sober and Fitzpatrick

Year Book of Diagnostic Radiology®: Drs. Bragg, Hendee, Keats, Kirkpatrick, Miller, Osborn, and Thompson

Year Book of Digestive Diseases®: Drs. Greenberger and Moody

Year Book of Drug Therapy®: Drs. Hollister and Lasagna

Year Book of Emergency Medicine®: Dr. Wagner

Year Book of Endocrinology®: Drs. Bagdade, Braverman, Halter, Horton, Korenman, Kornel, Metz, Molitch, Morley, Robertson, Rogol, Ryan, and Vaitukaitis

Year Book of Family Practice®: Drs. Rakel, Avant, Driscoll, Prichard, and Smith

Year Book of Geriatrics and Gerontology: Drs. Beck, Abrass, Burton, Cummings, Makinodan, and Small

Year Book of Hand Surgery®: Drs. Dobyns, Chase, and Amadio

Year Book of Hematology: Drs. Spivak, Bell, Ness, Quesenberry, and Wiernik

Year Book of Infectious Diseases®: Drs. Wolff, Barza, Keusch, Klempner, and Snydman

Year Book of Medicine®: Drs. Rogers, Des Prez, Cline, Braunwald, Greenberger, Wilson, Epstein, and Malawista

Year Book of Neurology and Neurosurgery®: Drs. DeJong, Currier, and Crowell

Year Book of Nuclear Medicine®: Drs. Hoffer, Gore, Gottschalk, Sostman, Zaret, and Zubal

Year Book of Obstetrics and Gynecology®: Drs. Mishell, Kirschbaum, and Morrow

Year Book of Ophthalmology®: Drs. Ernest and Deutsch

Year Book of Orthopedics®: Dr. Coventry

Year Book of Otolaryngology–Head and Neck Surgery®: Drs. Bailey and Paparella

Year Book of Pathology and Clinical Pathology®: Drs. Brinkhous, Dalldorf, Grisham, Langdell, and McLendon

Year Book of Pediatrics®: Drs. Oski and Stockman

Year Book of Perinatal/Neonatal Medicine: Drs. Klaus and Fanaroff

Year Book of Plastic and Reconstructive Surgery®: Drs. McCoy, Brauer, Haynes, Hoehn, Miller, and Whitaker

Year Book of Podiatric Medicine and Surgery®: Dr. Jay

Year Book of Psychiatry and Applied Mental Health®: Drs. Freedman, Lourie, Meltzer, Talbott, and Weiner

Year Book of Pulmonary Disease: Drs. Green, Ball, Menkes, Michael, Peters, Terry, Tockman, and Wise

Year Book of Rehabilitation: Drs. Kaplan and Szumski

Year Book of Sports Medicine®: Drs. Shepard and Torg, Col. Anderson, and Mr. George

Year Book of Surgery®: Drs. Schwartz, Jonasson, Peacock, Shires, Spencer, and Thompson

Year Book of Urology®: Drs. Gillenwater and Howards

Year Book of Vascular Surgery: Drs. Bergan and Yao

Editor-in-Chief

Robert C. Schlant, M.D.

Professor of Medicine (Cardiology), Division of Cardiology, Department of Medicine, Emory University School of Medicine, Atlanta, Georgia

Editors

John J. Collins, Jr., M.D.

Professor of Surgery, Harvard Medical School; Vice Chairman, Department of Surgery, Director, Sub-Department of Thoracic and Cardiac Surgery, Brigham and Women's Hospital, Boston, Massachusetts

Mary Allen Engle, M.D.

Stavros S. Niarchos Professor of Pediatric Cardiology, Professor of Pediatrics, Director of Pediatric Cardiology, The New York Hospital–Cornell Medical Center, New York, New York

Robert L. Frye, M.D.

Chairman, Department of Medicine, Rose M. and Maurice Eisenberg Professor, Mayo Clinic, Rochester, Minnesota

Norman M. Kaplan, M.D.

Professor of Internal Medicine, Chief, Hypertension Division, University of Texas Southwestern Medical Center, Dallas, Texas

Robert A. O'Rourke, M.D.

Charles Conrad and Anna Sahm Brown Professor of Medicine, Director, Cardiology Division, The University of Texas Health Science Center, San Antonio, Texas

1988

The Year Book of CARDIOLOGY®

Editor-in-Chief
Robert C. Schlant, M.D.

Editors
John J. Collins, Jr., M.D.
Mary Allen Engle, M.D.
Robert L. Frye, M.D.
Norman M. Kaplan, M.D.
Robert A. O'Rourke, M.D.

Year Book Medical Publishers, Inc.
Chicago • London • Boca Raton

Printed in U.S.A.

International Standard Book Number: 0-8151-4207-2

International Standard Serial Number: 0084-4145

Editorial Director, Year Book Publishing: Nancy Gorham
Sponsoring Editor: Bonnie R. Meyers
Manager, Medical Information Services: Laura J. Shedore
Assistant Director, Manuscript Services: Frances M. Perveiler
Associate Managing Editor, Year Book Editing Services: Linda H. Conheady
Production Manager: H.E. Nielsen
Proofroom Supervisor: Shirley E. Taylor

Table of Contents

The material covered in this volume represents literature reviewed up to November 1987.

Journals Represented

Year Book Medical Publishers subscribes to and surveys more than 700 U.S. and foreign medical and allied health journals. From these journals, the Editors select the articles to be abstracted. Journals represented in this YEAR BOOK are listed below.

Acta Medica Scandinavica
American Heart Journal
American Journal of Cardiology
American Journal of Diseases of Children
American Journal of Epidemiology
American Journal of Medicine
American Journal of Noninvasive Cardiology
American Journal of Pathology
American Journal of Physiology
Anesthesiology
Annals of Internal Medicine
Annals of Surgery
Annals of Thoracic Surgery
Archives of Disease in Childhood
Archives of Internal Medicine
British Heart Journal
British Medical Journal
Canadian Family Physician
Cardiovascular Research
Chest
Chinese Medical Journal
Circulation
Circulation Research
Clinical Pharmacology and Therapeutics
Critical Care Medicine
Current Problems in Cardiology
Hypertension
International Journal of Cardiology
Journal of the American College of Cardiology
Journal of the American Medical Association
Journal of Applied Physiology: Respiratory, Environmental and Exercise Physiology
Journal of Cardiovascular Surgery
Journal of Chronic Diseases
Journal of Clinical Investigation
Journal of Clinical Pharmacology
Journal of Hypertension
Journal of Nuclear Medicine
Journal of Pediatrics
Journal of Surgical Research
Journal of Thoracic and Cardiovascular Surgery
Klinische Wochenschrift
Lancet
Mayo Clinic Proceedings
Medical Journal of Australia
Nephron
New England Journal of Medicine
Pediatric Cardiology

Pediatrics
Postgraduate Medical Journal
Presse Medicale
Psychosomatic Medicine
Quarterly Journal of Medicine
Surgery

Publisher's Preface

We welcome Norman Kaplan, M.D., as an Editor of the YEAR BOOK OF CARDIOLOGY. Dr. Kaplan, a Professor of Internal Medicine and Chief of the Hypertension Division at the University of Texas Southwestern Medical Center in Dallas, selected and commented on material related to hypertension.

Introduction

This 1988 YEAR BOOK OF CARDIOLOGY is the 28th in the series. The volume continues the objectives and formats of its predecessors. We are pleased to welcome Norman M. Kaplan to the Editorial Board, where he will have responsibility for hypertension. As before, all section editors have complete freedom to select the articles for inclusion in their areas. Articles are selected for abstracting throughout the year, and occasionally another fine article on the same or a similar subject is published later in the year. In this situation, the editors attempt to refer to the later article in their comments whenever possible and appropriate.

All of the section editors again thank the staff at Year Book Medical Publishers for their assistance, patience, and understanding. In particular, we are indebted to Ms. Nancy Gorham and Ms. Bonnie Meyers.

Robert C. Schlant, M.D.

1 Normal and Altered Cardiovascular Function

Introduction

Clinically relevant, recently published articles concerning cardiovascular physiology, myocardial metabolism, commonly used noninvasive methods, and newer diagnostic and therapeutic techniques are reviewed in this section of the YEAR BOOK OF CARDIOLOGY. Both experimental animal and clinical studies are abstracted and discussed; a list of additional references is provided at the end of each subsection.

In the first subsection on ventricular hypertrophy, the effects of chronic pressure overload or hormonally induced left ventricular hypertrophy on direct ventricular interaction, echocardiographically determined left ventricular mass, rest and exercise myocardial blood flow, myocyte microtubule reorganization, myosin heavy chain isozyme transitions, and left ventricular diastolic function are detailed. The unanswered question concerning the desirability of reversing left ventricular hypertrophy with antihypertensive therapy is again addressed.

The subsection on ventricular diastolic function includes reports on the various determinants of left ventricular isovolumic relaxation, the effects of aging on left ventricular diastolic function, and the direct and indirect effects of calcium entry blocking drugs on left ventricular relaxation. Areas of controversy are highlighted in the editors' comments and in the additional references listed.

The ventricular systolic function subsection provides further detailed information on the left ventricular end-systolic pressure-volume relationship (ESPVR) and the limitations of ESPVR as a sensitive, load-independent indicator of the inotropic state or changes in the inotropic state, particularly when applied in clinical patient studies. Other reports in this subsection concern the effects of verapamil, endurance training, cyclic AMP phosphodiesterase, and aortic valve disease on left ventricular systolic performance; the sympathetic nerve activity during dynamic exercise; and abnormal calcium handling in myocardium from patients with end-stage heart failure.

The subsection on experimental myocardial ischemia/infarction contains several reports on the pathogenesis and pathophysiology of the "stunned" myocardium; the effects of myocardial ischemia on regional myocardial function and stiffness; and the role of granulocytes and oxygen radical formation in myocardial ischemia/infarction and reperfusion injury. The importance of defining the left ventricular region at risk by noninvasive or invasive means when assessing an agent's beneficial effects on "infarct size" is stressed and the use of isopotential surface mapping for detecting experimental right ventricular infarction is detailed. Additional reports concern the detection of myocardial necrosis with Indium-III antimyosin Fab; the detrimental effect of frequent ventricular ectopy on the extent of infarction; and the ability to produce successful coronary thrombolysis in experimental animals by the early intramuscular administration of human tPA with selected absorption enhancers.

The subsection on coronary artery spasm and stenosis details studies concerning a miniature swine model of coronary spasm produced by balloon denudation of regional coronary artery endothelium and the effects of leukotrienes C_4 and D_4 and of a thromboxane A_2 analogue on coronary artery vasomotor tone. Additional information concerning the mechanism by which calcium blockers induce preferential coronary artery dilation (α_1 adrenergic blockade) is described, and the usefulness of high-frequency epicardial echocardiography and quantitative angiographic methods for assessing the extent of coronary atherosclerosis is reviewed.

The noninvasive testing subsection includes reports on ECG exercise tests in the detection of asymptomatic myocardial ischemia; the usefulness of Doppler echocardiography for measuring cardiac output, stenotic valve areas, and left ventricular diastolic function; and the role of nuclear cardiology methods in defining patients needing catheterization and for assessing the results of coronary thrombolysis in patients with acute myocardial infarction.

The final subsection on newer diagnostic and therapeutic techniques describes the potential usefulness of ultrafast computed tomography for quantitating regional myocardial perfusion; the accuracy of nuclear magnetic resonance imaging (NMRI) for quantitating aortic and mitral regurgitation in patients; the possible use of NMRI for early detection of adriamycin toxicity; and the potential application of NMRS for detecting cardiac allograft rejection. Additional animal studies of clinical importance concern the safe and effective catheter ablation of the atrioventricular junction using radio frequency energy and the lack of myocardial injury produced by multiple defibrillating shocks in dogs undergoing serial testing of the efficacy of an automatic implantable cardioverter/defibrillator.

Robert A. O'Rourke, M.D.

Ventricular Hypertrophy

Chronic Pressure Overload Hypertrophy Decreases Direct Ventricular Interaction

Bryan K. Slinker, Antonio Carlos, P. Chagas, and Stanton A. Glantz (Univ. of California, San Francisco)

Am. J. Physiol. 253:H347–H357, August 1987 1–1

Right ventricular volume can influence left ventricular volume through series interaction, as the right heart output becomes the left heart input, and through direct interaction of the shared interventricular septum. Disease states that alter direct ventricular interaction will complicate assessment of left ventricular function. In hypertrophied hearts, direct interaction has not been well characterized. Therefore, the relative importance of direct interaction at end diastole and end systole, with and without the pericardium, was studied in dogs with concentric hypertrophy induced by chronic renovascular hypertension.

At end diastole, direct interaction was only approximately 10% as important as series interaction in determining left ventricular size. At end systole, direct interaction was approximately 20% as important as the pressure-volume relationship in determining left ventricular size. After removal of the pericardium, direct interaction became even less important in determining left ventricular size.

Because of the changing role of direct ventricular interaction, the slope of the end-systolic pressure-volume relationship is not comparable between normal and hypertrophic hearts. This further complicates clinical application of the end-systolic pressure-volume relationship.

▶ Direct ventricular interaction normally causes both left ventricular end-diastolic and end-systolic pressure-volume relationships to deviate from what they would be if no direct interaction occurred. The effects of ventricular interaction are reduced when the pericardium is removed. The study by Slinker and associates indicates that the influence of direct interaction between the ventricles on assessment of left ventricular function is decreased significantly when the left ventricular hypertrophies. Moreover, since the magnitude of direct ventricular interaction is different in normal as compared with hypertrophied hearts, pressure-volume relationships from normal and hypertrophied hearts cannot be compared simply.—R.A. O'Rourke, M.D.

Echocardiographic Left Ventricular Mass and Function in the Hypertensive Baboon

Michael H. Crawford, Richard A. Walsh, David Cragg, Gregory L. Freeman, and Jacelyn Miller (Univ. of Texas, San Antonio)

Hypertension 10:339–345, September 1987 1–2

Cardiac anatomy of nonhuman primates is particularly close to the human situation, and larger animals are better adapted to sophisticated hemodynamic studies. Left ventricular (LV) mass was investigated in the baboon by M-mode echocardiography, and LV size and function in chronic renal hypertension was characterized (Fig 1–1). Chronic hypertension of gradual onset was produced by either the two-kidney, one-clip Goldblatt procedure or by bilateral cellophane-wrap perinephritis.

Autopsy studies validated echographic estimates of LV mass. The reproducibility of echographic LV mass estimation was quite good. Body weight and heart rate were similar in hypertensive and normotensive animals, but peak systolic LV pressure was greater in the hypertensive animals, as was end-diastolic LV posterior wall thickness. The LV cross-

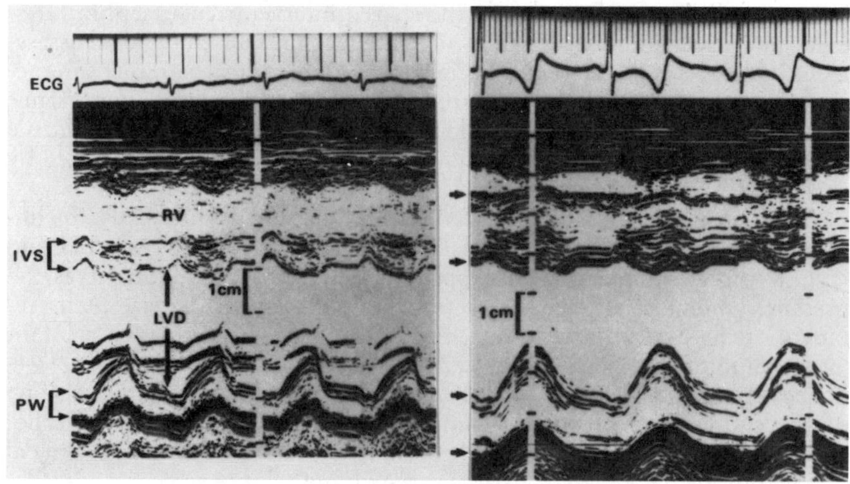

Fig 1–1.—M-mode echocardiograms of the left ventricle in a normotensive control baboon (**left**) and a hypertensive animal (**right**). *ECG,* electrocardiogram; *RV,* right ventricle; *IVS,* interventricular septum; *LVD,* left ventricular dimension: *PW,* posterior wall. *Arrows* indicate wall thickness. (Courtesy of Crawford, M.H., et al.: Hypertension 100:339–345, September 1987.)

sectional area and calculated mass were 44% greater in hypertensive animals, despite similar LV cavity dimensions. Rates of LV dimensional change and wall-thickness change in systole and diastole were about 25% less in hypertensive than in normotensive animals, despite matched heart rates and LV stress values. The overall percent change in cavity dimension and wall thickness in systole was not significantly altered in the hypertensive group.

The biochemical basis for load-independent changes in LV function resulting from hypertensive pressure-overload hypertrophy in higher mammals requires further study. M-mode echocardiography appears to be a useful means of following LV performance in a nonhuman primate model of pressure-overload hypertrophy.

▶ This study shows the feasibility of using M-mode echocardiography for the serial noninvasive assessment of left ventricular size and performance in the nonhuman primate with experimentally produced renal hypertension. Echocardiographically determined left ventricular mass accurately estimated postmortem left ventricular weight, and the echocardiographic measurement of mass was highly reproducible. Factors contributing to the hypertrophy process, such as altered myocardial contractility, relaxation, or material properties, may have accounted for the abnormal left ventricular chamber performance observed in this animal model. The depressed rates of LV chamber emptying and filling observed in these hypertrophied baboons are consistent with those of other studies of experimental renal hypertension.—R.A. O'Rourke, M.D.

Myocardial Blood Flow in Left Ventricular Hypertrophy Developing in Young and Adult Dogs

Robert J. Bache, David Alyono, Eugene Sublett, and Xue-Zheng Dai (Univ. of Minnesota)
Am. J. Physiol. 251:H949–H956, November 1986 1–3

It is well established that the pressure-overloaded, hypertrophied left ventricle has increased vulnerability to ischemia. Most investigators have reported normal or near normal values for blood flow during resting conditions in subjects with left ventricular hypertrophy. However, vasodilator reserve capacity has been found to be impaired during pharmacologically induced coronary vasodilation. It is thought that this abnormality is related to inadequate growth of coronary vasculature as hypertrophy occurs, so that coronary cross-sectional area fails to increase in proportion to the increase in myocardial mass. The present study was designed to test the hypothesis that growth of coronary vasculature would be facilitated if myocardial hypertrophy occurred during the period of normal body growth rather than in mature adult animals.

The authors caused left ventricular hypertrophy by banding the ascending aorta in 8 young dogs, 7 weeks of age, and in 9 adult dogs. The adult dogs were investigated 2 months after aortic banding, and the young dogs were allowed to grow to adulthood before study. The ratios of left ventricular weight to body weight were increased to 6.88 ± 0.36 gm/kg in the young dogs and to 6.64 ± 0.47 gm/kg in adult dogs; both values were markedly greater than those of 7 normal control animals (4.32 ± 0.05). The myocardial blood flow per gram, determined using microspheres during resting conditions, was substantially higher in young dogs with left ventricular hypertrophy than in normal dogs (Fig 1–2). The myocardial blood flow rates during maximum coronary vasodilation with adenosine were similar in all three groups; however, since mean coronary perfusion pressure was higher in the dogs with aortic banding, the minimum coronary vascular resistance per gram of myocardium was

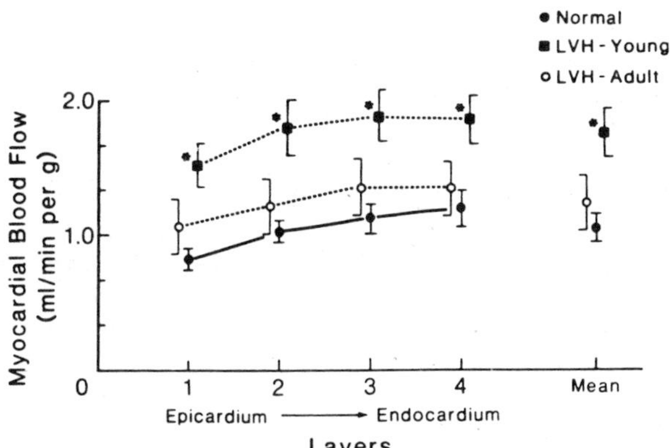

Fig 1–2.—Left ventricular myocardial blood flow during sinus rhythm to 4 transmural layers from epicardium to endocardium in 7 normal dogs, 8 dogs with left ventricular hypertrophy (LVH) produced by banding ascending aorta as puppies (LVH-Young), and 9 dogs in which LVH was produced by banding ascending aorta in adult dogs (LVH-Adult). **P*<.05 in comparison with normal dogs. (Courtesy of Bache, R.J., et al.: Am. J. Physiol. 251:H949–H956, November 1986.)

markedly higher in both young (21.1 ± 3.1 mm Hg/ml/min/gm) and adult dogs with left ventricular hypertrophy (21.8 ± 2.2) than in the normal dogs (16.8 ± 3.1). Finally, the mean coronary vascular resistance for the total left ventricle was similar in all three groups of animals, indicating that growth of coronary vasculature did not occur as the myocardium underwent hypertrophy.

These results suggest that left ventricular hypertrophy beginning at 7 weeks of age and continuing through the subsequent period of normal body growth leads to an impairment of minimum coronary vascular resistance similar to that seen when hypertrophy begins after the animals have reached adulthood.

▶ The importance of this study by Bache and associates is that left ventricular hypertrophy produced by pressure overload results in the impairment of minimum coronary vascular resistance per gram of myocardium regardless of whether hypertrophy develops during the period of normal body growth or after the animal has reached adulthood. The results are similar and consistent with previous studies by the same investigators showing impairment in myocardial blood flow during exercise but not at rest in adult dogs with pressure-overload hypertrophy produced by renovascular hypertension. It is likely that the decreased ratio of subendocardial to subepicardial blood flow observed during maximum coronary vasodilation in the hypertrophied heart is a result of a greater decrease in vascular density in the subendocardium.—R.A. O'Rourke, M.D.

Microtubule Reorganization Is Related to Rate of Heart Myocyte Hypertrophy in Rat

Jane-Lyse Samuel, Françoise Marotte, Claude Delcayre, and Lydie Rappaport (Hôpital Lariboisière, Paris, France)

Am. J. Physiol. 251:H1118–H1125, December 1986 1–4

Microtubules have been shown to increase in number both during the early phase of postnatal development and during active or compensatory hypertrophy. The authors contend that to substantiate the reports that microtubules have a role in the process of heart myocyte hypertrophy, it must be established whether the alterations occurring in the microtubule pattern are invariably related to this process, regardless of the type of growth stimulus applied. They sought to verify that the microtubule network in heart myocytes densified during postnatal growth in euthyroid rats and in hypothyroid rats whose growth was stimulated by 4 μg per day of L-thyroxine (T_4).

To carry out these studies, tubulin, the constituent protein of microtubules, was immunolabeled in myocytes isolated at various times after birth. The authors evaluated myocyte hypertrophy by myocyte size, the number of nuclei per cells and isomyosin expression. It was found that in hypothyroid rats, the microtubule network, which was underdeveloped, was most dense around the nucleus. In addition, during the phase of fast myocyte hypertrophy observed in euthyroid rats during late postnatal development and in hypothyroid rats after T_4 administration, transient microtubule densification occurred in a myocyte subpopulation in which size was mainly determined by the rate of myocyte hypertrophy. The densification process and its kinetics were similar to those observed when heart hypertrophy was induced by pressure overload.

In rat heart myocytes undergoing hypertrophy, microtubule densification might be related to fast sarcomerogenesis, whether the stimulus is mechanical (e.g., pressure overload) or hormonal (e.g., T_4).

▶ The data reported in this study indicate a link between increased microtubule density and rapid myocyte hypertrophy in models of postnatal rat heart development with different growth weights due to a thyroxine imbalance. When considered relative to data previously obtained in mechanically hypertrophied hearts, these results provide evidence that the reorganization of microtubules in cardiac myocytes is related to the onset of hypertrophy, whether these cells are stimulated mechanically or hormonally.—R.A. O'Rourke, M.D.

Myosin Heavy Chain Messenger RNA and Protein Isoform Transitions During Cardiac Hypertrophy: Interaction Between Hemodynamic and Thyroid Hormone-Induced Signals

Seigo Izumo, Anne-Marie Lompré, Rumiko Matsuoka, Gideon Koren, Ketty Schwartz, Bernardo Nadal-Ginard, and Vijak Mahdavi (Harvard Med. School and Beth Israel Hosp., Boston and Institut Natl. de la Sante et de la Recherche Med. Hosp. Lariboisiere, Paris)

J. Clin. Invest. 79:970–977, March 1987 1–5

Both hormonal stimuli and hemodynamic loading regulate expression of the cardiac myosin isozymes during development. The authors studied levels of expression of the alpha and beta isoforms of myosin heavy chain (MHC) during cardiac hypertrophy in the rat. Significant hypertrophy was produced by constricting the abdominal aorta. Analyses of MHC mRNA and myosin isozymes were carried out.

Alpha-MHC mRNA predominated in the ventricular myocardium of normal rats and sham-operated animals. Rapid induction of β-MHC mRNA followed aortic coarctation, and comparable levels of β-MHC protein ensued as left ventricular weight increased (Fig 1–3). Administration of thyroxine to animals with aortic coarctation led to rapid deinduction of β-MHC and induction of α-MHC, at both the mRNA and protein levels. Left ventricular hypertrophy nevertheless progressed.

These findings suggest that hemodynamic overload leads to induction of the β-MHC gene in the presence of physiologic levels of thyroid hormone. Isozyme transition during overload apparently is regulated chiefly by pretranslational mechanisms, as evidenced by the close correlation between relative levels of MHC mRNAs and the corresponding proteins. Many pathophysiologic states such as exercise, diabetes, and starvation can modulate the cardiac MHC isozyme distribution. It remains to be

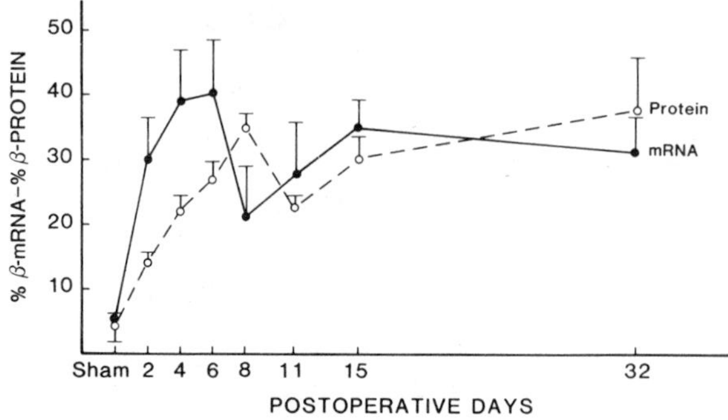

Fig 1–3.—β-MHC gene expression during aortic coarctation. The time courses of the relative amounts of the β-MHC mRNA *(solid circles)* and corresponding protein *(open circles)* in the left ventricles are shown. (Courtesy of Izumo, S., et al.: J. Clin. Invest. 79:970–977, March 1987.)

learned whether such stimuli act independently on the expression of MHC genes, or whether their effects are mediated by some common biochemical signal.

▶ Using gene-specific DNA probes, the authors assessed the regulation of myosin heavy chain (MHC) isozyme transitions that are observed during left ventricular hypertrophy. Left ventricular hypertrophy caused by coarctation of the aorta produced a shift of MHC isoforms both at the mRNA and protein levels. When L-thyroxine was administered daily before the operation and continued after the coarctation the induction of the β-MHC gene was prevented at both the mRNA and protein levels. While thyroid hormone appears to regulate the expression of MHC genes at the transcriptional level, it is not known whether its regulation is direct, presumably mediated by T_3-nuclear receptor bound to the regulatory regions of the MHC genes, or indirect, acting through the modulation of secondary intracellular signals.—R.A. O'Rourke, M.D.

Is Reversal of Cardiac Hypertrophy a Desirable Goal of Antihypertensive Therapy?

Robert C. Tarazi and Edward D. Frohlich (Cleveland Clinic Found. and Alton Ochsner Med. Found., New Orleans)
Circulation 75 (Suppl. I):I-113–I-118, January 1987 1–6

Several studies have demonstrated in both man and experimental animals that cardiac hypertrophy may regress toward normal with certain forms of antihypertensive therapy. However, whether this regression or reduction in cardiac mass constitutes an independent therapeutic goal of antihypertensive therapy is unknown. Nor is it known whether this reduction in cardiac mass influences cardiac performance and prognosis, and whether it may actually be deleterious.

In the absence of clinical trials or epidemiologic data regarding the impact of left ventricular hypertrophy (LVH) reversal on the evolution of hypertension, the consequences of that reversal can be evaluated only from any associated changes in cardiac function, e.g., cardiac pumping ability and myocardial contractility. Animal studies have demonstrated that regression of hypertrophy causes a return to normal of the cardiac function curve. However, in hypertensive patients, such indexes of ventricular performance as ejection fraction or velocity of LV circumferential shortening were unchanged after regression of LVH.

With regard to pumping ability, experiments in animals showed that improvement in pumping ability appears to result more from blood pressure reduction. In hypertensive patients there was no reported deterioration in LV performance at rest with reduction in LV mass; however, in these studies blood pressure also was reduced. There have been many echocardiographic studies that have revealed a close and significant correlation between LV end-systolic stress and LV performance as estimated by percent decrease in LV shortening. However, these results are still inadequate to permit conclusions concerning the value or disadvantages of a reduction in ventricular mass. Also, although reduction in cardiac mass has not been associated with deterioration in cardiac function, it is important not to consider the matter decided.

Another important consequence of reversal of LVH on coronary circulation is the influence of the ratio of the driving head of pressure to the ventricular mass (P/LV ratio). Coronary vascular reserve in hypertensive rats remains within normal range when the pressure load on the heart, the degree of LVH, and the driving head of pressure for the coronary circulation are closely related. However, when the coronary arterial pressure and the degree of LVH are dissociated, the coronary vascular reserve is related to the P/LV ratio. If these results are confirmed in man, they may have important clinical implications, because coronary flow reserve after antihypertensive therapy would remain normal if the decrease in blood pressure were associated with a parallel regression of hypertrophy.

▶ The successful reduction of the blood pressure in animals and patients with hypertension commonly causes regression or reduction in cardiac mass when the hypertension is reduced by drugs that either decrease or prevent a reflex elevation in catecholamines. There is considerable controversy as to whether the regression of left ventricular hypertrophy in animals or patients with hypertension is associated with an improvement, a decrease, or no change in myocardial contractility. One of the problems in patients being assessed for such changes in ventricular performance following the treatment of hypertension is that the usual systolic ejection phase indices of left ventricular performance are affected by changes in afterload as well as by changes in myocardial contractility per se.

As indicated by the authors, additional studies are necessary to determine whether or not the regression or reduction of left ventricular hypertrophy in patients being treated successfully for hypertension has a favorable or detrimental effect on left ventricular performance. Studies are needed of left ventricular hypertrophy regression with measurements of ventricular performance before and after regression made at similar afterloads. Also important are studies of groups of animals where a similar reduction in systolic blood pressure is produced with and without regression of hypertrophy, the difference in effect on left ventricular performance of blood pressure control, with and without regression, being assessed in an equivalent manner.—R.A. O'Rourke, M.D.

Left Ventricular Diastolic Function in Hypertensive Patients

Fetnat M. Fouad (Cleveland Clinic Found.)

Circulation 75:I-48–I-55, January 1987 1–7

Indices of left ventricular (LV) filling may be used to noninvasively assess abnormalities in diastolic left ventricular function in hypertensive patients. Such abnormalities are a common and early finding and may be present before other evidence of cardiac involvement in hypertension. Heart rate differences must be taken into account when studying alterations in diastolic indices.

Increased sympathetic drive enhances LV relaxation. Hypertensive patients with hyperkinetic circulation have normal LV filling, while those with essential hypertension do not. The effects of myocardial perfusion on LV diastole in hypertensive patients have not been directly studied, but studies of patients with coronary artery disease suggest a reduced peak rate of LV filling, which is corrected by successful bypass surgery. The complex interaction of cardiac inotropy with ventricular relaxation

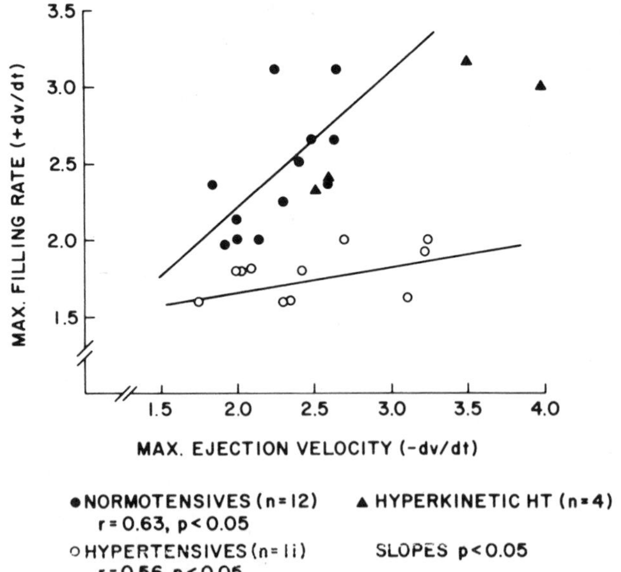

Fig 1–4.—Relationships between left ventricular maximum ejection and filling rates showing reduced left ventricular filling rate in untreated hypertensive patients (○) but not in age-matched normal volunteers (●). Values for hypertensive patients with hyperkinetic circulation (▲) fell closer to those for the normal group. (Courtesy of Fouad, F.M.: Circulation 75:I-48–I-55, January 1987.)

and early filling makes it difficult to determine whether abnormal LV diastolic function is primary or dependent on changes in inotropic state (Fig 1–4). Drug effects on LV filling also are difficult to interpret because of frequent multisystemic actions.

Studies of hypertensive patients using a normalized index, the filling rate/emptying rate ratio, indicated that increased peripheral resistance on head-up tilting is blunted in patients with reduced LV filling. Abnormal diastolic function in hypertension, therefore, may have a role in cardiovascular regulation through altering the sensitivity of cardiopulmonary reflexes. For similar degrees of reduced cardiac output, patients with abnormal LV filling apparently are unable to mobilize equal degrees of adrenergic vasoconstrictor response.

▶ It has been well documented by many investigators that altered left ventricular diastolic function frequently precedes impairment of systolic function in patients with left ventricular hypertrophy resulting from hypertension. Diastolic abnormalities in patients with hypertension include those related to LV relaxation and early filling, and to altered passive pressure-volume characteristics and reduced LV compliance. In this review, the author defines the factors contributing to disturbed early diastolic filling and hypertension, discusses calcium kinetics and abnormalities of early LV diastolic function in hypertension, and concludes that abnormalities of the diastolic function of the left ventricle are a frequent and early feature of hypertension. Impaired diastolic function is important because it can influence evolution of hypertension by influencing systolic performance and by modulating cardiovascular reflex and by affecting hemodynamic responses and changes to intravascular volume.—R.A. O'Rourke, M.D.

Additional recent publications to provide information concerning left ventricular hypertrophy include the following:

1. Meidell, R.S., Sen, A., Henderson S.A., et al.: α_1-Adrenergic stimulation of rat myocardial cells increases protein synthesis. *Am. J. Physiol.* 251(Heart Circ. Physiol.):H1076–H1084, 1986.
2. Parmacek, M.S., Magid, N.M., Lesch, M., et al.: Cardiac protein synthesis and degradation during thyroxine-induced left ventricular hypertrophy. *Am. Physiol. Soc.* (Cell Physiol. 20):C727–C736, 1986.
3. Nagai, R., Pritzl, N., Low, R.B., et al.: Myosin isozyme synthesis and mRNA levels in pressure-overloaded rabbit hearts. *Circ. Res.* 60:692–699, May 1987.
4. Schaible, T., Malhotra, A., Ciambrone, G., et al.: Effect of hypertension on hearts of rats trained by swimming. *J. Appl. Physiol.* 62:328–334, 1987.
5. Coleman, B., Cothran, L.V., Ison-Franklin, E.L., et al.: Estimation of left ventricular mass in conscious dogs. *Am. J. Physiol.* 251(Heart Circ. Physiol. 20):H1149–H1157, 1986.
6. Broughton, A., Korner, P.I.: Left ventricular pump function in renal hypertensive dogs with cardiac hypertrophy. *Am. J. Physiol.* 251(Heart Circ. Physiol. 20):H1260–H1266, 1986.

7. Bache, R.J., Dia, X.Z., Alyono, D., et al.: Myocardial blood flow during exercise in dogs with left ventricular hypertrophy produced by aortic banding and perinephritic hypertension. *Circulation* 76:835–842, 1987.
8. Breisch, E.A., White, F.C., Nimmo, L.E., et al.: Cardiac vasculature and flow during pressure-overload hypertrophy. *Am. J. Physiol.* 251(Heart Circ. Physiol. 20):H1031–H1037, 1986.

Ventricular Diastolic Function

Time Course of Systolic Loading Is an Important Determinant of Ventricular Relaxation

Frank J. Zatko, Paul Martin, and Robert C. Bahler (Case Western Reserve Univ. and Mt. Sinai Med. Ctr., Cleveland)
Am. J. Physiol. 252:H461–H466, March 1987 1–8

In the past decade, there has been increased interest in ventricular relaxation, in part because relaxation abnormalities occur clinically and may precede systolic dysfunction. However, the determinants of relaxation in the intact heart are not well understood, and investigators disagree about physiologic mechanisms that potentially affect relaxation. The effects of increases in systolic load on relaxation in the intact heart were examined.

The authors measured the dependency of left ventricular relaxation on the timing of an abrupt increase in systolic load. The study used ten canine isolated heart-lung preparations, in which a load step of 15 mm Hg was imposed at specific intervals throughout systole, and the time of loading was defined as the interval from the R wave to the completion of the load step (R-load interval). The authors held preload constant and paced the right atrium at a cycle length of 450 msec. The decay of the left ventricular pressure during isovolumic relaxation was described by a single exponential time contrast (T_{exp}), and load effects on isovolumic relaxation were expressed as a percent change in T_{exp} as compared with T_{exp} of the beat preceding the load intervention. Loads imposed early in systole consistently prolonged T_{exp}, and load changes late in systole consistently abbreviated T_{exp}. The transition from augmentation to diminution of T_{exp} always occurred when the R-load interval was 120–130 msec. The mean time interval of electromechanical systole for the test beats was not different from that of the control beats.

The effects of abrupt increases in systolic load on isovolumic relaxation are dependent on the timing of the load.

▶ Many isolated cardiac muscle studies clearly demonstrate the importance of the timing of contraction load steps on diastolic relaxation. This study in the canine isolated heart-lung preparation is consistent with prior studies in isolated muscle showing that load changes late in systole abbreviate the time constant of isovolumic relaxation, which is prolonged by load changes imposed earlier in systole.—R.A. O'Rourke, M.D.

Load-Dependent Relaxation With Late Systolic Volume Steps: Servo-Pump Studies in the Intact Canine Heart

Yoram Ariel, William H. Gaasch, Daniel K. Bogen, and Thomas A. McMahon (Harvard Univ., Tufts Univ., and VA Med. Ctr., Boston)

Circulation 75:1287–1294, June 1987 1–9

An abrupt increase in load in the latter part of contraction leads to premature, more rapid relaxation in isolated heart muscle. An attempt was made to learn whether this load-dependent relaxation can be observed in the intact heart. Left ventricular responses to abrupt increments in load throughout the cardiac cycle were studied using a microcomputer-controlled servo-pump attached to the cardiac apex. Use of a single-beat basis for the studies made it possible to minimize reflex and other feedback mechanisms that might influence the results.

In ejecting beats, an early volume step immediately after aortic valve opening led to a 3% increase in duration of systole. A late volume step just before aortic valve closure led to a 7% decrease in the duration of systole. In nonejecting beats with aortic occlusion, early volume steps led to an increase in duration of systole, whereas later steps decreased the duration of systole.

Load-dependent relaxation is observed in the intact canine heart. Changes in the mechanisms underlying this phenomenon might explain disordered relaxation in clinical and experimental studies of the diastolic properties of the left ventricle. The inability of cardiac muscle to bear a late systolic load increment could limit the use of late systolic pressure volume data in assessing left ventricular contractility.

▶ The results of this study in the intact ejecting canine heart are consistent with the results abstracted above. Importantly, a volume step immediately after aortic valve opening led to a 3% increase in the duration of systole, while the volume step just before the aortic valve closure led to a 7% decrease in the duration of systole. The prolongation of isovolumic relaxation by a late systolic load increment could explain disorders of left ventricular relaxation occurring in various clinical and experimental cardiac diseases such as hypertension. Also, the inability of cardiac muscles to bear late systolic load increments may limit the use of late systolic pressure-volume data in assessing left ventricular systolic function (see the next abstract).—R.A. O'Rourke, M.D.

Atrial Kinetics and Left Ventricular Diastolic Filling in the Healthy Elderly

Rohit R. Arora, Josef Machac, Martin E. Goldman, Robert N. Butler, Richard Gorlin, and Steven F. Horowitz (The Mount Sinai Med. Ctr., New York)

J. Am. Coll. Cardiol. 9:1255–1260, June 1987 1–10

A delay of left ventricular isovolumic relaxation and decrease in myocardial compliance may result in a decline of measured early filling rates in elderly subjects. However, previous studies of diastolic function have

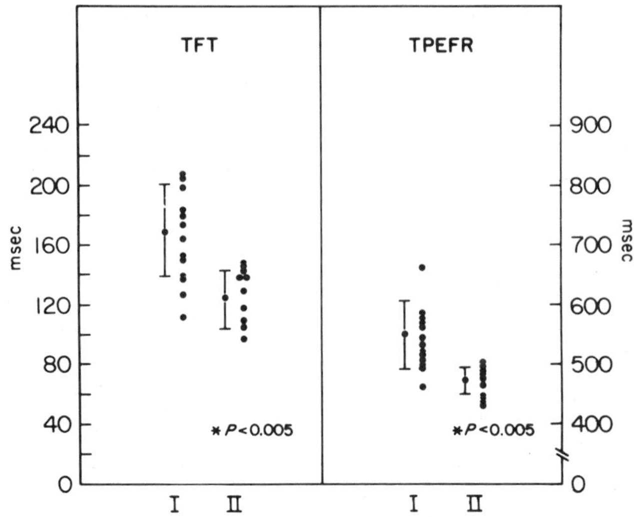

Fig 1–5.—Comparison of time to peak early filling rate (TPEFR) and time of first third filling (TFT) in the elderly (group I) and the younger subjects (group II), showing statistically significant differences in both parameters. (Courtesy of Arora, R.R., et al.: J. Am. Coll. Cardiol 9:1255–1260, June 1987.)

not excluded occult coronary artery disease or addressed the contribution of atrial contraction to diastole. The kinetics of early and late diastolic filling were evaluated in 13 healthy elderly volunteers, aged 75 ± 6 years, using high temporal resolution gated blood pool scintigraphy. These subjects had no symptoms or risk factors for coronary disease and demonstrated normal findings on stress ECG, stress gated blood pool imaging, and two-dimensional echocardiogram.

In the healthy elderly, peak early diastolic filling rate was decreased and both the time of peak early filling and the time to first third of diastolic filling were delayed compared with values obtained from 10 healthy young volunteers, aged 26 ± 5 years (Fig 1–5). The peak late filling rate and percent atrial filling volume were augmented in the elderly.

Both atrial filling velocities and atrial volume are augmented in the healthy elderly, together with declining early peak filling velocities of the left ventricle. Possibly, the atrial changes are an adaptive response of the atria to diminished left ventricular compliance.

▶ Previous noninvasive and invasive studies of diastolic function in both aging humans and experimental animals indicate a progressive decline in diastolic functioning with increasing age. A progressive increase in systolic blood pressure and left ventricular wall thickness with a decrease in left ventricular compliance has been documented in the elderly. In this study, high temporal resolution radionuclide ventricular scintigraphy was used to assess diastolic filling in elderly volunteers with no other evidence of cardiac disease.

Although the noninvasive technique utilized has some limitations in defining left ventricular diastolic function, the data indicate that atrial contribution to left ventricular filling increases with aging, with the reduced early filling velocities suggesting abnormal isovolumetric relaxation, reduced compliance of the ventricle or both. Interestingly, the wall thickness measured by ultrasound was normal in these patients; however, the serial assessment of wall thickness during many studies over several decades may be necessary to show a change during the aging process.—R.A. O'Rourke, M.D.

Effects of Verapamil, Nifedipine, and Dilazep on Left Ventricular Relaxation in the Conscious Dog

Massimo Pagani, Paolo Pizzinelli, Raffaello Furlan, Stefano Guzzetti, Ornella Rimoldi, and Giulia Sandrone (Univ. of Milan)

Cardiovasc. Res. 21:55–64, January 1987 1–11

Recently, there has been much interest in calcium channel blocking drugs because of their clinical efficacy in common pathophysiologic situations including coronary artery disease and hypertension. However, the effects of calcium channel blockers on myocardial relaxation have been investigated less extensively. The goal of the study was to determine the cardiac systolic and diastolic effects of the two major calcium channel blocking drugs, verapamil and nifedipine, and to compare them with the effects of dilazep, a relatively new vasodilator with calcium channel blocking abilities.

The study was carried out using conscious instrumented dogs to avoid the complications of anesthesia and recent surgery. The mean arterial pressure was reduced by nifedipine and dilazep but not by verapamil. In contrast, peak left ventricular pressure was reduced only by dilazep and verapamil. There was consistent tachycardia, with the highest rate observed with nifedipine and the lowest rate observed with dilazep. The left ventricular dP/dt was not changed by dilazep, was reduced by verapamil, and was increased by nifedipine; however, this increase was no longer seen after β-adrenergic blockade. When ventricular relaxation was assessed calculating the time relaxation constant, tau, it was found that verapamil significantly increased tau only after β-adrenergic blockade, whereas nifedipine and dilazep reduced it both before and after β-adrenergic blockade.

Reflex β-adrenergic mechanisms may modulate the effects of calcium channel blockers on both systolic and diastolic performance.

▶ In this study, the effects of three calcium entry blocking drugs, when given intravenously, on the time constant of isovolumic relaxation were assessed, the effects on isovolumic being closely linked to alterations in the preceding left ventricular systole. In previous comparative studies of the effect of the three calcium blockers on isovolumic relaxation in the conscious dog when given intravenously (affecting systolic pressure, heart rate, and myocardial contractility) and when given intracoronary (producing only regional decreases in myocardial contractility), the direct effect of these drugs is to prolong isovolumic relaxation. The direct effect is masked by changes in systolic hemodynamics produced by these drugs when they are given systemically (Walsh, R.A., O'Rourke, R.A.: *JCI* 75:1426–1434, 1985).

Consistent with the study by Pagani et al., verapamil caused the greatest prolongation of isovolumic relaxation, an effect that was significantly potentiated by β-blockade. In our prior studies, verapamil in equal hypotensive doses to nifedipine and diltiazem produced the greatest depression of left ventricular systolic function.—R.A. O'Rourke, M.D.

Additional interesting publications concerning left ventricular diastolic function include the following:

1. Pasipoularides, A., Mirsky, I., Hess, O.M., et al.: Myocardial relaxation and passive diastolic properties in man. *Circulation* 74:991–1001, November 1986.
2. Junemann, M., Smiseth, O.A., Refsum, H., et al.: Quantification of effect of pericardium on LV diastolic PV relation in dogs. *Am. J. Physiol.* 252(Heart Circ. Physiol. 21):H963–H968, 1987.
3. Assanelli, D., Lew, W.Y.W., Shabetai, R., et al.: Influence of the pericardium on right and left ventricular filling in the dog. *J. Appl. Physiol.* 63:1025–1032, 1987.
4. Wexler, L.F., Weinberg, E.O., Ingwall, J.S., et al.: Acute alterations in diastolic left ventricular chamber distensibility: Mechanistic differences between hypoxemia and ischemia in isolated perfused rabbit and rat hearts. *Circ. Res.* 59:515–528, 1986.
5. Lecarpentier, Y., Waldenstrom, A., Clergue, M., et al.: Major alterations in relaxation during cardiac hypertrophy induced by aortic stenosis in guinea pig. *Circ. Res.* 61:107–116, 1987.
6. Toma, Y., Matsuda, Y., Moritani, K., et al.: Left atrial filling in normal human subjects: Relation between left atrial contraction and left atrial early filling. *Cardiovasc. Res.* 21:255–259, April 1987.
7. Zoghbi, W.A., Rokey, R., Limacher, M.C., et al.: Assessment of left ventricular diastolic filling by two-dimensional echocardiography. *Am. Heart J.* 113:1108–1113, 1987.
8. Friedman, B.J., Drinkovic, N., Miles, H., et al.: Assessment of left ventricular diastolic function: Comparison of Doppler echocardiography and gated blood pool scintigraphy. *J. Am. Coll. Cardiol.* 8:1348–1354, 1986.
9. Seals, A.A., Verani, M.S., Tadros, S., et al.: Comparison of left ventricular diastolic function as determined by nuclear cardiac probe, radionuclide angiography, and contrast cineangiography. *J. Nucl. Med.* 27:1908–1915, 1986.

Ventricular Systolic Function

The End-Systolic Pressure-Volume Relationship in Conscious Dogs

John A. Spratt, George S. Tyson, Donald D. Glower, James W. Davis, Lawrence H. Muhlbaier, Craig O. Olsen, and J. Scott Rankin (Duke Univ.)
Circulation 75:1295–1309, June 1987 1–12

Previous studies indicate that the end-systolic pressure-volume relation (ESPVR) is insensitive to changes in afterload but sensitive to alterations

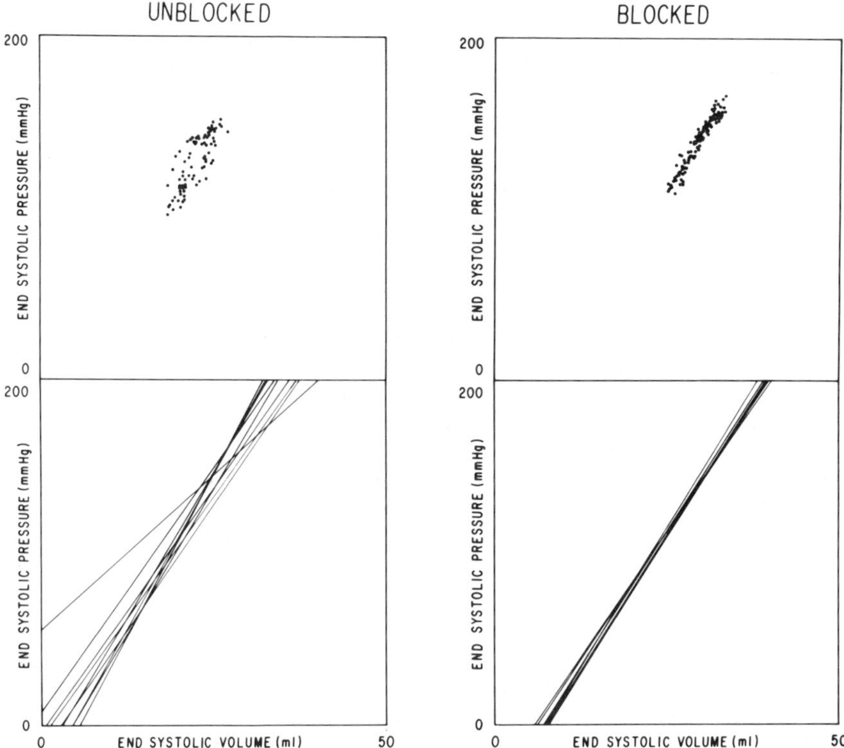

Fig 1–6.—Representative raw data from dogs in the unblocked state and during autonomic blockade. Raw data points are shown in the *upper panels,* and the individual ESPVR regression lines are illustrated in the *lower panels.* (Courtesy of Spratt, J.A., et al.: Circulation 75:1295–1309, June 1987.)

in inotropic state in the isolated heart. The effects of changes in afterload, heart rate, intravascular volume, inotropy, and autonomic tone on ESPVR now have been studied in conscious dogs. The relationship was studied by micromanometer records of left ventricular and pleural pressures and ultrasonic estimation of LV volume, during caval occlusions, with pharmacologic afterload interventions in the baseline state and following autonomic blockade.

All estimates of ESPVR in conscious animals involved large extrapolations to estimate the intercept of the ESPVR regression line. Repeat determinations of slope at baseline differed significantly in most animals but not after autonomic blockade (Fig 1–6). Alterations in heart rate and volume loading had minimal effects on the ESPVR. Increases in inotropy with calcium or dobutamine led to parallel shifts in the ESPVR at baseline. After autonomic blockade, the slope increased with increased inotropy, while the intercept was unchanged. Slope and afterload were not significantly related.

It appears that the ESPVR is valid in the conscious dog, but that significant variability with afterload hampers measurements with an intact cardiovascular system. The autonomic nervous system magnifies baseline variability. Use of the ESPVR in the intact circulation requires control of autonomic tone and consideration of the problems of statistical extrapolation and reproducibility.

▶ The left ventricular end-systolic pressure-volume relation (ESPVR) was developed in the isolated heart to define myocardial contractility relatively independent of changes in afterload and preload and has been verified in multiple experimental studies to be a relatively sensitive index of changes in myocardial contractility. The important study by Spratt and associates indicates, as do several of the studies referenced below, that ESPVR is more difficult to measure accurately in intact animals, that repeated measurements in the intact circulation vary significantly, and that measures of ESPVR are less reproducible in the autonomically intact animal.

This study and the studies of Kass et al. (*Circulation* 76:1422–1436, 1987) and Freeman and associates (*Circulation* 74:1107–1113, 1986) indicate that the wide application of ESPVR to studies of patients with heart disease may be premature, that ESPVR in the intact animal is not very sensitive in detecting changes in the inotropic state, and that the ESPVR obtained is highly dependent on the drugs or other techniques utilized to increase or decrease the arterial pressure.—R.A. O'Rourke, M.D.

Frequency-Dependent Myocardial Depression Induced by Verapamil in Conscious Dogs

Robert J. Applegate, Richard A. Walsh, and Robert A. O'Rourke (Univ. of Texas Health Sci. Ctr. and Audie Murphy VA Hosp. at San Antonio)

Am. J. Physiol. 253:H487–H492, September 1987 1–13

Verapamil depresses resting myocardial contractility, as do other calcium entry blockers. However, verapamil may have different effects on cardiac muscle force generation during increased stimulation frequency. The effects of incremental left atrial pacing were examined during verapamil, diltiazem, and nifedipine administration under equivalent loading conditions in seven conscious preinstrumented dogs. These animals were pretreated with propranolol to eliminate reflex sympathetic stimulation effects.

Prior to atrial pacing, peak positive left ventricular pressure development [$(+)dP/dt_{max}$] was similar for all three drugs. At 150 beats per minute peak paced heart rate under equivalent loading conditions, $(+)dP/dt_{max}$ was significantly reduced only after verapamil (2,392 ± 416 mm Hg per second to 2,131 ± 415 mm Hg per second). There was no significant linear relation between stimulation frequency and $(+)dP/dt_{max}$ during atrial pacing, during atrial pacing plus β-blockade alone or during β-blockade combined with diltiazem or nifedipine. A significant negative force-frequency relation was detected during incremental atrial pacing after verapamil administration.

In contrast to diltiazem or nifedipine, verapamil produces myocardial depression by a frequency-dependent mechanism that is independent of ventricular loading conditions. Excitation-contraction coupling is altered in the intact animal only after verapamil administration.

▶ This study is consistent with previous reports concerning the development of cardiac muscle tension with higher frequency of contraction before and after verapamil in isolated papillary muscles and in isolated perfused rabbit ventricle. The results indicated that verapamil, unlike other types of calcium blockers, reverses the positive force-frequency relation usually observed with increased stimulation rates. This is the first demonstration of this singular "negative staircase" property of verapamil in the intact circulation.—R.A. O'Rourke, M.D.

Hemodynamic Effects of Endurance Training on Canine Left Ventricle
Pauliina Rämö, Raimo Kettunen, and Leo Hirvonen (Univ. of Oulu, Finland)
Am. J. Physiol. 252:H7–H13, January 1987 1–14

It is known that pump performance of the heart may be increased either by enhancing the intrinsic contractile properties of the myocardium or by extracardiac adaptations that have secondary effects on performance. Repetitive exercise has been demonstrated to modify both heart

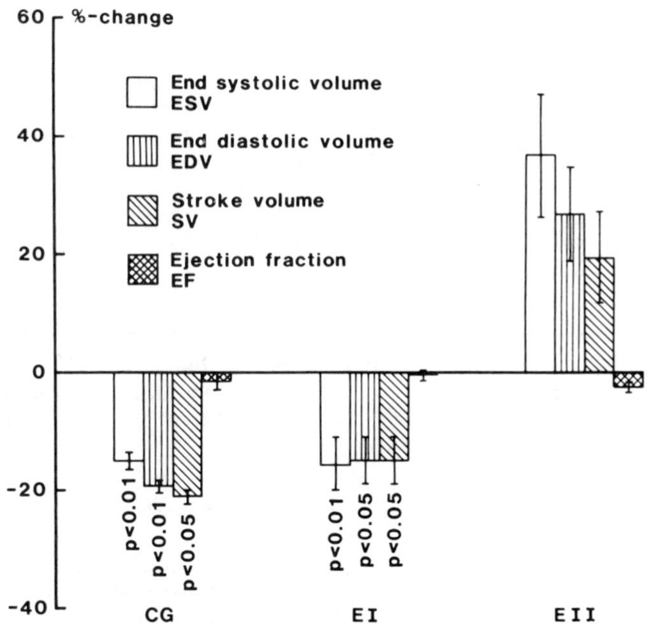

Fig 1–7.—Percentage changes of zero-time values in left ventricular volumes and ejection fraction (ESV, EDV, SV, and EF) after 7.5-min isoproterenol infusion in control group (CG) and in exercise group before (EI) and after (EII) experimental period. Statistical differences are calculated between CG and EII and between EI and EII (means ± SE). (Courtesy of Rämö, P., et al.: Am. J. Physiol. 252:H7–H13, January 1987.)

rate and stroke volume. However, it is not known whether physical training exerts any influence on intrinsic myocardial function. The effects of endurance training on myocardial performance were studied.

The authors used 14 beagle dogs; 7 dogs were trained by treadmill running for 6–7 weeks (exercise group), and the other 7 animals served as controls. Before and after the experimental period, both groups underwent a standard submaximal exercise test (SMT), and hemodynamic status was checked during anesthesia by catheterization technique exposing the animals to different loadings: pacing, volume loading, and isoproterenol infusion. The increase in heart rate during SMT was about 30 beats per minute less in the exercise group than in controls. There was a highly linear relationship between stroke work and end-diastolic volume within the groups, but the slope of the regression line obtained for the exercise group appeared to be markedly greater. In the exercise group, isoproterenol induced increases in end-diastolic (27%), end-systolic (37%), and stroke volumes (19%); conversely, in controls, isoproterenol led to decreases of these volumes (19%, 15%, and 22%, respectively) (Fig 1–7). There was no change in the ejection fraction for either the exercise group or controls. Ventricular stroke work was markedly greater in the exercise group, and systemic vascular resistance decreased in the exercise group in every loading test.

These findings indicate an improved pump performance, which is related not only to the heterometric autoregulatory adjustments but also to extracardial adaptations.

▶ In the past there has been considerable controversy as to whether physical training exerts any influence on intrinsic myocardial function. Both improvement and impairment of myocardial muscle mechanics have been reported. The data from this study by Rämö and associates suggest that long-term endurance training improves the pump performance of the heart by improving the filling properties of the left ventricle and optimizing its Frank-Starling relationship.—R.A. O'Rourke, M.D.

Differential Control of Heart Rate and Sympathetic Nerve Activity During Dynamic Exercise: Insight From Intraneural Recordings in Humans

Ronald G. Victor, Douglas R. Seals, and Allyn L. Mark, with the technical assistance of Joan Kempf (Univ. of Iowa)

J. Clin. Invest. 79:508–516, February 1987 1–15

It has been proposed that dynamic exercise leads to a generalized, uniform activation of sympathetic vasoconstrictor outflow and tachycardia, with widespread reflex vasoconstriction resulting. It also is said that central command and muscle afferent reflexes are redundant control mechanisms acting on the same neural circuits in the brain stem, and producing comparable autonomic effects. Microelectrode recordings of sympathetic nerve activity were made from the peroneal nerve in the leg during arm exercise in conscious individuals. Responses to rhythmic handgrip, with and without forearm vascular occlusion, were recorded, and two-arm cycling was carried out at graded intensities.

Both nonischemic rhythmic handgrip exercise and mild arm cycling produced graded increases in heart rate and arterial pressure but did not increase muscle sympathetic nerve activity. Ischemic handgrip exercise and moderate arm cycling increased muscle sympathetic nerve activity to a substantial degree, but with a slow onset of action. Muscle sympathetic nerve activity remained elevated when forearm ischemia continued after ischemic handgrip, but the heart rate returned to normal.

The onset of sympathetic activation of nonexercising skeletal muscle and the heart is delayed when dynamic exercise begins. Both central neural and peripheral reflex mechanisms are involved in maintaining arterial pressure, but central command and muscle chemoreflexes do not have comparable effects on sympathetic and parasympathetic responses.

▶ Marked increases in sympathetic activity have been used to explain many of the hemodynamic changes occurring in exercise such as increased heart rate, redistribution of blood flow to exercising muscles, and increased ventricular performance. The studies by Victor and associates utilized a unique microelectrode technique for recording sympathetic nerve activity in nonexercised muscle in conscious subjects performing arm exercise. They have demonstrated (1) that the onset of dynamic exercise is associated with a delay in the sympathetic activation of nonexercising the delta muscle in activation to the heart and nonexercising skeletal muscle and (2) that peripheral reflex mechanisms and central neural control are both involved in the complex control of heart rate, arterial pressure, and muscle sympathetic nerve activity.—R.A. O'Rourke, M.D.

Subclasses of Cyclic Amp-Specific Phosphodiesterase in Left Ventricular Muscle and Their Involvement in Regulating Myocardial Contractility

Ronald E. Weishaar, Dianne C. Kobylarz-Singer, Robert P. Steffen, and Harvey R. Kaplan (Warner-Lambert/Parke Davis Pharmaceutical Research, Ann Arbor, Mich.)

Circ. Res. 61:539–547, Oct. 5, 1987 1–16

Ventricular muscle contains a low K_m, cyclic AMP-specific form of phosphodiesterase (PDE III), which is believed to be the site of action of several cardiotonic agents, including imazodan, amrinone, cilostamide, and enoximone. Species differences in the inotropic response to these agents have been described. In this study, PDE III was isolated from dog, guinea pig, and rat left ventricular muscle to examine the source of these differences.

Canine left ventricular muscle contains two subclasses of PDE III. One form is sensitive to imazodan and is membrane bound. The other form of PDE III is imazodan-insensitive, soluble, and inhibited by Ro 20–1724 and rolipram. Guinea pig left ventricular muscle also contains an

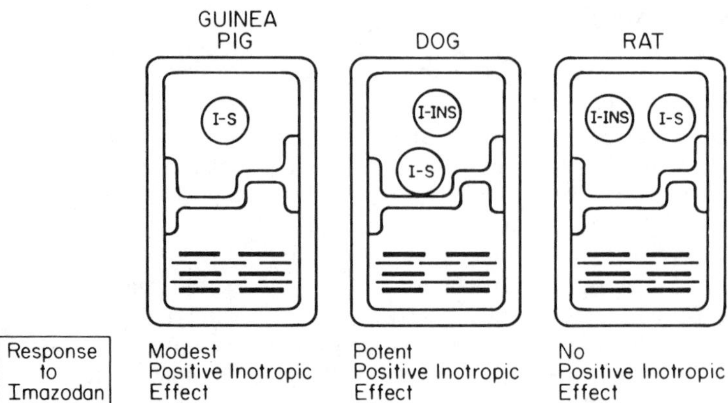

Fig 1–8.—Relation between the intracellular location of the imazodan-sensitive cAMP-specific phosphodiesterase and the positive inotropic response to imazodan. For this figure, I-S refers to the imazodan-sensitive cAMP-specific phosphodiesterase and I-INS refers to the imazodan-insensitive cAMP-specific phosphodiesterase. (Courtesy of Weishaar, R.E., et al.: Circ. Res. 61:539–547, Oct. 5, 1987.)

imazodan-sensitive PDE III, which is soluble. In rat left ventricle, there are imazodan-sensitive and insensitive forms of PDE III and both are soluble. Imazodan has a potent inotropic effect in the dog, where the imazodan-sensitive subclass of PDE III is membrane bound, but not in the other two species. Inhibitors of the soluble subclass of PDE III did not have this effect in the dog.

Functional subclasses of PDE III exist in ventricular muscle. The imazodan-sensitive subclass of PDE III is important in the positive inotropic response to several cardiotonic agents. The species differences that have been detected in response to imazodan can be accounted for by the differences in localization of the imazodan-sensitive subclass of PDE III among these species (Fig 1–8).

▶ During the past 10 years many new positive inotropic agents have been undergoing development and testing for treatment of moderate to severe congestive heart failure. The positive inotropic activity of the selective phosphodiesterase inhibitors has been attributed to their selective inhibitory effects on cAMP-specific form of phosphodiesterase (PDE III), which has been identified in ventricular muscle from several species. However, species differences in inotropic response to these agents have raised questions about the relationship between PDE III inhibition and cardiotonic activity. This study demonstrates that these differences can be accounted for by the presence of two subclasses of PDE III in ventricular muscle and variation in the intracellular localization of these two enzymes. The results demonstrate that functional subclasses of PDE III exist in ventricular muscle and suggest that species differences in the positive inotropic response to imazodan and related drugs can be attributed to the proper intracellular localization of the imazodan-sensitive subclass of PDE III.—R.A. O'Rourke, M.D.

Abnormal Intracellular Calcium Handling in Myocardium From Patients With End-Stage Heart Failure

Judith K. Gwathmey, Linda Copelas, Roderick MacKinnon, Frederick J. Schoen, Marc D. Feldman, William Grossman, and James P. Morgan (Charles A. Dana Research Inst., Beth Israel Hosp., Brigham and Women's Hosp., Children's Hosp. Med. Ctr., and Harvard Univ., Boston)

Circ. Res. 61:70–76, July 1987 1–17

Calcium plays a role in the process of excitation-contraction coupling in the heart. Therefore, abnormalities in calcium metabolism may be involved in cardiac failure. The intracellular calcium transients of hearts, isolated from nine patients with end-stage heart failure, were compared with those from eight organ donors with healthy hearts to assess the role of calcium metabolism in cardiac failure.

Myopathic muscles had prolonged isometric tension development, delayed relaxation, increased action potential duration, and prolonged calcium transients, compared to controls. Calcium dose-response curves were performed. In myopathic muscles only, increased calcium led to increased prolongation of the isometric twitch, and in five of nine patients an increase in the end-diastolic levels of light and tension.

The results of these experiments indicate abnormal calcium processing by myopathic cardiac heart muscle. This inability to maintain calcium homeostasis may be a cause of contractile failure.

▶ These studies of myocardium from patients with end-stage heart failure, using aequorin to indicate intracellular calcium transients, suggest that abnormal Ca^{++} handling by the sarcolemma and sarcoplasm of myopathic muscle may be a primary cause of systolic and diastolic dysfunction in humans.—R.A. O'Rourke, M.D.

Influence of Aortic Valve Disease on Systolic Stiffness of the Human Left Ventricular Myocardium

Thomas Wisenbaugh, Jonathan L. Elion, and Steven E. Nissen (VA Med. Ctr., Lexington, Ky., and Univ. of Kentucky)

Circulation 75:964–972, May 1987 1–18

The concept of systolic myocardial stiffness was applied to the study of ejection mechanics in aortic valve disease. Studies were done in nine controls catheterized to evaluate chest pain not typical of angina, as well as in eight patients with isolated aortic regurgitation and nine with fixed aortic valve or discrete subvalvular stenosis and no more than 2+ regurgitation. Frame-by-frame analysis of stress and volume was carried out for differently loaded beats during simultaneous cineangiography and micromanometry. Maximal myocardial stiffness was defined as the slope of the end-systolic stress-strain relationship.

Maximum myocardial stiffness was preserved in persons with aortic regurgitation and increased in those with aortic stenosis. It appeared that contractile force per unit myocardium was maintained in both groups. However, the theoretical "unloaded" shortening fraction was depressed in aortic stenosis but preserved in aortic regurgitation. The values were inversely related to maximum myocardial stiffness, indicating a disparity between shortening potential and force potential. In patients with aortic stenosis and a normal ejection fraction, stiffness approached the maximum earlier in ejection than in normal persons or in patients with aortic regurgitation.

Chronic myocardial hypertrophy produces more complex changes in the end-systolic stress-volume relationship than do short-term inotropic interventions. Hypertrophy may be an adaptation to hemodynamic loading in which contractile force per unit of myocardium is maintained, but shortening ability may be depressed in patients having aortic stenosis and regurgitation.

▶ Clinical symptoms, natural history, hemodynamic findings, and left ventricular mechanics vary in patients with isolated aortic regurgitation, or predominant aortic stenosis as compared to normals. In this clinical study, the authors assessed maximum myocardial stiffness, defined as the slope of the end-systolic stress-strain relationship in two groups of patients with aortic valve disease as compared to normals. Interestingly, maximum myocardial stiffness was preserved in patients with aortic regurgitation but increased significantly in those with aortic stenosis. The contractile force per unit of myocardial was maintained in both groups, however. The data indicate that alterations in ES stress-volume relationship with chronic hypertrophy are more complex than with short term inotropic interventions and that maximum, myocardial stiffness may be less sensitive to long term changes in contractility than are shortening indices.—R.A. O'Rourke, M.D.

Other interesting publications concerning left ventricular systolic performance include the following:

1. Freeman, G.L., Little, W.C., O'Rourke, R.A.: The effect of vasoactive agents on the left ventricular end-systolic pressure-volume relation in closed-chest dogs. *Circulation* 74:1107–1113, 1986.
2. McKay, R.G., Miller, M.J., Ferguson, J.J., et al.: Assessment of left ventricular end-systolic pressure-volume relations with an impedance catheter and transient inferior vena cava occlusion: use of this system in the evaluation of the cardiotonic effects of dobutamine, milrinone, posicor and epinephrine. *J. Am. Coll. Cardiol.* 8:1152–1160, 1986.
3. Igarashi, Y., Goto, Y., Yamada, O., et al.: Transient vs. steady end-systolic pressure-volume relation in dog left ventricle. *Am. J. Physiol.* 252(Heart Circ. Physiol. 21):H998–H1004, 1987.
4. Freeman, G.L., Little, W.C., O'Rourke, R.A.: Influence of heart rate on left ventricular performance in conscious dogs. *Circ. Res.* 61:455–464, 1987.
5. Crottogini, A.J., Willshaw, P., Barra, J.G., et al.: Inconsistency of the slope and the volume intercept of the end-systolic pressure-volume relationship as individual indexes of inotropic state

in conscious dogs: Presentation of an index combining both variables. *Circulation* 76:1115–1126, 1987.
6. Lee, J-D., Tajimi, T., Widmann, T.F., et al.: Application of end-systolic pressure-volume and pressure-wall thickness relations in conscious dogs. *Am. Coll. Cardiol.* 9:136–146, 1987.
7. Mirsky, I., Tajimi, T., Peterson, K.L.: The development of the entire end-systolic pressure-volume and ejection fraction-afterload relations: A new concept of systolic myocardial stiffness. *Circulation* 76:343–356, 1987.
8. Latson, T.W., Hunter, W.C., Burkhoff, D., et al.: Time sequential prediction of ventricular-vascular interactions. *Am. J. Physiol.* 251(Heart Circ. Physiol. 20):H1341–H1353, 1986.
9. Waldman, L.K., Covell, J.W.: Effects of ventricular pacing on finite deformation in canine left ventricles. *Am. J. Physiol.* 252(Heart Circ. Physiol. 21):H1023–H1030, 1987.
10. Suga, H., Goto, Y., Nozawa, T., et al.: Force-time integral decreases with ejection despite constant oxygen consumption and pressure-volume area in dog left ventricle. *Circ. Res.* 60:797–803, 1987.
11. Slinker, B.K., Glantz, S.A.: End-systolic and end-diastolic ventricular interaction. *Am. J. Physiol.* 251(Heart Circ. Physiol. 20):H1062–H1075, 1986.

Experimental Myocardial Ischemia/Infarction

Preconditioning With Ischemia: A Delay of Lethal Cell Injury in Ischemic Myocardium

Charles E. Murry, Robert B. Jennings, and Keith A. Reimer (Duke Univ.)
Circulation 74:1124–1136, November 1986 1–19

A previous study showed that a brief episode of ischemia slowed the rate of adenosine triphosphate (ATP) depletion during subsequent ischemic episodes. In addition, potentially harmful catabolites that accumulated during ischemia were washed out following intermittent reperfusion. These effects suggest that multiple, brief ischemic episodes may actually protect the heart from a subsequent sustained ischemic insult. To test this hypothesis, adult dogs were randomized into a preconditioned group that included preconditioning with four 5-minute circumflex occlusions, each separated by 5 minutes of reperfusion, and a control group in two studies.

In the first study, the preconditioned group underwent the preconditioning protocol followed by a 40-minute occlusion while the control-group received a single 40-minute occlusion. In the second study, the preconditioned group underwent the same preconditioning protocol followed by a 3-hour sustained occlusion, and the control group received sustained 3-hour occlusion. Animals were allowed 4 days of reperfusion thereafter. Histologic infarct size was measured and correlated to the major baseline predictors of infarct size, including the anatomical area at risk and collateral blood flow.

In the 40-minute study, reconditioning significantly limited the infarct

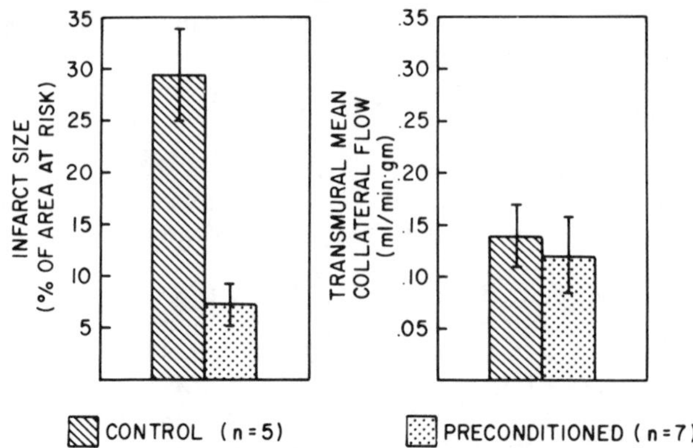

Fig 1–9.—Infarct size and collateral blood flow in the 40-min study. **Left,** infarct size, as a percentage of the anatomical area at risk, in the control *(striped bar)* and preconditioned *(stippled bar)* hearts. Infarct size in control animals averaged 29.4% of the area at risk. Infarct size in control hearts averaged only 7.3% of the area at risk (preconditioned vs. control, $P<.001$). Transmural mean collateral blood flow (**right**) was not significantly different in the two groups. Thus, the protective effect of preconditioning was independent of the two major baseline predictors of infarct size, area at risk and collateral blood flow. Bars represent group means ± SEM. (Courtesy of Murry, C.E., et al.: Circulation 74:1124–1136, November 1986.)

size to 25% of that seen in the control group (Fig 1–9). Collateral blood flow to the subendocardium (zone of infarction) or as a transmural mean midway through the 40-minute occlusion was not significantly different between groups. Histologically, preconditioned animals showed multiple small foci of necrosis, scattered within predominantly viable myocardium, and viable and necrotic cells frequently interspersed in the necrotic foci, whereas control animals exhibited solid infarcts. In the 3-hour study, infarct size and collateral blood flow to the subepicardium and as a transmural average did not differ significantly in the two groups.

Brief, intermittent episodes of ischemia have a protective effect on the myocardium that is later subjected to a 40-minute occlusion, possibly because of reduction in ATP depletion and/or to reduced catabolite accumulation during the sustained occlusion. However, preconditioning serves only to delay cell death since it fails to limit infarct size after 3 hours of sustained occlusion. Although these results should be extrapolated in clinical situations with caution, it appears that multiple anginal episodes that often precede myocardial infarction in man may delay cell death after coronary occlusion, and thereby may allow for greater salvage of myocardium through reperfusion therapy.

▶ Previous studies have shown that repeated brief episodes of ischemia do not have accumulative deleterious effects. The results of this interesting study show that brief, intermittent episodes of myocardial ischemia have a protective effect when the myocardium is later subjected to a sustained bout of ischemia of 40 minutes duration. The two mechanisms postulated by the authors to explain these data include (1) slowing of ATP depletion, or (2) limitation of catabolite accumulation during the terminal episode of ischemia. The possible clinical implication is that patients who experience repeated episodes of angina may similarly precondition their myocardium and alter the time course of cell death after the onset of a sustained coronary occlusion, providing a longer window of timing in which it might be possible to salvage myocardium.—R.A. O'Rourke, M.D.

Pathophysiology and Pathogenesis of Stunned Myocardium: Depressed Ca^{2+} Activation of Contraction as a Consequence of Reperfusion-Induced Cellular Calcium Overload in Ferret Hearts

Hideo Kusuoka, James K. Porterfield, Harlan F. Weisman, Myron L. Weisfeldt, and Eduardo Marban (The Johns Hopkins Univ.)

J. Clin. Invest. 79:950–961, March 1987 1–20

Although reperfusion after myocardial ischemia of brief duration does not induce necrosis, it does lead to prolonged contractile dysfunction. This phenomenon of myocardial stunning is manifested clinically in the sluggish recovery of pump function after coronary revascularization after brief periods of ischemia. The authors hypothesize that this contractile dysfunction could result from a decrease in the intracellular free $[Ca^{2+}]$ transient during each beta, a decrease in maximal Ca^{2+}-activated force, or a shift in myofilament Ca^{2+} sensitivity. This hypothesis was tested in the present study.

The authors measured developed pressure (DP) at several $[Ca]_o$ (0.5–7.5 mM) in isovolumic Langendorff-perfused ferret hearts at 37C after 15 min of global ischemia (stunned group, n = 13), or in a nonischemic control group (n = 6). It was found that at all $[Ca]_o$, DP was depressed in the stunned group; however, maximal Ca^{2+}-activated pressure (MCAP), measured from tetani after exposure to ryanodine, was decreased after stunning. Normalization of the DP-$[Ca]_o$ relationship by corresponding MCAP (Ca_o sensitivity) demonstrated a shift to higher $[Ca]_o$ in stunned hearts. To assess whether cellular Ca overload initiates stunning, the authors reperfused with low-$[Ca]_o$ solution (0.1–0.5 mM; n = 8). It was shown that DP and MCAP in the low-$[Ca]_o$ group were comparable to control and higher than in the stunned group. The myocardial [ATP] observed by phosphorous NMR did not correlate with functional recovery.

It is concluded that contractile dysfunction in stunned myocardium is the result of a decline in maximal force, and a shift in Ca_o sensitivity (which may reflect either decreased myofilament Ca^{2+} sensitivity or a decrease in the $[Ca^{2+}]$ transient). These results suggest that calcium entry on reperfusion plays a major role in the pathogenesis of myocardial stunning.

► In this study myocardial "stunning" is defined as the sluggish recovery of pump function after coronary revascularization following brief periods of ischemia. The results described by Kusuoka and associates indicate that a "stunned" myocardium likely is due to a depressed maximal calcium-activated pressure and a decrease of cardiac muscle twitch to changes in extracellular calcium. The observations made in this report indicate that the primary determination of stunning is not ischemia but rather reperfusion. The authors conclude that reperfusion with calcium solutions may be useful in improving the recovery of cardiac performance in clinical settings such as angioplasty or cardiac surgery in which the reperfusate could be modified selectively.—R.A. O'Rourke, M.D.

Effects of Myocardial Ischemia on Regional Function and Stiffness in Conscious Dogs

Jun Amano, John X. Thomas, Jr., Michel Lavallee, Israel Mirsky, David Glover, W. Thomas Manders, Walter C. Randall, and Stephen F. Vatner (Harvard Univ. and Brigham and Women's Hosp., Boston, New England Regional Primate Research Ctr., Southborough, Mass., and Stritch School of Medicine, Loyola Univ., Maywood, Ill.)

Am. J. Physiol. 252:H110–H117, January 1987 1–21

Cardiac transplantation is being used increasingly, and because of this it is important to understand the pathophysiology of the transplanted heart in the absence of its extrinsic innervation. It is also crucial to elucidate the consequences of myocardial ischemia in the denervated heart. The goal of the present study was to determine the extent to which cardiac nerves influence responses of regional ventricular function to acute myocardial ischemia.

The authors used conscious dogs with intact cardiac innervation (N) and dogs with chronic cardiac denervation (D). After coronary artery occlusion (CAO), it was found that left ventricular (LV) end-diastolic pressure increased more in D than in N dogs, whereas heart rate increased more in N than in D dogs. In nonischemic zones of D dogs there were more marked increases, in end-diastolic segment length, systolic segment shortening, and velocity of shortening than in N dogs. In ischemic zones, the authors also observed significantly greater increases in end-diastolic segment length in the D group, but saw similar reductions in segmental shortening in both N and D dogs. There was no difference in the time constant of isovolumic relaxation in the two groups. However, in ischemic zones of N dogs, the myocardial stiffness constant *(k)* was found to increase by 109 ± 24 from 33 ± 4.9, and end-diastolic stiffness (E_{ed}) rose by 1,527 ± 310 from 253 ± 34 mm Hg, whereas *k* increased significantly less in D dogs. E_{ed} of ischemic zones also increased markedly less in D dogs.

In conscious dogs, chronic D does not attenuate depression of LV function in ischemic zones but is associated with enhanced regional function of nonischemic myocardium through the Frank-Starling mechanism and delayed increases in myocardial stiffness in the ischemic zone, despite larger increases in LV end-diastolic pressure.

▶ This interesting study by Amano and associates indicates the total cardiac denervation does not exert a protective effect on regional ischemic zones following coronary artery occlusion in the conscious animal. By blocking the initial tachycardia following coronary artery occlusion, cardiac denervation allows greater use of the Frank-Starling mechanism to augment regional function in the nonischemic zones. Importantly, cardiac denervation delays the increase in regional myocardial stiffness in ischemic zones following coronary occlusion indicating that the augmented rise in LV end-diastolic pressure is not due to increased myocardial stiffness.—R.A. O'Rourke, M.D.

Granulocytes Cause Reperfusion Ventricular Dysfunction After 15-Minute Ischemia in the Dog

Robert Engler and James W. Covell (VA Med. Ctr. Research Serv. and Univ. of California at San Diego, La Jolla)

Circ. Res. 61:20–28, July 1987 1–22

After 15 minutes of ischemia, regional ventricular dysfunction (myocardial stunning) persists for several hours after reperfusion. One of the mechanisms of this injury appears to be superoxide radical-induced damage. The importance of granulocytes to this process was tested in a dog model.

After 15 minutes of ischemia, coronary perfusion was returned either extracorporeally through Leukopak filters, agranulocytic reperfusion, or

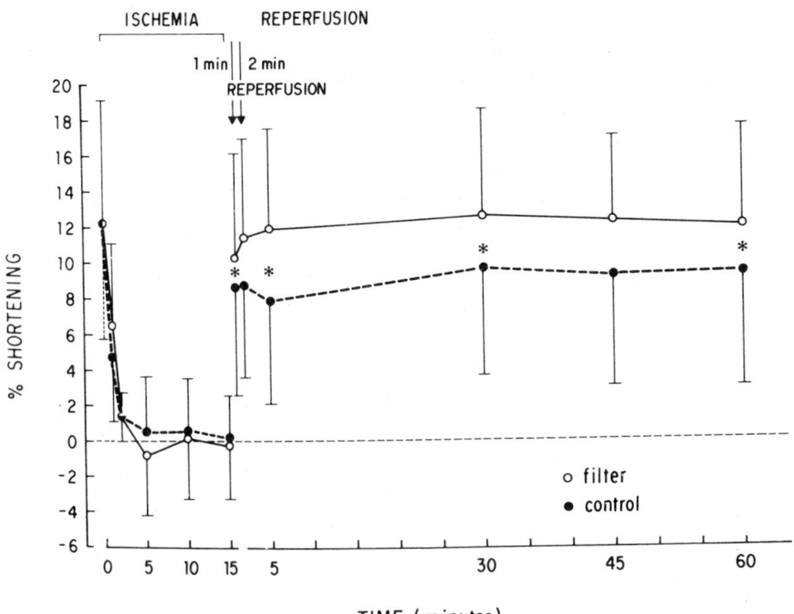

Fig 1–10.—Segment shortening in anterior ischemic area at preischemia (time = 0), during 15 minutes of ischemia, and 60 minutes of reperfusion during agranulocytic perfusion (filter) and after filter removal in same animals (control). %SS, (end-diastolic length − end-systolic length)/end-diastolic length. ANOVA performed at preischemia and 1, 5, 30, and 60 minutes reperfusion only. $*P < .05$ from preischemia. Mean ± SEM. (Courtesy of Engler, R., and Covell, J.W.: Circ. Res. 61:20–28, July 1987.)

without filters, granulocytopenic reperfusion. Flow reduction, reperfusion flow, preload, afterload, and inotropic stimulation were the same during both reperfusions. During agranulocytic reperfusion, 100% of preischemic function returned, and stunning did not occur. During granulocytopenic reperfusion, only 76% of preischemic function returned by 60 minutes (Fig 1–10).

Another group of dogs had extracorporeal perfusion and replete granulocyte perfusion. All of these animals had less than 75% return of function. This indicated that it was the presence of granulocytes and not the extracorporeal method of reperfusion that prevented stunning.

Granulocytes are a direct cause of the injury in stunned myocardium in the reperfused ischemic dog model. They appear to be the main source of superoxide radicals in this system.

▶ These dog studies indicate the granulocytes have a major effect on regional ventricular function following 15 minutes of acute myocardial ischemia and reperfusion. They also show that edema formation, arrhythmias, and blood flow during the first hour of ischemia are all improved dramatically by agranulocytosis. They suggest that ischemia initiates a cascade reaction including mechanical capillary obstruction by granulocytes, oxygen-radical formation and perhaps other inflammatory events that markedly increase the myocardial injury.—R.A. O'Rourke, M.D.

Neutrophil Accumulation in Experimental Myocardial Infarcts: Relation With Extent of Injury and Effect of Reperfusion

Pascal Chatelain, Jean-Gilles Latour, Duc Tran, Michel de Lorgeril, Georges Dupras, and Martial Bourassa (Montreal Heart Inst., Montreal)

Circulation 75:1083–1090, May 1987 1–23

Coronary reperfusion is a promising approach to limiting the extent of myocardial necrosis after transmural infarction, but if neutrophil accumulation and resultant inflammation is enhanced, the beneficial effects of restoring blood flow may be countered. Accumulation of ^{111}In-labeled neutrophils in reperfused and control myocardial infarcts was studied in dogs having occlusion of the left anterior descending coronary artery for 3 hours, followed by 21 hours of reperfusion. Autologous neutrophils sometimes were injected at the time of coronary occlusion, whereas other animals were made leukopenic by antineutrophil serum. Digitized scintigraphy of heart slices was done to quantify radioactivity.

An 80% increase in neutrophil accumulation was noted in the infarct region following reperfusion, compared with animals having permanent coronary occlusion. The accumulation ratio was highest in the subendocardial central zone of the infarct. Flow in the previously occluded vessel was higher in leukopenic animals 30 minutes after reperfusion, but no difference from preocclusion flow was noted in a study without leukopenia. Infarct size and the area of myocardium at risk were similar in all groups.

Reperfusion after coronary occlusion markedly increased accumulation of neutrophils in this canine model of myocardial infarction. Histologic study confirmed leukocyte plugging after reperfusion. The finding of higher coronary flow during reperfusion in leukopenic animals suggests a role for neutrophil accumulation in persistent impairment of the coronary microcirculation. Leukopenia did not, however, limit infarct size.

▶ Relative to the preceding report, the authors studied the effect of reperfusion on myocardial accumulation neutrophil using ^{111}In-labeled autologous neutrophils and digitized scintigraphy in a canine preparation with a 3-hour coronary occlusion followed by 21 hours of reperfusion. Any reperfusion after a 3-hour occlusion of the left anterior descending coronary artery markedly increased the accumulation of labeled neutrophils compared with nonreperfused myocardium, the increase being limited to the subendocardium. Coronary blood flow during reperfusion was higher in the presence of leukopenia, suggesting a role of neutrophil accumulation in persistent impairment of the microcirculation. —R.A. O'Rourke, M.D.

Free Radical-Producing Enzyme, Xanthine Oxidase, Is Undetectable in Human Hearts

Lynne J. Eddy, James R. Stewart, Harold P. Jones, Todd D. Engerson, Joe M. McCord and James M. Downey (Univ. of South Alabama, Mobile, and Vanderbilt Univ., Nashville)

Am. J. Physiol. 253:H709–H711, September 1987 1–24

One proposed source of injurious oxygen free radicals in the reperfused ischemic heart is xanthine oxidase. However, the xanthine oxidase content in human heart has not yet been defined. Therefore, the xanthine oxidase content of heart samples obtained from two surgical patients and two organ donors was determined by the standard spectrophotometric assay and by a more sensitive spectrofluorometric method.

No activity was detected in any of these four samples. Therefore, human heart must contain less than 2.0 nU/gm of activity.

Xanthine oxidase does not appear to be an important source of oxygen free radicals in the ischemic human heart. Therefore, xanthine oxidase inhibitors will be of limited therapeutic value in reperfused hearts.

▶ As indicated above, manipulation of granulocyte function following longer periods of ischemia has been shown by several (but not all) investigators to salvage ischemia myocardium. Oxygen radical formation has been found to play a role in myocardial necrosis following ischemia. Since the xanthine oxidase is proposed to be the source of injurious oxygen free radicals in the reperfused ischemic heart, the applicability of the xanthine oxidase hypothesis to myocardial ischemia depends on whether the human heart contains xanthine oxidase.

Interestingly, using both the conventional spectrophotometric assay and a more sensitive fluorometric assay to determine the content of xanthine oxidase in four human hearts, the investigators could not define activity in any of the samples utilized. The importance of oxygen free radicals in promoting myocardial injury during acute myocardial infarction remains debated and attempts to salvage myocardium by blocking oxygen free radicals have led to conflicting results.—R.A. O'Rourke, M.D.

Attenuation of Dysfunction in the Postischemic 'Stunned' Myocardium by Dimethylthiourea

Roberto Bolli, Wei-Xi Zhu, Craig J. Hartley, Lloyd H. Michael, John E. Repine, Michael L. Hess, Rakesh C. Kukreja, and Robert Roberts (Baylor College of Medicine, Houston, Univ. of Colorado Health Science Ctr., Denver, and Med. College of Virginia, Richmond)

Circulation 76:458–468, August 1987 1–25

After reversible regional ischemia, reperfused myocardium can suffer from contractile dysfunction. Myocardium in this state is referred to as "stunned." It has been suggested that free radicals may be involved in this process. The role of the hydroxl radical was assessed in a canine model involving 15 minutes of occlusion followed by 4 hours of reperfusion in the presence of the hydroxyl radical scavenger, dimethylthiourea (DMTU) or in the presence of saline. An epicardial Doppler probe was used to assess wall thickening as a measure of regional myocardial function.

The two groups were comparable prior to experimental manipulations. During ischemia, both groups experienced dyskinesis. However, after reperfusion, wall thickening was significantly greater in treated dogs. At 1 hour of reperfusion, the level in treated dogs was 53 ± 9% of baseline, while in the control group it was 9 ± 14%. At 4 hours, the treated group was at 67 ± 5% of baseline, while the control group was at 36 ± 13%.

Administration of DMTU enhanced recovery of contractile function in reperfused myocardium. Because DMTU did not scavenge either hydrogen peroxide or superoxide ions in vitro, these results suggest that myocardial stunning may be partly mediated by the hydroxyl radical.

▶ In this study dimethylthiourea (DMTU), a compound that is more effective than traditional ·OH scavangers, produced a persistent improvement in recovery of myocardial function after regional reversible ischemia. These results suggest that ·OH may contribute to the myocardial dysfunction that follows prolonged global ischemia in the arrested heart perfused with artificial solutions. This is one of the first studies to implicate the ·OH radical in the myocardial "stunning" seen in the working, blood-perfused heart following brief, reversible regional ischemia.—R.A. O'Rourke, M.D.

The Importance of Defining Left Ventricular Area at Risk In Vivo During Acute Myocardial Infarction: An Experimental Evaluation With Myocardial Contrast Two-Dimensional Echocardiography

Sanjiv Kaul, William Glasheen, Terrence D. Ruddy, Natesa G. Pandian, Arthur E. Weyman, and Robert D. Okada (Univ. of Virginia and Harvard Univ.)
Circulation 75:1249–1260, June 1987 1–26

It seems best to consider thrombolytic therapy or coronary angioplasty for those patients with acute infarction who are at risk of developing larger infarcts. The left ventricular (LV) area at risk was related to hemodynamic variables and to LV systolic function, and changes in area at risk over time were assessed in dogs. Progressively larger areas of myocardium were made ischemic in two to five stages by occluding the LAD or left circumflex coronary artery successively more proximally.

Hemodynamics became abnormal when the area at risk was 25% to 40% of the left ventricle, and the LV ejection fraction was abnormal when the area at risk was 18%. Normalized cardiac output (Fig 1–11) and LV ejection fraction were closely related inversely to the area at risk, but normalized mean arterial pressure was not. The circumferential endocardial extent of the area at risk closely predicted the extent of infarction, and it did not change significantly over 6 hours after coronary occlusion.

Left ventricular ejection fraction may be a better indicator of the area

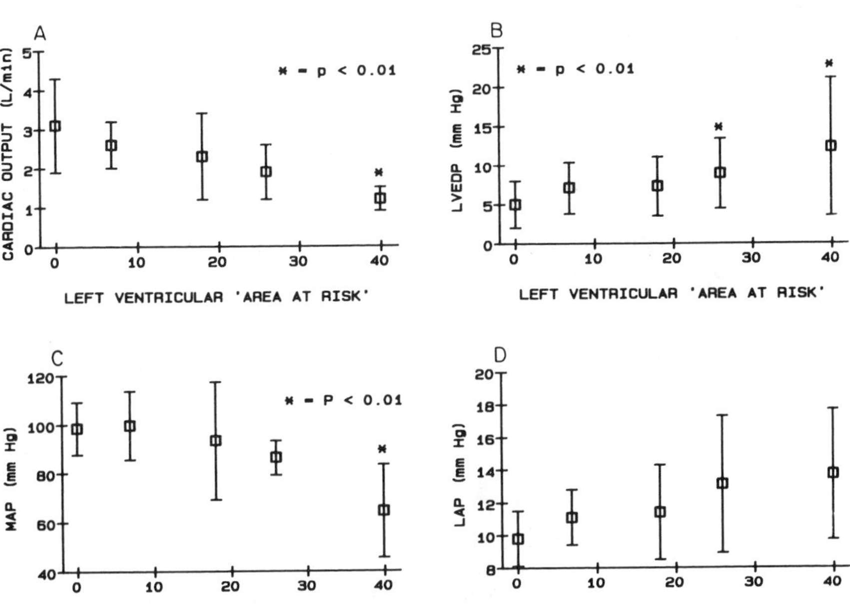

Fig 1–11.—**A**, relationship of cardiac output and area at risk. Interstage difference in cardiac output is significant only when the mean area at risk is approximately 40%. **B**, relationship of left ventricular end-diastolic pressure (LVEDP) and area at risk. The LVEDP rises significantly only when area at risk is about 25% of the left ventricle. **C**, relationship between mean arterial pressure (MAP) and area at risk. The MAP was maintained at near normal or higher levels until area at risk was approximately 40% of the left ventricle. **D**, relationship between mean left atrial pressure (LAP) and area at risk. There is no significant difference in the mean LAP for different sizes of risk area. (Courtesy of Kaul, S., et al.: Circulation 75:1249–1260, June 1987.)

of myocardium at risk after coronary occlusion than are hemodynamic variables. A direct method of estimating area at risk, such as myocardial contrast echocardiography, would be very helpful in planning management. It might be possible to obtain left heart opacification by injecting contrast intravenously, making possible studies in the emergency room or coronary care unit.

▶ The purpose of the dog studies described in this report was to determine whether current methods of assessing left ventricular function during acute myocardial infarction reflect the true size of the "area at risk" as measured by myocardial contrast echocardiography (MCE). Various hemodynamic variables, the left ventricular ejection fraction and MCE results were assessed in four groups of dogs undergoing proximal left coronary artery occlusion for a variable duration. Results indicate that measurements of hemodynamic variables and the left ventricular ejection fraction do not preclude the necessity for a direct method of measuring the "area at risk" such as by MCE, the latter correlating-well with the ultimate infarct size observed by histology at both 3 and 6 hours after occlusion.—R.A. O'Rourke, M.D.

Effect of Frequent Ventricular Ectopy on Myocardial Infarct Size in Dogs

Stanley Nattel, Scott Beau, and Gary McCarragher (McGill Univ. and Montreal Gen. Hosp., Montreal)

Cardiovasc. Res. 21:286–292, April 1987 1–27

It is known that a substantial proportion of patients admitted to the hospital for acute myocardial infarction have frequent premature ventricular complexes. However, there has been considerable controversy about the value of prophylactic antiarrhythmic drug treatment in this population. Although tachycardia has been shown to increase the size of an evolving myocardial infarction, the effect of frequent ventricular extrasystoles is unknown. The goal of the present study was to determine the effect of frequent ventricular extrasystoles on the size of an evolving myocardial infarction.

The study was carried out on mongrel dogs that were allocated to a control group ($n = 15$), or to groups of dogs with electrically induced ventricular bigeminy. The authors used ventricular extrasystoles with short coupling intervals (mean, 251 msec) to simulate interpolated premature complexes in 10 dogs, and extrasystoles with long coupling intervals (mean, 606 msec) resulting in compensatory pauses were applied in 10 additional dogs. Each dog underwent single stage left anterior descending coronary artery ligation followed by a 6 hour monitoring period. The premature stimulation was started at the time of coronary artery occlusion and continued throughout the observation period. The ratio of myocardial infarct size to the region at risk of infarction was markedly larger in dogs with electrically induced, closely coupled extrasystoles than in control dogs or in dogs with widely coupled induced extrasystoles (Fig 1–12).

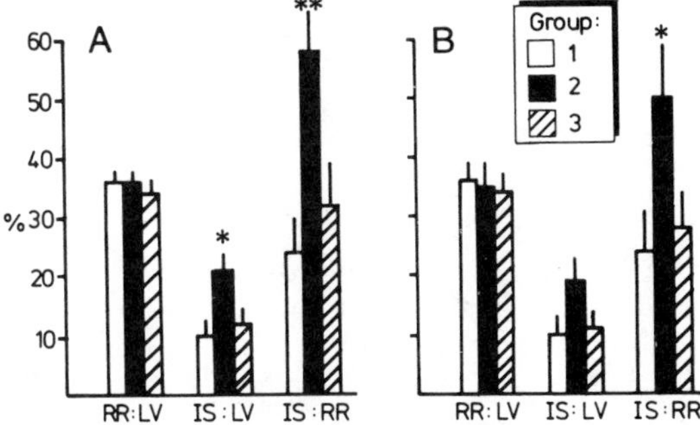

Fig 1–12.—Risk region (RR) and infarct size (IS) expressed as a percentage of left ventricular mass (LV), and infarct size as a percentage of risk region for all three groups of dogs. Values are mean (SEM). **A** shows results obtained from all 35 dogs studied; **B,** results obtained by excluding dogs with sustained spontaneous ventricular arrhythmias (1 in group 1, 3 in group 2, and 1 in group 3). $^*P<.05$, $^{**}P<.01$ vs. control (group #1) dogs. (Courtesy of Nattel, S., et al.: Cardiovasc. Res. 21:286–292, April 1987.)

Frequent closely coupled ventricular extrasystoles can increase the size of an evolving acute myocardial infarction.

▶ In this interesting dog study, the ratio of myocardial infarction size to the region at risk of infarction was substantially larger in dogs with electrically induced, closely coupled extrasystoles than in the control dogs or in dogs with widely coupled, electrically induced extrasystoles, suggesting that frequent ventricular ectopy at the time of myocardial infarction may actually increase the "infarct size" of an evolving acute injury.—R.A. O'Rourke, M.D.

Intramuscular Administration of Human Tissue-Type Plasminogen Activator in Rabbits and Dogs and Its Implications for Coronary Thrombolysis

Burton E. Sobel, Jeffrey E. Saffitz, Larry E. Fields, Donald W. Myears, Stanley J. Sarnoff, Alice K. Robison, Dwain A. Owensby, and Keith A.A. Fox with the technical assistance of John Botz, Denise Nachowiak, Richard Rodriguez, and Joseph R. Williamson (Washington Univ., St. Louis)

Circulation 75:1261–1272, June 1987 1–28

The feasibility of intramuscular administration of tissue-type plasminogen activator (t-PA) for coronary thrombolysis was examined in rabbits and dogs. An attempt was made to elicit functionally active, therapeutic blood levels of t-PA that were sustained for several hours after intramuscular injection.

When t-PA was directly injected into exposed rabbit muscle, followed by local electrical stimulation, early absorption was much increased by adding methylamine plus hydroxylamine to the excipient. These enhancers also were effective with percutaneous injections in the absence of local electrical stimulation, and no adverse local or systemic effects were noted. The same substances induced local egress of intravascular labeled albumin within the injection site in rats. In dogs, percutaneous intramuscular injection of t-PA without enhancers did not produce early increases

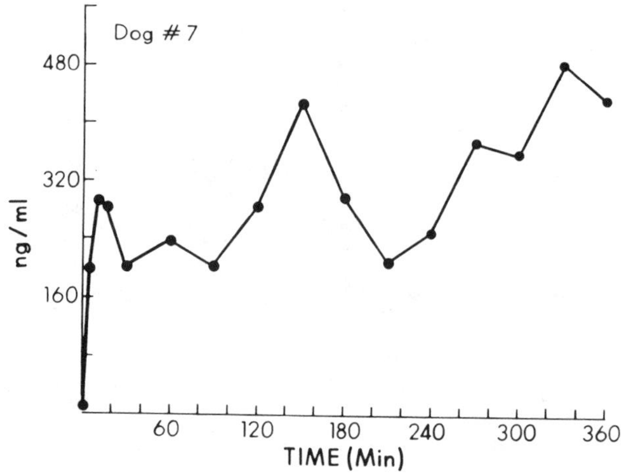

Fig 1–13.—Concentrations of plasma t-PA as a function of time after intramuscular injection in a dog given percutaneous intramuscular injections of t-PA (10 mg/kg) in injection media constituted with 0.63 M methylamine plus 0.079M hydroxylamine. (Courtesy of Sobel, B.E., et al.: Circulation 75:1261–1272, June 1987.)

in plasma levels, but late elevations occurred. When enhancers were used, early elevations were observed (Fig 1–13). Coronary angiography showed thrombolysis following induced coronary thrombosis.

Intramuscular administration of t-PA with enhancers of absorption is a practical means of rapidly inducing fibrinolysis.

▶ Although coronary thrombolytic agents with low toxic to therapeutic ratios are currently available for coronary thrombolysis, its clinical efficacy is dependent under the rapidity with which it can be induced after the onset of thrombosis and ischemia. In this important study, intramuscular injections of human tissue-type plasminogen activator (tPA) with enhancers of absorption were given to a large number of rabbits and 13 dogs. When the enhancers were used, early elevation of human tPA was observed in the plasma of both species and sequential coronary arteriography showed thrombolysis after experimentally induced thrombosis. This exciting information suggests that intramuscular administration of tPA with selected enhancers of absorption is a feasible approach in inducing fibrinolysis.—R.A. O'Rourke, M.D.

Detection of Experimental Right Ventricular Infarction by Isopotential Body Surface Mapping During Sinus Rhythm and During Ectopic Ventricular Pacing

David M. Mirvis (VA Med. Ctr. and Univ. of Tennessee, Memphis)
J. Am. Coll. Cardiol. 10:157–163, July 1987 1–29

Right ventricular necrosis often accompanies left ventricular infarction. To define ECG abnormalities associated with right ventricular necrosis, latex was injected into the right coronary artery of dogs (Fig 1–14). The ECG results were examined by body surface isopotential mapping.

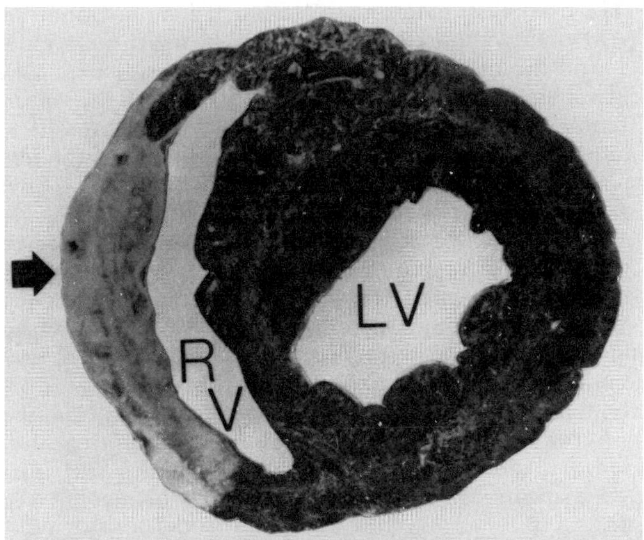

Fig 1–14.—Heart slice stained with triphenyltetrazolium chloride after latex embolization of the right coronary artery. The unstained region of necrosis *(arrow)* is limited to the right ventricular (RV) free wall. LV = left ventricle. (Courtesy of Mirvis, D.M.: J. Am. Coll. Cardiol. 10:157–163, July 1987.)

During sinus rhythm, right ventricular necrosis produced abnormal negative potentials over the right hemithorax throughout the QRS complex. There was a loss of R waves and a deepening or new development of Q and S waves. Compared with 13 control dogs, there was a right-sided abnormal minimum throughout the QRS complex.

Right ventricular necrosis produces QRS complex changes over the right torso. An abnormal right-sided minimum was seen regardless of the pattern of ventricular inactivation. This suggests that a supplementary path for current to reenter the heart was provided by the area lost to right ventricular necrosis.

▶ Electrocardiographic detection of right ventricular infarction is more clearly defined than for infarction of the left ventricle. In this dog study infarction was limited to the right ventricle and ECG alterations were evaluated by isopotential body surface mapping. The results indicate that the polarity of voltage recorded over the lesion is negative regardless of the activation sequence and the persistence of negativity throughout the QRS complex is consistent with the dense transmural lesion producing complete electrical silence.—R.A. O'Rourke, M.D.

Myocardial Damage Delineated by Indium-111 Antimyosin Fab and Technetium-99m Pyrophosphate

Ban An Khaw, H. William Strauss, Richard Moore, John T. Fallon, Tsunehiro Yasuda, Herman K. Gold, and Edgar Haber (Massachusetts Gen. Hosp., Boston)
J. Nucl. Med. 28:76–82, January 1987 1–30

Both ^{99m}Tc-pyrophosphate and ^{111}In-labeled monoclonal antimyosin antibody (AM) Fab were used to estimate myocardial infarct size in a canine model, and the results were compared with histochemical estimates of infarct size in reperfused infarcts. The mixture of radiopharmaceuticals was administered by the intracoronary or intravenous (IV) route after 15 minutes of reperfusion and a 3-hour occlusion of the left anterior descending (LAD) coronary artery. Pathologic infarct size was determined by staining with triphenyl tetrazolium chloride (TTC).

Mean infarct size delineated by pyrophosphate was larger than that obtained with antimyosin, and the latter was greater than estimates made by TTC staining. Overestimates occurred regardless of the route by which the radiopharmaceuticals were given. Good correlation was, however, obtained between the pyrophosphate and antimyosin estimates of infarct size in both the intracoronary and IV groups.

It is likely that differences in estimated areas of myocardial damage delineated by pyrophosphate and antimyosin reflect the area of viable but compromised myocardium. If this is the case, studies with these agents may provide a means of identifying severely ischemic but recoverable myocardium.

▶ Technetium-99m pyrophosphate (PYP), when administered simultaneously with antimyosin in a canine model of acute myocardial infarction with reperfusion, is taken up by a significantly larger volume of myocardium whether the tracers are given by intracoronary or intravenous routes. Also, a greater percentage of injection antimyosin localizes in the infarct relative to PYP. The authors' suggestion that the combination of the agents to provide a marker for severely ischemic but recoverable myocardium (PYP uptake minus antimyosin localization) merits additional investigation.—R.A. O'Rourke, M.D.

Additional recent relevant publications concerning myocardial ischemia/infarction include the following:

1. Borgers, M., Shu, L.G., Xhonneux, R., et al.: Changes in ultrastructure and Ca^{2+} distribution in the isolated working rabbit heart after ischemia: A time-related study. *Am. J. Pathol.* 126:92–102, 1987.
2. Greenfield, R.A., Swain, J.L.: Disruption of myofibrillar energy use: Dual mechanisms that may contribute to postischemic dysfunction in stunned myocardium. *Circ. Res.* 60:283–289, 1987.
3. Guth, B.D., Huesch, G., Seitelberger, R., et al.: Mechanism of beneficial effect of beta-adrenergic blockage on exercise-induced myocardial ischemia in conscious dogs. *Circ. Res.* 60:738–746, 1987.
4. Simpson, P.J., et al.: Prostacyclin protects ischemic reperfused myocardium in the dog by inhibition of neutrophil activation. *Am. Heart J.* 113:129–137, 1987.
5. Bjornsson, O.G., Kobayashi, K., Williamson, J.R.: Interaction between leukotriene D_4 and adenosine or iloprost in the isolated working guinea-pig heart. Department of Biochemistry and Biophysics, Univ. of Pennsylvania, Philadelphia, U.S.A. *Eur. J. Clin. Invest.* 17:146–155, 1987.
6. Ambrosio, G., Weisfeldt, M.L., Jacobus, W.E., et al.: Evidence for a reversible oxygen radical-mediated component of reperfusion injury: Reduction by recombinant human superoxide dismutase administered at the time of reflow. *Circulation* 75:282–291, 1987.

7. Campbell, C.A., Kloner, R.A., Alker, K.J., et al.: Effect of verapamil on infarct size in dogs subjected to coronary artery occlusion with transient reperfusion. *J. Am. Coll. Cardiol.* 8:1169–1174, 1986.
8. Kolodgie, F.D., Dawson, A.K., Roden, D.M., et al.: Effect of fluosol-DA on infarct morphology and vulnerability to ventricular arrhythmia. *Am. Heart J.* 112:1192–1201, 1986.
9. Heller, G.V., et al.: Intercoronary thallium-201 scintigraphy after thrombolytic therapy for acute myocardial infarction compared with 10 and 100 day intravenous thallium-201 scintigraphy. *J. Am. Coll. Cardiol.* 9:300–307, 1987.

Coronary Artery Spasms and Stenosis

Pathogenesis of Coronary Artery Spasm in Miniature Swine With Regional Intimal Thickening After Balloon Denudation

Yusuke Yamamoto, Hitonobu Tamoike, Kensuke Egashira, Tadashi Kobayashi, Takayuki Kawasaki, and Motoomi Nakamura (Kyushu Univ., Fukuoka, Japan)
Circ. Res. 60:113–121, January 1987 1–31

A previous study showed that coronary artery spasm can be provoked in Göttingen miniature pigs and can be documented angiographically. Using this swine model, the pathogenesis of coronary artery spasm induced by histamine was studied angiographically in in vivo and in vitro conditions.

Endothelial balloon denudation was performed on the left circumflex and left anterior descending coronary arteries, and the animals were fed laboratory chow for 3 months. Thereafter, coronary artery spasm was repeatedly provoked by histamine (10 μg/kg) given intracoronarily. Coronary artery spasm was documented in vivo by selective coronary arteriography, and the resulting myocardial ischemia was confirmed by electrocardiographic ST segment changes. Histamine more significantly reduced the diameter of the coronary artery in the denuded area than in the nondenuded area (63 ± 3 vs. 26 ± 2%).

An in vitro study was undertaken to evaluate coronary artery spasm without the influence of blood constituents and neural control and to quantitate the pharmacophysiologic characteristics of histamine-induced coronary constriction in the coronary spasm. The same heart used in the in vivo study was isolated and perfused with Krebs-Henseleit solution under a constant perfusion pressure of 90 mm Hg. Histamine (10^{-5} M) caused a significant dose-response reduction in the diameter of the coronary artery of the isolated heart in the denuded area compared with that in the nondenuded area (29 ± 4 vs. 67 ± 3%), similar to that observed in vivo. The constriction of the denuded areas in response to histamine was topologically the same in vivo and in vitro. Also, the degree of focal constriction induced by histamine, defined as percent of stenoses from the mean diameter of the areas proximal and distal to the spastic site, was similar in vivo and in vitro.

Percent luminal reduction caused by potassium chloride and phenylephrine was similar in the denuded and nondenuded areas. There was no significant influence of neurotransmitter blockade with guanethidine, atropine, and tetradotoxin, on the dose-response relation of the coronary artery to histamine. There was absence of enhanced constriction in the denuded areas by histamine in a calcium-free perfusate. Pretreatment with mepyramine, an H_1-receptor blocker, abolished the histamine-induced augmented constriction. Histologically, the intima was invariably thickened along the spastic portion and was coated by endothelial cells.

Histamine-induced augmented constriction can be reproduced in a similar degree and area as that observed angiographically in vivo in isolated pig hearts perfused with electrolyte solution containing 2.6 mM of calcium. These results suggest that enhanced influx of Ca^{2+} via H_1 receptors at the denuded area plays a major role in coronary artery spasm.

▶ This study in a swine model of coronary artery vasoconstriction provides important information concerning the possible pathogenesis of coronary artery spasm. These investigations of histamine-induced coronary vasospasm suggest that the enhanced influx of calcium through H_1 receptors at the denuded vessel plays a major role in the initiation of coronary artery spasm. Further studies in vitro using the same hearts in which coronary artery spasm occurred in vivo should provide additional important information concerning this interesting cause of myocardial ischemia.—R.A. O'Rourke, M.D.

Leukotriene C_4- and D_4-Induced Diffuse Peripheral Constriction of Swine Coronary Artery Accompanied by ST Elevation on the Electrocardiogram: Angiographic Analysis

Hitonobu Tomoike, Kensuke Egashira, Akira Yamada, Yasuo Hayashi and Motoomi Nakamura (Kyushu Univ., Higashi-ku, Fukuoka, Japan)

Circulation 76:480–487, August 1987 1–32

Leukotriene (LT) C_4 and LTD_4 have a potent constrictive effect on vascular smooth muscle and have been presumed to be involved in coronary artery spasm. The effect of these two leukotrienes on coronary artery spasm was investigated angiographically in 15 Göttingen miniature pigs. These pigs were subjected to endothelial balloon denudation of the left circumflex coronary artery, then 11 were fed a 2% cholesterol diet, and the rest were fed a regular diet. Three months later the denuded area of the coronary artery was reduced by 94 ± 2% and the nondenuded area by 43 ± 5% by the administration of 10 μg/kg histamine after pretreatment with 60 mg/kg intravenous cimetidine.

Administration of LTC_4 or LTD_4 in doses of 1 and 10 μg caused elevations in the ST segment on the ECG. There was delayed filling of the-contrast medium in the peripheral coronary artery. However, there were no increased constrictions. Diphenhydramine, a histamine H_1-receptor blocker, eliminated the histamine-induced coronary spasm. FPL-55712, an LTC_4 and LTD_4 receptor blocker, eliminated the LT-induced myocardial ischemia but not the histamine-induced coronary spasm.

In a swine model of coronary artery spasm, LTC_4 and LTD_4 constricted small vessels and caused ischemia. However, they did not play an important role in histamine-induced arterial spasm.

▶ Using the same swine model of histamine-induced coronary artery vasoconstriction discussed above, these investigators assess the effects of leukotriene (LT) C_4 and LTD_4 on coronary spasm in atherosclerotic miniature pigs as examined arteriographically. These compounds did not augment constriction at any site of the epicardial coronary arteries; however, their administration produced elevations in the ST segments on the ECG and delayed filling of the contrast medium in the peripheral coronary arteries. Thus, LTC_4 + LTD_4 appear to constrict the coronary arteries at the level of small vessels, rendering the perfused myocardial ischemia without producing epicardial coronary artery spasm.—R.A. O'Rourke, M.D.

Thromboxane A_2 Analogue Induced Coronary Artery Vasoconstriction in the Rabbit

Yoshiki Yui, Keiji Sakaguchi, Takashi Susawa, Ryuichi Hattori, Yoshiki Takatsu, Natsuko Yui, and Chuichi Kawai (Kyoto Univ., Japan)

Cardiovasc. Res. 21:119–123, February 1987 1–33

The role of thromboxane A_2, a strong platelet aggregator and vasoconstrictor, in coronary artery vasospasm remains to be fully defined. A study was conducted in the rabbit to determine whether the thromboxane A_2 analogue, 9,11-epithio-11,12-methano thromboxane A_2 (STA_2) could provoke coronary artery vasoconstriction and to determine the role of extracellular calcium in STA_2-induced vasoconstriction.

Injection of 25 μg/kg STA_2 into the left main trunk resulted in complete occlusion of the left anterior descending artery and narrowing of the left circumflex artery. The right coronary artery was also temporarily occluded by an injection of 25 $\mu g/kg^{-2}$ STA_2. The diameter of the coronary artery returned to the control value two minutes after injection. These findings were similar to the diffuse vasoconstriction seen clinically. Injection of STA_2 caused a significant increase in left ventricular end diastolic pressure and ST segment elevation. The STA_2-induced vasoconstriction was prevented by the preadministration of the calcium antagonist, diltiazem, 25 μg/kg, or a thromboxane A_2 receptor antagonist, ONO 3708 ($n = 10$).

The role of calcium in the STA_2-induced vasoconstriction was evaluated in vitro using isolated left circumflex artery. Administration of STA_2, 50 μg/L to 0.5 mg/L, produced a dose-dependent contraction of helical strips of the artery, which was suppressed by diltiazem, likewise, in a dose-dependent fashion (Fig 1–15). Reduction of the concentration of calcium in the incubation medium from 2.54 to 1.0 mmole/L significantly reduced the STA_2-induced contraction. Administration of STA_2 to a calcium-free medium failed to produce contraction, whereas the addition of calcium to the medium caused an abrupt contraction. Pretreatment of the coronary artery with ONO 3708 caused a significant

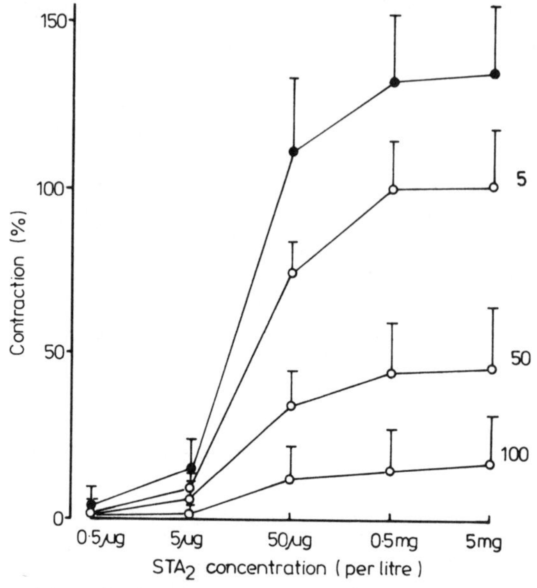

Fig 1–15.—Control dose-related contraction after STA_2 (●) and its gradual suppression by diltiazem (○) (doses in gm/L^{-1}) (n = 5). (Courtesy of Yui, Y., et al.: Cardiovasc. Res.: 21:119–123, February 1987.)

dose-related rightward and downward shift of the dose-response curve, whereas the serotonin antagonist, α-blocker, and angiotensin II analogue had no effect on the STA_2-induced vasoconstriction.

These results suggest that STA_2 induces transmembrane calcium influx into the smooth muscle cells, which leads to the vasoconstriction. The administration of a calcium antagonist or a thromboxane A_2 receptor antagonist may be useful in preventing vasoconstrictions caused by an increase in thromboxane A_2 concentrations.

▶ This study in rabbits provides important information concerning the possible role of thromboxane A_2 as a possible mediator of coronary vasospasm. The results of this study suggest that thromboxane A_2 can provoke coronary artery vasoconstriction, which could be documented arteriographically, and that the presence of extracellular calcium is an obligatory requirement for thromboxane A_2-induced vasoconstriction, indicating that the mechanism is likely related to increased transmembrane calcium influx.—R.A. O'Rourke, M.D.

Calcium Channel Blockers Induce Preferential Coronary Vasodilation by an α_1- Mechanism

Delvin R. Knight and Stephen F. Vatner (Harvard Univ. and Brigham and Women's Hosp., Boston, and New England Regional Primate Research Ctr., Southborough, Mass.)

Am. J. Physiol. 253:H604–H613, September 1987 1–34

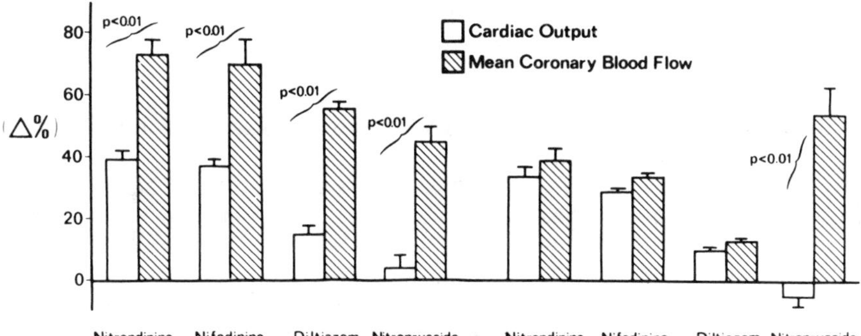

Fig 1–16.—Effects of nitrendipine, nifedipine, diltiazem, and nitroprusside on cardiac output *(open bars)* and mean coronary blood flow *(shaded bars)* are compared in presence of β-adrenergic and cholinergic receptor blockades (**left**) and following α_1-adrenergic receptor blockade in presence of β-adrenergic and cholinergic receptor blockades (**right**). Prior to α_1-adrenergic receptor blockade, nitrendipine, nifedipine, diltiazem, and nitroprusside induced significantly greater increases in coronary blood flow than cardiac output. After α_1-adrenergic receptor blockade preferential vasodilation in coronary bed was abolished for all three calcium channel blockers but not nitroprusside. (Courtesy of Knight, D.R., and Vatner, S.F.: Am. J. Physiol. 253:H604–H613, September 1987.)

The calcium channel blocker nitrendipine, which has high affinity for vascular smooth muscle, was used to determine to what extent these drugs dilate the coronary vessels and to what degree this effect is dependent on reflex β-adrenergic and cholinergic receptor mechanisms. Conscious mongrel dogs were utilized. Studies also were done with another dihydropyridine, nifedipine, and with a benzothiazepine, diltiazem.

Nitrendipine decreased late diastolic left circumflex coronary resistance significantly more than total peripheral resistance. This effect persisted after propranolol and atropine administration. After prazosin, however, nitrendipine no longer had this differential effect on coronary resistance. Nifedipine and diltiazem also reduced late diastolic coronary resistance more than total peripheral resistance, before but not after α_1-adrenergic receptor blockade with prazosin. Sodium nitroprusside reduced coronary resistance more than total peripheral resistance both before and after α_1-adrenergic blockade (Fig 1–16).

It appears that calcium channel blockers preferentially increase coronary blood flow and lower late diastolic coronary resistance in the conscious dog, compared with changes in total peripheral resistance and cardiac output. As this preferential effect is abolished by prazosin, an α_1-adrenergic mechanism may be involved.

► The preferential vasodilation of the coronary arteries in comparison with changes in cardiac output and total peripheral resistance induced by calcium entry blockers is even more prominent after the elimination of the reflex increase in heart rate and myocardial contractility secondary to the fall in arterial pressure and persists after α_1-adrenergic receptor blockade. However, the preferential effects on the coronary bed compared with the systemic circulation were abolished by α-adrenergic receptor blockade. The data suggests that the calcium blockers either interfere with baroreceptor reflex control or α_1-adrenergic receptor control of the systemic circulation in general and the coronary circulation in particular.—R.A. O'Rourke, M.D.

Delineation of the Extent of Coronary Atherosclerosis by High-Frequency Epicardial Echocardiography

David D. McPherson, Loren F. Hiratzka, Wade C. Lamberth, Berkely Brandt, Michelle Hunt, Robert A. Kieso, Melvin L. Marcus, and Richard E. Kerber (Univ. of Iowa)

N. Engl. J. Med. 316:304–309, Feb. 5, 1987 1–35

Postmortem studies suggest that coronary angiography does not always accurately predict the severity of coronary artery disease. A new technique—high-frequency epicardial echocardiography—allows direct imaging of the coronary arterial wall and lumen intraoperatively. High-frequency epicardial echocardiography was used to quantify the extent of coronary atherosclerosis in 37 patients at the time of cardiac surgery by measuring the ratio of the diameter of the lumen of the coronary artery to the thickness of its wall.

Eleven patients had no angiographic evidence of coronary disease in any coronary artery (group I); the mean luminal diameter/wall thickness ratio was 6. Twenty-one patients had angiographic evidence of coronary disease (more than 50% narrowing) at the site evaluated by echocardiography (group II); the mean ratio was 2, reflecting encroachment into the arterial lumen by atherosclerotic plaque. Fifteen patients had arterial segments that were angiographically normal but had arterial stenoses elsewhere in the coronary tree (group III); the mean ratio was 4, with marked overlap with the values in group II patients.

Group means in groups II and III were significantly lower than the mean of group I and were different from each other. Arterial segments in group II were compared with matching segments in group III. Many of the segments in group III had luminal dimater/wall thickness ratios equal to or lower than their corresponding segments in group II, rather than being higher, which would be expected if the segments in group III were truly normal. In addition, many group III segments showed maximal wall thickness well above the normal (group I) range.

These findings indicated the presence of arterial wall thickening not demonstrated by angiography. Thus, in living human hearts, diffuse intimal atherosclerosis is often present even when coronary angiography reveals only discrete stenoses, indicating that coronary angiography often underestimates the severity and extent of coronary disease.

▶ Since selective coronary arteriography does not always accurately indicate the severity of coronary artery disease, other techniques, particularly noninvasive methods, have been sought for imaging the coronary arteries. This study shows the usefulness of high-frequency epicardial echocardiography for measuring the ratio of the diameter of the coronary artery lumen to the thickness of its wall. These studies indicate the frequent presence of diffuse intimal coronary atherosclerosis when coronary arteriography only reveals discrete coronary artery stenosis, indicating the need for improved methods of appropriately estimating the severity and extent of coronary artery disease.—R.A. O'Rourke, M.D.

Prediction of the Physiologic Significance of Coronary Arterial Lesions by Quantitative Lesion Geometry in Patients With Limited Coronary Artery Disease

Robert F. Wilson, Melvin L. Marcus, and Carl W. White (Univ. of Iowa and VA Hosp., Iowa City)

Circulation 75:723–732, April 1987 1–36

Studies in animals with normal coronary arteries have demonstrated that coronary flow reserve can be predicted by angiographic measurements of arterial stenosis. In contrast, studies in humans suggest that even quantitative analysis of coronary angiograms cannot predict the physiologic significance of individual coronary lesions. However, these later studies were carried out in patients with either widespread diffuse coronary artery disease or by measurement techniques that tend to underestimate maximal coronary flow reserve. The relationship between coronary arterial stenosis and coronary flow reserve (CFR) was studied in patients with discrete limited coronary atherosclerosis.

The study included 50 patients with a single discrete coronary stenosis in only one or two vessels. The authors determined that the minimum coronary arterial cross-sectional area (mCSA), percent area stenosis (%AS), and percent diameter stenosis in the left and right anterior oblique projections were determined by the Brown/Dodge method of quantitative coronary angiography. They placed a No. 3F coronary Doppler catheter immediately proximal to the lesion and measured CFR by intracoronary administration of papaverine in doses sufficient to provide maximal arteriolar vasodilation. A translesional pressure gradient was obtained with an angioplasty catheter in 25 patients. The authors measured the CFR in patients with coronary artery disease and compared it with that in 13 patients with normal coronary vessels.

The CFR of normal patients averaged 5.0 ± 0.6 (peak/resting velocity ratio). In patients with limited coronary artery disease, CFR was observed to be closely correlated with %AS, mCSA, and the translesional pressure gradient. In addition, the most severe percent diameter stenosis in either the left or right oblique view was also highly correlated with CFR. All arteries with 2.5 sq mm mCSA had CFR of over 3.5.

In contrast to the poor correlation of percent area and percent diameter stenosis to CFR measured in patients with multivessel coronary artery disease, CFR measured at angiography in patients with discrete, limited coronary artery disease correlates closely with luminal stenosis determined precisely with quantitative coronary angiography. The authors suggest that differences in the extent of diffuse arterial narrowing may account for these differences.

▶ The findings of this study in patients with single discrete coronary artery stenosis involving only one or two vessels differ from those of two previous studies from the same laboratory. They demonstrate an important relationship between both visual and quantitative estimates of coronary luminal stenosis and intraoperative measurements of coronary flow reserve, in contrast to results obtained in patients with more widespread coronary artery disease. In this study, precisely measured percent area stenosis and minimum cross-sectional area predicted the coronary flow reserve of individual coronary arteries in patients with limited discrete atherosclerosis, facilitating the assessment of the physiologic significance of coronary artery lesions in the catheterization laboratory.—R.A. O'Rourke, M.D.

Additional important references concerning coronary artery vasoconstriction and the physiologic significance of coronary artery stenoses are listed below:

1. Kanmura, Y., Itoh, T., Kuriyama, H.: Mechanisms of vasoconstriction induced by 9,11-Epithio-11, 12-methano-thromboxane A_2 in the rabbit coronary artery. *Circ. Res.* 60:402–409, 1987.
2. Ashton, J.H., et al.: Inhibition of cyclic flow variations in stenosed canine coronary arteries by thromboxane A_2/prostaglandin H_2 receptor antagonists. *Circ. Res.* 59:568–578, 1986.
3. Young, M.A., Vatner, S.F.: Regulation of large coronary arteries. *Circ. Res.* 59:579–596, 1986.
4. McEwan, J., et al.: Calcitonin gene-related peptide: A potent dilator of human epicardial coronary arteries. *Circulation* 74:1243–1247, 1986.
5. Sasaguri, T., Itoh, T., Hirata, M., et al.: Regulation of coronary artery tone in relation to the activation of signal transductors that regulate calcium homeostasis. *J. Am. Coll. Cardiol.* 9:1167–1175, 1987.
6. Zijlstra, F., van Ommeren, J.V., Reiber, J.H.C., et al.: Does the quantitative assessment of coronary artery dimensions predict the physiologic significance of a coronary stenosis? *Circulation* 75:1154–1161, 1987.

Noninvasive Testing

Frequency of Painless Myocardial Ischemia During Exercise Tolerance Testing in Patients With and Without Diabetes Mellitus

Stuart R. Chipkin, David Frid, Joseph S. Alpert, Stephen P. Baker, James E. Dalen, and Neil Aronin (Univ. of Massachusetts)
Am. J. Cardiol. 59:61–65, Jan. 1, 1987 1–37

The prevalence of painless myocardial ischemia in patients with diabetes mellitus compared with other patients with coronary artery disease is not well known. To investigate this, all patients with positive exercise tolerance test responses, defined by at least 2 mm of ST depression, during a 2-year period were examined.

Of the 211 patients with exercise-induced myocardial ischemia, 101 (48%) had no chest pain during the ischemic period. Patients with painless myocardial ischemia reported prior episodes of chest pain and were taking nitrates less often than were patients who reported pain. Lack of pain did not correlate with age (mean, 59 years), gender, presence of systemic hypertension, previous myocardial infarction, coronary artery bypass grafting, cigarette smoking, or use of β-blocking or calcium-channel blocking drugs. Twenty-six patients (12%) had diabetes mellitus; 14 (54%) did not have chest pain. This prevalence did not differ significantly from that in nondiabetic patients who had painless ischemia during exercise testing (47%).

Diabetic patients had significantly more hypertension and were likely to be referred for exercise testing because of claudication than were nondiabetic patients. The duration of exercise was shorter in diabetics and in patients who had pain with myocardial ischemia. No significant difference in age, gender, use of nitrates, β-blocking or calcium-channel blocking drugs, history of myocardial infarction, angina pectoris, or cigarette smoking was found between diabetic and nondiabetic patients. Neither diabetes mellitus nor painless myocardial ischemia correlated with the number of narrowed coronary arteries or average calculated ejection fraction at cardiac catheterization.

Painless myocardial ischemia is common among patients with positive exercise tolerance test responses. Its frequency, however, is similar in diabetic and nondiabetic patients.

▶ Asymptomatic or "silent" myocardial ischemia has been recognized with increased frequency recently because of currently available noninvasive techniques, and diabetes is known to be associated frequently with myocardial infarction in the absence of chest pain or discomfort. It has been suggested that myocardial ischemia without infarction is also far more prevalent in diabetics as compared to nondiabetics. Interestingly, the authors found a 48% incidence of silent myocardial ischemia during exercise-induced ECG changes in 211 patients. There was no difference in the incidence of asymptomatic episodes of significant ST segment depression in nondiabetics as compared to diabetic patients. These data suggest the changes in the autonomic nervous system associated with diabetes mellitus do not result in a higher incidence of exercise-induced myocardial ischemia without chest pain. However, the number of patients studied is relatively small and may be insufficient for detecting an actual difference.—R.A. O'Rourke, M.D.

Comparison of Pulsed Doppler and Thermodilution Methods for Measuring Cardiac Output in Critically Ill Patients

Karl D. Donovan, Geoffrey J. Dobb, Mark A. Newman, Bernard E.S. Hockings, and Mark Ireland (Royal Perth Hosp., Western Australia)

Crit. Care Med. 15:853–857, September 1987 1–38

The most common method of measuring cardiac function in intensive and coronary care units is thermodilution. A noninvasive technique would be useful. In this study, pulsed Doppler echocardiography is compared with the thermodilution technique in the assessment of cardiac function in 38 critically ill patients.

The mean thermodilution cardiac ouput (TD_{co}) was 5.7 ± 1.87 L per minute. The mean pulsed Doppler cardiac output was 5.16 ± 1.66 L per minute. The mean difference between these two measurements was 0.51 ± 1.6 L per minute. The overall coefficient of correlation between these two methods was only .58. In all types of patients examined, the standard deviation of the difference between the measurements with these two methods was greater than 1 L per minute.

The noninvasive pulsed Doppler technique was not able to accurately predict thermodilution cardiac output in critically ill patients.

▶ This and the subsequent three abstracts concern the use of Doppler echocardiography, a frequently used non-invasive technique for detecting various kinds of information in patients with suspected or definite cardiac disease.

Pulse Doppler echocardiography has been used frequently for the serial noninvasive measurements of cardiac output in critically ill patients. Although many reports show a good correlation between cardiac output estimated by Doppler and then estimated by other methods, a few studies show a poor correlation. The technique utilized is extremely important, and an accurate measurement of the aortic diameter is essential for Doppler cardiac output determination. Importantly, the study above failed to demonstrate that the Doppler-measured cardiac output accurately predicted thermodilution cardiac output in critically ill patients.—R.A. O'Rourke, M.D.

When Should Doppler-Determined Valve Area be Better Than the Gorlin Formula?: Variation in Hydraulic Constants in Low Flow States

Jerome Segal, Daniel J. Lerner, D. Craig Miller, R. Scott Mitchell, Edwin A. Alderman, and Richard L. Popp (Stanford Univ.)

J. Am. Coll. Cardiol. 9:1294–1305, June 1987 1–39

Aortic stenosis is typically assessed hemodynamically by the Gorlin formula. The Gorlin formula underestimates valve area in low flow states. Unsteady flow was investigated in a pulsatile pump model and in a dog model. Valve areas were calculated from pressure and flow data using a modified Gorlin formula with constants for hydraulic discharge coefficient (C_d) and coefficient for orifice contraction (C_c), a corrected formula with C_d and C_c values obtained from steady state data or from the continuity equation with constant C_c. Flow velocities were measured by ultrasound Doppler catheter.

Both the corrected formula and the continuity equation were highly predictive of the actual valve area in the pump model. The modified Gorlin equation tended to underestimate valve areas, especially at low flow rates. Both the corrected and continuity equations predicted valve area in the dog model more accurately than the modified Gorlin formula.

In patients with low cardiac output, the Gorlin formula and other hemodynamic formulas, which assume a constant value for C_d, appear to be less accurate than formulas that use either a corrected C_d value or Doppler-determined flow velocity and mean systolic flow.

▶ Doppler velocity recordings are frequently used for the noninvasive assessment of the degree of valvular stenosis noninvasively, particularly in patients with aortic valve stenosis and in those with mitral stenosis. While the peak or instantaneous pressure gradient can be estimated by the Bernoulli principle and is $4V^2$, it is important to know the actual valve orifice size rather than just the peak or instantaneous pressure gradient across the valve.

In this study, unsteady flow was examined in a pulsatile pump model and in a dog model. K velocities were measured using a newly designed ultrasound Doppler catheter. The data from multiple experiments indicate that the Gorlin formula, which assumes a constant value for the hydraulic discharge coefficient (C_d), may be less accurate than formulas that contain only a coefficient for orifice contraction, along with velocity and flow measurements. The Doppler-determined mean jet velocity used with several possible methods for measuring mean systolic flow may improve the accuracy of assessing valve areas in patients with low cardiac output.

There has frequently been a disparity between the aortic valve area estimated at the time of cardiac catheterization using the Gorlin formula and the area of the valve found at corrective surgery in patients where the severity of the aortic stenosis is dependent upon a low cardiac output and long ventricular ejection time with a moderate pressure gradient across the valve.—R.A. O'Rourke, M.D.

Doppler Transmitral Flow Velocity Parameters: Relationship Between Age, Body Surface Area, Blood Pressure and Gender in Normal Subjects

Julius M. Gardin, Mary K. Rohan, Dennis M. Davidson, Ali Dabestani, Mark Sklansky, Raymond Garcia, Margaret L. Knoll, Donald B. White, Susan K. Gardin, and Walter L. Henry (VA Med. Ctr., Long Beach, Calif., and Univ. of California, Irvine Med. Ctr., Orange, Calif.)

Am. J. Noninvas. Cardiol. 1:3–10, January–February 1987 1–40

Previous studies at necropsy and using M-mode echocardiography have demonstrated thicker left ventricular walls and alterations in the mitral valve echogram with aging. More recently, Doppler studies of mitral valve flow velocity have suggested that the Doppler technique might yield useful information about left ventricular diastolic filling. The effects of age, body surface area, gender, and blood pressure on pulsed Doppler transmitral flow velocity measurements were assessed.

The study group included 66 adult men and women, aged 21–78 years, without a history of hypertension or cardiovascular disease. The authors made measurements at the level of the mitral leaflet tips of early and late diastolic transmitral peak flow (filling) velocities, flow times and flow velocity integrals, and of early diastolic flow acceleration and deceleration. The mitral peak flow velocity in early diastole (PFVE) was markedly lower in the 61–70 year age decade (45 ± 10 cm per second) than in the 21–30 year age decade (66 ± 11 cm per second). In addition, the mitral peak flow velocity in late diastole (PFVA) was significantly greater in the 61–70 age decade (55 ± 11 cm per second) than in the 21–30 year age group (41 ± 7 cm per second). Furthermore, the mitral A/E ratio (i.e., PFVA/PFVE) was significantly higher in the oldest (1.2 ± 0.3) compared with the youngest (0.6 ± 0.1) age group. The early and late diastolic flow times increased with age, whereas the early diastolic deceleration decreased with age. Two Doppler parameters were discovered to be positively correlated with systolic blood pressure: mitral A/E ratio and late diastolic flow velocity integral. Finally, there was no significant relationship between any of the Doppler mitral flow parameters and body surface area, diastolic blood pressure, or gender.

Age-related changes in pulsed Doppler transmitral flow velocity parameters must be taken into account when evaluating patients with suspected alterations in left ventricular filling.

▶ A noninvasive method for the accurate serial reproducible assessment of left ventricular diastolic function would provide important information concerning a large number of patients who have symptoms of breathlessness. Most recently, high temporal resolution radionuclide ventricular cineangiography and pulsed Doppler echocardiography have been used for this purpose. Neither technique has been evaluated extensively, and the present study was conducted to assess the effects of age, body surface area, gender, and blood pressure on pulsed Doppler transmitral flow velocity measurements.

No significant relationship was found between any of the Doppler mitral flow parameters and body surface area, diastolic blood pressure or gender. Both mitral A/E ratio and late diastolic flow velocity integral correlated with systolic blood pressure. Also, early and late diastolic flow times increased with age, whereas early diastolic deceleration decreased with age. However, the various correlations, although significant, were only fair at best and standard errors of the estimate appear large. The results and multiple other studies indicate that considerable further work is necessary to validate Doppler transmitral flow velocity parameters as indicators of left ventricular diastolic function.—R.A. O'Rourke, M.D.

Evaluation of Diastolic Function With Doppler Echocardiography: The PDF Formalism

Sandor J. Kovacs, Benico Barzilai, and Julio E. Perez (Washington Univ.)
Am. J. Physiol. 252:H178–H187, January 1987 1–41

Clinical and experimental characterization of normal and abnormal ventricular diastolic function has an extensive history. Currently, Doppler echocardiography provides a quantitative noninvasive means by which cardiac hemodynamics and their coupling to ventricular function can be investigated. A parametrized diastolic filling (PDF) formalism was developed for evaluation of holodiastolic (left and right) ventricular function via Doppler echocardiography.

This formalism is motivated by the empiric observation that during diastole the heart behaves as a suction pump whose dynamics, in certain respects, are those of a damped harmonic oscillator. If the solution $x(t)$ of the linear differential equation that describes the motion of a forced, damped harmonic oscillator is differentiated, one can obtain an expression for elastic recoil (suction) initiated ventricular diastolic fluid inflow velocity $v(t)$. This expression is solved for "over-damped" motion, for zero initial velocity, and initial displacement = x_o cm. An explicit forcing term—$F(t) = F_o \sin(wt)$—was used to accout for late diastolic (atrial) filling. The quantitative parameters of the model include inertia, viscosity, source of stored energy for suction, and its initial displacement x_o, the amplitude and frequency of the (atrial) forcing term Fo,w. When clinical examples of normal and abnormal transmitral DVPs are compared with $v(t)$, calculated using the harmonic oscillator model, excellent agreement is obtained throughout diastole.

The model permits accurate qualitative and quantitative characterization of global ventricular diastolic behavior by noninvasive means in a variety of normal and abnormal stiffness-compliance states. Furthermore, it may serve as a prototype for a class of mathematical models that can encompass the essential dynamic elements of ventricular diastolic function that couple to flow and further enhance the role of the heart as a suction pump.

► This study shows another approach to the use of Doppler echocardiography for the noninvasive quantitative assessment of left ventricular diastolic function. A new parameterized diastolic filling formula (PDF) that defines holodiastolic ventricular function with Doppler echocardiography was applied to several clinical examples of normal and abnormal transmitral diastolic flow patterns. The PDF formulism may be extended to allow noninvasive computation of other time-dependent parameters of diastolic function.—R.A. O'Rourke, M.D.

Nuclear Scans: A Clinical Decision Making Tool That Reduces the Need for Cardiac Catheterization

Sylvia Wassertheil-Smoller, Richard M. Steingart, John P. Wexler, Jonathan Tobin, Nancy Budner, Joseph Wachspress, Lloyd Lense, and Susan Slagle (Albert Einstein College of Medicine and Montefiore Hosp. and Med. Ctr., New York)
J. Chron. Dis. 40:385–397, 1987 1–42

Cardiovascular nuclear medicine studies (CVNMS) are used to detect cardiovascular disease. The study reviewed in this article examined whether these tests have an impact on the physician's decision to catheterize in 439 patients with suspected ischemic heart disease.

There was a change in the clinician's decision regarding catheterization in 31% of the cases. Resting studies had relatively low impact, while exercise studies had significant impact. After a normal exercise study, catheterization was reduced by 82%. An interesting finding of this study was that men with abnormal exercise results were seven times as likely to have catheterization as women, regardless of age.

Resting CVNMS had limited impact on the physician's decision. Nevertheless, exercise CVNMS reduced the catheterization rate in men significantly.

It appears that the exercise studies are highly useful. The sex difference in CVNMS impact seen in these tests requires further investigation.

▶ Multiple logistic regression analysis indicated that the results of exercise (but not resting) cardiovascular nuclear medicine studies (exercise radionuclide ventriculography and/or thallium myocardial perfusion scintigraphy) made an independent contribution to the clinicians' decision to catheterize for men only in this observational study of patients with suspected myocardial ischemia. A decision change to no catheterization occurred in 61% of patients for whom catheterization was planned before cardiovascular nuclear medicine studies (CVNMS) were performed and in 14% of patients (CVNMS) resulted in a change to catheterization.

Interestingly, there was a sevenfold greater likelihood of men with abnormal CVNMS as compared to women with abnormal CVNMS being referred for subsequent cardiac catheterizations. The reasons for this discrepancy are not entirely clear but may represent the lower likelihood of coronary heart disease (CHD) in women, the greater prevalence of "false positive" tests in women, or bias toward a less aggressive therapeutic approach for women with CHD or a combination of factors.—R.A. O'Rourke, M.D.

Sex-Specific Criteria for Interpretation of Thallium-201 Myocardial Uptake and Washout Studies

Mark Rabinovitch, Samy Suissa, Jack Elstein, Howard Staniloff, Anwu Tang, Christopher Rush, Anne Aldis, Rosemonde Tannous, Michelle Turek, Abdul Addas, Christopher O'Brien, J.H. Burgess, and Leonard Rosenthall (McGill Univ., Montreal)

J. Nucl. Med. 27:1837–1841, December 1986 1–43

Criteria for abnormal exercise thallium scintigrams have been derived from mixed-gender groups of normal subjects, but breast attenuation may affect regional count densities. Sex-specific criteria were therefore developed in 49 normal subjects having exercise-redistribution thallium perfusion studies, 23 men and 26 women. Eleven subjects had atypical chest pain and negative or non-interpretable exercise ECGs. Maximal treadmill exercise was performed at scintigraphy.

Several regional uptake ratios were significantly lower in females than in males. Significant gender differences also were found in washout rates. The differences appeared to reflect proportionally reduced anterior and upper septal uptake in women, as well as faster washout in women.

Faster washout could not be attributed to either physiologic or artifactitious factors. The results obtained by two observers correlated very closely for 23 of 24 quantitative parameters.

Both thallium myocardial uptake and washout are influenced by gender to a significant degree. A prospective study is needed to learn whether sex-specific criteria will improve the predictive accuracy of exercise-redistribution myocardial perfusion scintigraphy in detecting and localizing coronary artery disease.

▶ In this study significant sexual differences were found in both regional thallum-201 uptake ratios and washout rates, reflecting a proportionally lesser anterior and upper septal myocardium uptake in women and faster washout in women. The authors recommend that postexercise thallum-201 images be checked immediately for a pattern of uptake suggestive of a breast shadow; repetition of a view with the breast taped upward and medially may resolve interpretation problems.—R.A. O'Rourke, M.D.

Role of Myocardial Perfusion Imaging in Evaluating Thrombolytic Therapy for Acute Myocardial Infarction

George A. Beller (Univ. of Virginia)

J. Am. Coll. Cardiol. 9:661–668, March 1987 1–44

Increasingly, myocardial thallium-201 scintigraphy is being used to assess myocardial ischemia and infarction noninvasively. Here clinical studies are summarized, limitations of the technique are reviewed, and recommendations for the future are given.

Studies have found that new thallium uptake, after intracoronary tracer administration following successful recanalization, indicates that nutrient blood flow has been successfully restored. It is presumed that there has been some myocardial salvage if thallium thus administered is transported intracellularly by myocytes with intact sarcolemmal membranes. If thallium is injected intracoronarily immediately after reperfusion, initial uptake in reperfused myocardium may represent mostly hyperemic flow. In this case, regional thallium counts may not be proportional to the mass of viable myocytes. Two separate thallium injections may be administered before and 24 hours after treatment with thrombolytic therapy.

The improvement in defect size on serial images predicts improvement in regional function and patency of the infarct-related vessel. Before discharge, patients treated with intravenous thrombolytic therapy for acute myocardial infarction may undergo exercise thallium-201 scintigraphy to stratify risk, detect residual ischemia, and determine subsequent management (Fig 1–17).

Thallium imaging has several limitations. If technique is faulty, image artifacts may be mistaken for defects. Absolute blood flow cannot be quantitated; only relative abnormalities can be detected. At present, accu-

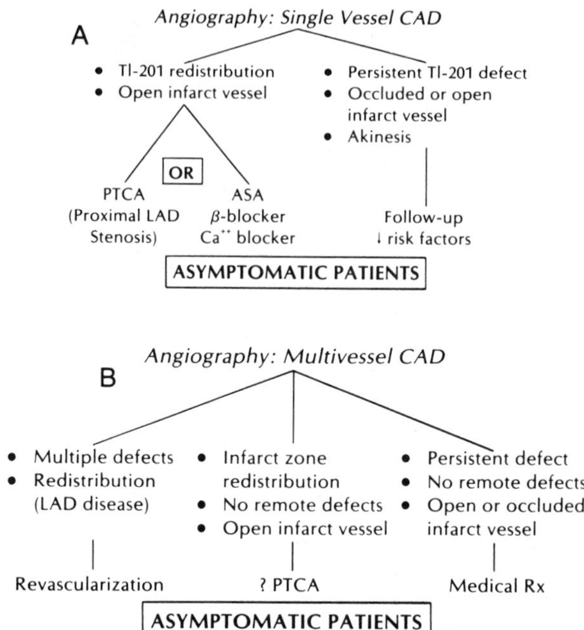

Fig 1–17.—**A,** potential approaches to management of postmyocardial infarction patients with single vessel coronary artery disease (CAD) who have undergone predischarge exercise thallium-201 (Tl-201) scintigraphy. **B,** potential approaches to management of patients undergoing thrombolytic therapy who have multivessel CAD and have undergone predischarge exercise Tl-201 scintigraphy. *ASA* = aspirin; *LAD* = left anterior descending artery; *PTCA* = percutaneous transluminal coronary angioplasty; *Rx* = treatment. (Courtesy of Beller, G.A.: J. Am. Coll. Cardiol. 9:661–668, March 1987.)

racy in quantitating infarct size is somewhat limited. Many technical drawbacks could be overcome with a technetium-99m-labeled perfusion agent that was also taken up by the myocardium in proportion to blood flow.

▶ Myocardial perfusion imaging, usually with thallium-201, is a potentially useful method for assessing patients with acute infarction undergoing coronary thrombolytic therapy. Initial defects that persist after thrombolysis suggest that the infarct-related artery is still occluded or that reflow to irreversibly injured myocardium has occurred; however, severe ischemia without substantial necrosis may also cause persistent defects. When rest imaging is performed 24 hours to 10 days after thrombolytic therapy, the extent of thallium-201 uptake in the reperfused zone is proportional to the amount of viable myocardium supplied by the infarct-related artery.

Exercise thallium-201 imaging may be useful for assessing the amount of residual jeopardized but viable myocardium in the perfusion zone of the infarct-related artery and in areas distant from the infarction. There are many limitations in the use of thallium scintigraphy, some of which will be overcome as newer myocardial perfusion imaging agents are developed for this purpose and undergo large-scale clinical testing.—R.A. O'Rourke, M.D.

Additional interesting publications concerning the usefulness of noninvasive techniques for measuring cardiac function and detecting evidence of myocardial ischemia are listed as follows:

1. Hancock, E.W., Norcini, J.J., Webster, G.D.: A standardized examination in the interpretation of electrocardiograms. *J. Am. Coll. Cardiol.* 10:882–886, 1987.
2. Mark, D.B., Hlatky, M.A., Lee, K.L., et al.: Localizing coronary artery obstructions with the exercise treadmill test. *Ann. Intern. Med.* 106:53–55, 1987.
3. Kuo, L.C., Bolli, R., Thornby, J., et al.: Effects of exercise tolerance, age, and gender on the specificity of radionuclide angiography: Sequential ejection fraction analysis during multistage exercise. *Curr. Cardiol.* 113:1180–1189, 1987.
4. Hatle, L.: Noninvasive measurements of intracardiac blood flow velocities with Doppler ultrasound. *Acta Med. Scand.* 221:133–136, 1987.
5. Meijboom, E.J., Rijsterborgh, H., Bot, H., et al.: Limits of reproducibility of blood flow measurements by Doppler echocardiography. *Am. J. Cardiol.* 59:133–137, 1987.
6. Dittmann, H., Voelker, W., Karsch, K-R., et al.: Influence of sampling site and flow area on cardiac output measurements by Doppler echocardiography. *J. Am. Coll. Cardiol.* 10:818–823, 1987.
7. Appel, P.L., Kram, H.B., Mackabee, J., et al.: Comparison of measurements of cardiac output by bioimpedance and thermodilution in severely ill surgical patients. *Crit. Care Med.* 14:933–935, 1986.
8. Veyrat, C., Gourtschiglouian, C., Dumora, P., et al.: A new noninvasive estimation of the stenotic aortic valve area by pulsed Doppler mapping. *Br. Heart J.* 57:44–50, 1987.
9. Switzer, D.F., Yoganathan, A.P., Nanda, N.C., et al.: Calibration of color Doppler flow mapping during extreme hemodynamic conditions in vitro: A foundation for reliable quantitative grading system for aortic incompetence. *Circulation* 75:837–846, 1987.
10. Sprecher, D.L., Adamick, R., Adams, D., et al.: In vitro color flow, pulsed and continuous wave Doppler ultrasound masking of flow by prosthetic valves. *J. Am. Coll. Cardiol.* 9:1306–1310, 1987.
11. Prigent, F., Maddahi, J., Garcia, E.V., et al.: Comparative methods for quantifying myocardial infarct size by thallium-201 SPECT. *J. Nucl. Med.* 28:325–333, 1987.
12. Granato, J.E., Watson, D.D., Flanagan, T.L., et al.: Myocardial thallium-201 kinetics and regional flow alterations with 3 hours of coronary occlusion and either rapid reperfusion through a totally patent vessel or slow reperfusion through a critical stenosis. *J. Am. Coll. Cardiol.* 9:109–118, 1987.
13. Okada, R.D., Bendersy, R., Strauss, H.W., et al.: Comparison of intravenous dipyridamole thallium cardiac imaging with exercise radionuclide angiography. *Am. Heart J.* 114:524–531, 1987.
14. Goldberg, H.L., Herrold, E., Hochreiter, C., et al.: Videodensitometric determination of right ventricular and left ventricular ejection fraction. *Am. J. Noninvas. Cardiol.* 1:18–23, 1987.
15. Helfant, R.H., Klein, L.W., Agarwal, J.B.: Role of cardiac testing in anera of proliferating technology and cost containment. *J. Am. Coll. Cardiol.* 9:1194–1198, 1987.

Newer Diagnostic and Therapeutic Techniques

Use of Ultrafast Computed Tomography to Quantitate Regional Myocardial Perfusion: A Preliminary Report

John A. Rumberger, Andrew J. Feiring, Martin J. Lipton, Charles B. Higgins, Stephen R. Ell, and Melvin L. Marcus (Univ. of Iowa and Univ. of California at San Francisco)

J. Am. Coll. Cardiol. 9:59–69, January 1987 1–45

The potential role for rapid acquisition computed axial tomography (CT) (Imatron C-100) to quantify regional myocardial perfusion was evaluated in six anesthetized, closed chest dogs. Myocardial and left ventricular (LV) cavity contrast clearance curves were constructed after injecting nonionic contrast into the inferior vena cava at a rate of 1 ml/kg for 2–3 seconds. Independent myocardial perfusion measurements were obtained by coincident injection of radiolabeled microspheres into the left atrium during control, intermediate, and maximal myocardial vasodilation with adenosine. At each flow state, 40 serial short-axis scans of the left ventricle were taken near end-diastole at the midpapillary muscle level. Contrast clearance curves were generated and analyzed from the LV cavity and posterior papillary muscle regions after excluding contrast recirculation and minimizing partial volume effects. The area under the curve (gamma variate function) was determined for a region of interest placed within the LV cavity.

High-quality contrast density data were generated by ultrafast CT in the LV cavity and posterior LV myocardium after injection of iodinated contrast. Myocardial perfusion values, as assessed by microspheres, varied from 30 ml/100 gm per minute to 450 ml/100 gm per minute (mean, 167 ml/100 gm per minute). Quantitative measurements of myocardial perfusion in the posterior papillary region included peak myocardial opacification, area under the contrast clearance curve, and a contrast clearance time defined by the full width/half maximal extent of the clearance curves. Two flow algorithms evaluating characteristics of the LV and myocardial contrast clearance curves correlated significantly with regional myocardial perfusion in the posterior papillary muscle region as assessed by microspheres: the ratio of the peak myocardial opacification from baseline to the area under the LV cavity curve ($r = 0.7$; SEE = 44.4 m/100 gm per minute), and the ratio of the LV cavity to posterior papillary muscle curve areas divided by the full width/half maximal contrast time in the region of the posterior papillary muscle ($r = 0.82$; SEE = 52.2 ml/100 gm per minute).

Regional myocardial perfusion in the posterior papillary muscle of the dog as assessed by microspheres correlates with indices derived from myocardial/LV cavity density versus time curves measured by ultrafast CT. These preliminary results suggest a promising approach to quantitation of regional myocardial perfusion and myocardial reserve flow in man, although technical, theoretical, and practical errors may occur during its application in man.

▶ Fast cine CT has been utilized at several centers for assessing left ventricular (LV) function, for measuring LV mass, and for evaluating coronary artery bypass grafts. Measurements of LV mass by this method correlate highly with direct measurements of LV mass in postmortem studies in experiment animals. In this preliminary report of six anesthetized, closed chest dogs, derived indices from myocardial/LV cavity density versus time curves measured by ultrafast CT correlate extremely well with microsphere measurements of myocardial perfusion in the posterior papillary muscle of the dog. The noninvasive studies require the injection of nonionic contrast into the systemic venous system. However, if reproducible results can be demonstrated in patients with coronary artery disease, this technique will provide an accurate method for assessing regional myocardial perfusion and myocardial reserve flow in man.—R.A. O'Rourke, M.D.

Magnetic Resonance Assessment of Aortic and Mitral Regurgitation

S.R. Underwood, R.H. Klipstein, D.N. Firmin, K.M. Fox, P.A. Poole-Wilson, R.S.O. Rees, and D.B. Longmore (The Natl. Heart and Chest Hosp., London)

Br. Heart J. 56:455–462, November 1986 1–46

Magnetic resonance imaging provides an accurate method for the measurement of left and right ventricular volume. The left to right ventricular stroke volume ratio was calculated from contiguous transverse magnetic resonance images to quantify the severity of regurgitation in 18 patients with aortic regurgitation and 10 patients with mitral regurgitation. The findings were compared with those obtained from radionuclide ventriculography and cardiac catheterization.

Cardiac anatomy was well demonstrated, allowing an assessment of relative chamber volumes and associated anatomical features. Although the mitral and aortic valves were visible in many patients, the details of valve abnormalities were not well shown. A weak correlation was evident between left ventricular end diastolic volume and stroke volume ratio as measured by magnetic resonance. Magnetic resonance measurements of mean stroke volume ratio increased significantly with severity of regurgitation as shown at cardiac catheterization, and all but the patients with trivial regurgitation differed significantly from normal. In addition, stroke volume ratio differed significantly between patients with trivial, mild, moderate, and severe regurgitation.

There was a good correlation between magnetic resonance and radionuclide measurements of left ventricular ejection fraction and stroke volume ratio (Fig 1–18), although the radionuclide technique consistently overestimated the stroke volume ratio. Correlation was worse for right ventricular ejection fraction, which was consistently underestimated by the radionuclide ventriculography.

Magnetic resonance imaging provides an accurate measure of ventricular volume, ejection fraction, and the left to right ventricular stroke volume ratio that can be used to quantify the severity of regurgitation in patients with isolated aortic and mitral regurgitation. It is a valuable

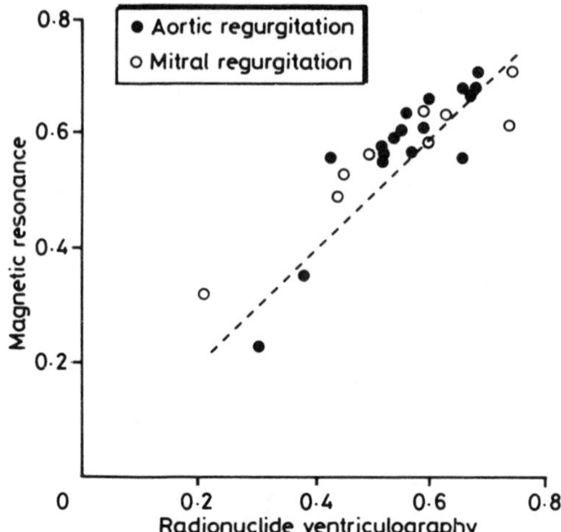

Fig 1–18.—Correlation between magnetic resonance and radionuclide measurements of left ventricular ejection fraction ($y = .73x + .16$, $r = .85$, $P<.001$, standard error of the estimate = .06). The *dotted line* is the line of identity. (Courtesy of Underwood, S.R., et al.: Br. Heart J. 56:455–462, November 1986.)

addition to the conventional methods of assessing valvar regurgitation and can serve as a suitable standard by which to judge their accuracy.

▶ In the past, the ratio of left ventricular stroke volume to right ventricular stroke volume, as determined by radionuclide ventriculography, has been used to measure quantitatively the severity of aortic and/or mitral regurgitation in patients. This is a fairly accurate technique but requires careful assignment of right and left ventricular regions of interest and is being replaced by Doppler echocardiography for the noninvasive assessment of left-sided valvular regurgitation in man. Since nuclear magnetic resonance imaging (MRI) can be used to measure left and right ventricular volumes accurately, the same information about the severity of regurgitation is obtainable by this technique as determined by radionuclide ventriculography or contrast left ventricular cineangiography in man. Although the results are promising, nuclear MRI is unlikely to replace more conventional measurements of valvular regurgitation that are less costly and more readily available.—R.A. O'Rourke, M.D.

Adriamycin Cardiotoxicity and Proton Nuclear Magnetic Resonance Relaxation Properties

Randall C. Thompson, Robert C. Canby, Edwin W. Lojeski, Adam V. Ratner, John T. Fallon, and Gerald M. Pohost (Massachusetts Gen. Hosp., Boston, and Univ. of Alabama at Birmingham)
Am. Heart J. 113:1444–1448, June 1987 1–47

Doxorubicin (Adriamycin) is a valuable chemotherapeutic agent for the treatment of a variety of solid tumors and hematologic malignancies.

However, doxorubicin and other anthracyclines may be cardiotoxic; chronic life-threatening cardiomyopathy that occurs most frequently with high cumulative doses is a major limitation of the efficacy of these agents. Present noninvasive techniques to detect Adriamycin toxicity rely on assessment of myocardial function rather than on direct observation of change in tissue characteristics. Whether proton nuclear magnetic resonance imaging (NMRI) can characterize the myocardium was investigated.

The relaxation properties T1 and T2 are related to certain biophysical properties of tissue, e.g., water and lipid and macromolecular content, and have considerable impact on the intensity observed in NMRI. In a model of chronic Adriamycin cardiotoxicity in rats, it was observed that the T1 values of excised hearts were elevated, relative to control, in rats with histologic evidence of chronic cardiotoxicity, and more so in rats with gross evidence of chronic cardiotoxicity or heart failure. There was no significant change in T2. This T1 prolongation increased as disease worsened, whereas water concentration did not change significantly.

These findings demonstrate that predictable prolongation in T1 occurs in association with cardiotoxicity. Proton NMRI may provide a new means of assessing Adriamycin cardiotoxicity.

▶ Many noninvasive techniques, including echocardiography and radionuclide ventriculography, have been utilized for the early detection of myocardial toxicity in patients undergoing treatment with doxorubicin for various tumors. Current techniques depend on measurement of ventricular function rather than on direct observation of changes in tissue characteristics during doxorubicin administration. The results of this study in rats suggest that the detection of an elevation relaxation time as compared to control occurs with doxorubicin induced myocardial disease, thus providing a potential new method for assessing toxic effects from this drug in man. However, the specificity of the findings and the applicability of this technique to man as compared to other methods for defining doxorubicin toxicity need further assessment.—R.A. O'Rourke, M.D.

Monitoring the Bioenergetics of Cardiac Allograft Rejection Using In Vivo P-31 Nuclear Magnetic Resonance Spectroscopy

Robert C. Canby, William T. Evanochko, Leslie V. Barrett, James K. Kirklin, David C. McGiffin, Ted T. Sakai, Michael E. Brown, Robert E. Foster, Russell C. Reeves, and Gerald M. Pohost (Univ. of Alabama at Birmingham)

J. Am. Coll. Cardiol. 9:1067–1074, May 1987 1–48

Endomyocardial biopsy is used to monitor human cardiac allograft rejection. A noninvasive method would be preferable. In vivo phosphorus-31 (P-31) nuclear magnetic resonance (NMR) spectroscopy was used to noninvasively assess bioenergetic processes that occur during cardiac allograft rejection using a rat model. Brown Norway rat hearts were transplanted subcutaneously into the neck of Lewis rat recipients (allografts). Lewis hearts were also transplanted into Lewis recipients (isografts). Phosphocreatine to inorganic phosphate (PCr/Pi), phosphocreatine to beta-adenosine triphosphate (PCr/ATPβ), beta-adenosine triphosphate to inorganic phosphate (ATPβ/Pi) ratios and the pH of the transplanted hearts were monitored by surface coil P-31 NMR spectroscopy at 4.7 tesla daily for 7 days. Day 2 measurements were used as the baseline.

The PCr/Pi remained unchanged or increased in the isografts but decreased in the allografts. This difference was significant by day 4 when compared to the allograft levels at baseline and by day 3 when compared to the isografts. PCr/ATPβ did not change in isografts, but decreased in allografts. This difference became significant by day 4. The ATPβ/Pi also became significantly different by day 4 between these two groups. Intracellular pH did not change in the isograft group. In the allograft group an initial alkaline shift was followed by acidosis.

This study suggests that the abnormal bioenergetics associated with cardiac allograft rejection and detected by P-31 spectroscopy may be a useful noninvasive method of monitoring rejection in cardiac transplant patients.

▶ There is considerable interest and need for the development of a noninvasive method for early detection of cardiac allograph rejection in transplant patients. This study in a rat indicates that P-31 nuclear magnetic resonance spectroscopy (NMRS) can discriminate between rejecting and nonrejecting cardiac tissue. However, the suitability, sensitivity, and specificity of this method for assessing patients undergoing cardiac transplantation are unknown, and the relationship of this potential technique to current clinical methods must be assessed before the ultimate clinical usefulness of NMRS for this purpose can be defined.—R.A. O'Rourke, M.D.

Closed Chest Catheter Desiccation of the Atrioventricular Junction Using Radiofrequency Energy: A New Method of Catheter Ablation

Shoei K. Huang, Seroja Bharati, Anna R. Graham, Maurice Lev, Frank I. Marcus, and Roger C. Odell (Univ. of Arizona, Deborah Heart and Lung Ctr, Brown Mills, N.J., and Valleylab, Boulder, Col.)

J. Am. Coll. Cardiol. 9:349–358, February 1987 1–49

The use of radiofrequency energy on ablation of the atrioventricular (AV) junction was explored in 13 dogs. A 750-kHz radiofrequency energy was generated from an electrosurgical generator in the bipolar mode. The radiofrequency output was delivered at varying power (watts) but constant pulse duration of 10 seconds between two distal electrodes (bipolar ablation) in 8 dogs and between the distal electrode and an external patch electrode (unipolar ablation) in 5 dogs.

Complete AV block was achieved in 11 dogs and second-degree AV block in 2. The site of block was supra-His in dogs with partial AV block; His bundle activity was absent in dogs with complete AV block. Within 4–7 days after ablation, complete AV block persisted in 9 of 11 dogs with initial complete AV block, whereas the other 2 had return of AV conduction, with a persistent 2:1 AV block in 1 and first-degree AV block in the other. Of the 2 dogs with initial second-degree AV block, complete AV block developed in 1, whereas the other had resumption of 1:1 AV conduction with a normal PR interval. Energy was delivered in 1–13 applications per dog. Total energy delivered ranged from 100–700 joules per application with bipolar ablation, and 10–100 joules with unipolar ablation. There was no ventricular tachyarrhythmia, asystole, or death associated with the procedure.

There was no catheter damage unless the catheter was used repeatedly in excess of 1,500 joules of total energy. Catheter damage also was observed with the 6F quadripolar electrode catheters with a stylet or with the 6F catheters with a 5-mm interelectrode distance. Pathologically, a well-delineated area of coagulation necrosis was observed at the AV junction with no surrounding hemorrhage or mural thrombus. Microscopically, the area of necrosis was well demarcated with a peripheral contrast zone of mononuclear infiltrate. Most injuries involved the AV node, approaches to the AV node, and the penetrating bundle.

Catheter ablation of the AV junction using radiofrequency energy is safe and effective, producing various degrees of AV block and focal coagulation necrosis at the site of ablation. Ablation by radiofrequency energy has several distinct advantages over catheter ablation with direct current or laser energy, including absence of ventricular tachyarrhythmias and mural thrombi, less catheter damage, and absence of myocardial perforation, hemorrhage, or microscopic cavitations.

▶ The use of catheter ablation of the AV junction in patients with refractory tachyarrhythmias has been a major therapeutic advance. In both experimental animals and man, catheter ablation has most commonly utilized direct current or laser energy. The present study in dogs indicates the potential usefulness of ablation of the AV junction using radiofrequency energy to produce varying degrees of AV block at the site of ablation. Successful induction of AV block occurred in all the animal studies and complications were minimal. This appears to be a safe and effective technique for potential use in selected patients with recurrent supraventricular tachyarrhythmias that are unresponsive to drug therapy.—R.A. O'Rourke, M.D.

Internal Cardiac Defibrillation: Histopathology and Temporal Stability of Defibrillation Energy Requirements

Eric S. Fain, Margaret Billingham, and Roger A. Winkle (Stanford Univ.)

J. Am. Coll. Cardiol. 9:631–638, March 1987 1–50

The automatic implantable cardioverter/defibrillator is usually tested at the time of implantation to assure its effectiveness. However, this process requires a number of induced fibrillation-defibrillation trials that have a potential for inducing myocardial injury. In addition, it is possible that energy requirements at the time of implantation may also change over the years. To address these issues, the temporal stability of defibrillation energy requirements and the histopathologic effects of multiple defibrillating shocks were studied in 12 dogs chronically instrumented with an internal spring-patch lead system identical to that used in human beings. The animals were studied on days 1, 11, 18, 25, and 32, and sacrificed on day 32 for pathologic studies.

The animals received a mean of 209 shocks using energies ranging from 1–24 joules, for a mean total cumulative dose of 1,524 joules. A significant decrease in energy requirements for successful cardiac defibrillation was observed from day 1 to day 11. The energy required for 50% successful defibrillation decreased significantly from a mean of 7 joules to 5 joules, and the energy associated with 80% success decreased from a mean of 8.5 joules to 6 joules. Energy requirements thereafter remained stable. In no animal was there evidence of pathologic change in the myocardium or coronary vessels, either grossly or microscopically, other than changes associated with the implantation itself. These alterations consisted of a fibrous plaque developing beneath the patch electrodes, at times containing an area of patchy hemorrhage or mixed inflammatory infiltrate accompanying the hemorrhage. Endothelialization of the spring electrode with mild right atrial endocardial fibrosis also was observed.

The energy requirements for successful defibrillation decrease during the first 11 days after surgical implantation and then remain stable. In addition, multiple closely spaced defibrillating shocks applied through the spring-patch electrode system do not cause myocardial damage or changes other than those associated with implantation.

► Multiple defibrillating shocks are necessary to assess the effectiveness of the automatic implantable cardioverter/defibrillator at the time of implantation. This study in dogs examined the histopathologic effects and energy requirements for testing this device during the first month following implantation. The results indicate that the energy requirements for successful defibrillation decrease during the first 11 days then become stable and that testing defibrillating shocks can be applied without causing myocardial damage. This is important information relevant to patients with refractory recurrent arrhythmias requiring such long-term therapy.—R.A. O'Rourke, M.D.

Additional important publications concerning special cardiovascular techniques that have recently been developed and are being used in studies of experimental animals or man are included below:

1. Zhu, W.X., Myers, M.L., Hartley, C.J., et al.: Validation of a single crystal for measurement of transmural and epicardial thickening. *Am. J. Physiol.* 251(Heart Circ. Physiol. 20):H1045–H1055, 1986.
2. Rees, M.R., MacMillan, R.M., Fender, B., et al.: Demonstration of mitral and aortic valves by ultrafast computed tomography. *J. Comput. Tomogr.* 11:190–192, 1987.
3. Bittl, J.A., Balaschi, J.A., Ingwall, J.S.: Contractile failure and high-energy phosphate turnover during hypoxia: ^{31}P-NMR surface coil studies in living rat. *Circ. Res.* 60:871–878, 1987.
4. Gastfriend, R.J., Van De Water, J.M., Leonard, M.L., et al.: Imped-

2 Cardiovascular Disease in Infants and Children

Introduction

Among many interesting and thought-provoking articles in the general field of pediatric cardiology, those in the section that follows are particularly instructive.

Physiologic response of the normally formed heart is reported in response to dynamic and also to isometric exercise in trained swimmers and wrestlers who are adolescents.

In the general field of congenital cardiovascular malformations, the Noras' article takes another look at maternal transmission of congenital heart disease. A large prospective study from West Germany describes the pattern of extracardiac malformations in children without and in those with a malformation syndrome such as Down's syndrome. A population-based survey of more than 1,000 people with Down's syndrome in British Columbia showed that over the past three decades of progress in cardiovascular medicine and surgery there has been remarkably little evidence of improved survival in these children who commonly have congenital heart disease.

Concerning specific common anomalies, there is more information on another of the spontaneously developing changes in hearts with ventricular septal defect, and there are two more selections on coarctation of the aorta. The first of these provides information on the longstanding hypothesis that the ductus is involved in the coarctation process. The second reports on an animal model that mimics human coarctation.

The length of the section on diagnostic techniques reflects the rapid growth in the field of imaging, especially in echo-Doppler methodology and applications.

Increasingly, the cardiac catheter is being used not only to obtain physiologic data and anatomical details but also to relieve obstructions. Several articles address the benefits and complications during the learning curve of this therapy. Two papers provide anatomical analyses of congenital pulmonary valvular stenosis and the outflow tract of the right ventricle, important information for those embarking on or already involved in this form of therapy.

The section on cardiac surgery includes some long-term observations after repair or palliation of congenital heart disease and presents the results of two approaches to aftercare in children with artificial valves.

A contribution to understanding the significance of arrhythmias in children is the report of 24-hour ambulatory monitoring in healthy children. Reports of new antiarrhythmic agents and of atrial-tracking pacemakers should also be helpful in management of patients.

Additional cardiac conditions in children are dealt with in reviews or reports on congestive heart failure and on acquired heart disease. The Task Force Report on Hypertension provides standards of blood pressure measurements and guidelines. Particularly disturbing are the outbreaks of acute rheumatic fever following very mild and often unrecognized antecedent illness. In Kawasaki syndrome, we find guidance in evaluating abnormalities in coronary arteries and we learn to be alert to the development of coronary aneurysms in young children who do not fulfill all the criteria for diagnosis of the mucocutaneous lymph node syndrome.

The section on cardiovascular disease in infants and children concludes with studies on cardiac performance in children with sickle cell anemia and anorexia nervosa and takes a look at what pediatricians are thinking about prevention of heart disease.

Mary Allen Engle, M.D.

Physiology

'Athlete's Heart' in Prepubertal Children

Thomas W. Rowland, Brian C. Delaney, and Steven F. Siconolfi (Baystate Med. Ctr. and Springfield College, Springfield, Mass.)
Pediatrics 79:800–804, May 1987

2–1

Adults who engage in endurance training have cardiac findings that may resemble some findings of heart disease, but which presumably reflect a beneficial adaptation to chronic exercise stress. It is not clear whether the "athlete's heart" is observed in prepubertal children who undergo endurance training. The physical, ECG, and echocardiographic findings were reviewed in 14 prepubertal boys, with an average age of 11 years, who were competitive swimmers. Nineteen healthy boys of similar age served as a control group.

The swimmers were taller than the control boys and had a greater percent of body fat and a greater body surface area. Systolic blood pressure was higher in the swimmers. The PR interval was slightly longer than in control subjects. No athlete had electrocardiographic ventricular hypertrophy. Left ventricular end-diastolic dimensions and left atrial size were greater in the athletes. Left ventricular posterior wall and ventricular septal thicknesses also were greater in the swimmers. Left systolic shortening fraction was significantly higher in the athletes.

Prepubertal children who participate in intensive endurance training have many features of athlete's heart. None of the present subjects had left ventricular hypertrophy, and only one had a possible significant finding, first-degree atrioventricular block. Further studies are needed to determine whether these changes are an adaptive response, or are inherited characteristics that allow superior athletic performance.

▶ Swimming involves dynamic isometric exercise, while wrestling involves isotonic exercise, training, and competition. This study in 14 prepubertal competitive swimmers, in training for about 3 years, showed some features on echocardiography that were similar to those found in teenaged elite wrestlers. In comparison with 19 control boys, the swimmers had lower resting heart rates and greater left ventricular end-diastolic and left atrial dimensions along with an increase in septal and left ventricular posterior wall thickness, and they had higher left ventricular shortening fraction. Their physical examinations revealed a higher systolic blood pressure, mean of 116 versus a mean of 106 in the nonswimmers, and they also had a greater body surface area. These two were thought to be related. On ECG the swimmers had slightly longer PR intervals.

The conclusion was that features of the adult "athlete's heart" begin in childhood with intensive endurance training.—M.A. Engle, M.D.

Cardiac Structure and Function of Elite High School Wrestlers

Craig R. Cohen, Hugh D. Allen, Jack Spain, Gerald R. Marx, Robert W. Wolfe, and John S. Harvey (Univ. of Colorado, Denver, and Univ. of Arizona, Tucson)

Am. J. Dis. Child. 141:576–581, May 1987 2–2

In adults, there are functional differences between the effects of dynamic and isometric training. The effects of isometric training were assessed by Doppler echocardiography in 17 successful high school wrestlers. Ten nonathletic, age-matched control subjects also were studied. Isometric exercise was performed with a hand dynamometer. The average duration of competitive wrestling was nearly 9 years. Nearly 60% of training time was spent wrestling, 21% in running, and 12% in weight training. Most of the athletes had deliberately lost weight.

The resting diastolic blood pressure was lower in wrestlers than in control subjects, and resting heart rates were lower. Both groups had a marked rise in heart rate on handgrip exercise. Pulmonary artery diameter but not aortic diameter was greater in the athletes. Resting left ventricular posterior wall and septal dimensions were greater in the wrestlers, as was the change in dimensions with exercise. Resting aortic stroke volume was higher in the athletes than in control subjects. Cardiac indices were similar at rest, and did not change significantly on exercise. Stroke volume fell significantly on exercise in the wrestlers.

The hearts of elite high school wrestlers differ structurally and functionally from those of nonathletes. There are similarities to adults undergoing combined isometric and dynamic training. The high school athlete's heart responds more efficiently to isometric exercise than does the nonathlete's heart. The adaptation is not limited to the heart, but involves the great vessels and peripheral vascular system as well.

▶ This interesting study by echocardiography provides insight into the effects on the heart and the vessels of from 4 to 12 years of training for and involvement in competitive wrestling by 17 star high school wrestlers compared with

10 nonathletic, untrained controls. The wrestlers had no difference in systolic pressure but had lower diastolic pressure, slower resting heart rate, greater pulmonary artery diameter, larger dimensions of left ventricular posterior wall and internal dimensions and of interventricular septum with greater change from rest to exercise than did the controls. Wrestler's stroke volume was higher but fell more during isometric exercise.—M.A. Engle, M.D.

Congenital Anomalies of the Cardiovascular System

Maternal Transmission of Congenital Heart Diseases: New Recurrence Risk Figures and the Questions of Cytoplasmic Inheritance and Vulnerability to Teratogens

James J. Nora and Audrey Hart Nora (Univ. of Colorado, Denver)
Am. J. Cardiol. 59:459–463, February 1987 2–3

In 1982 Whittemore et al. (*Am. J. Cardiol.* 50:641–651) published the results of a study which suggested that recurrence risks for congenital heart disease in offspring were much higher than previously appreciated. The data differed from that in other published reports because the affected parents of affected offspring were, by design, all women, and the offspring were carefully examined from the newborn period through the first 3 years of life.

The authors have hypothesized that cytoplasmic inheritance may play a role in congenital heart disease in some families. To investigate this hypothesis, they reviewed the results of eight studies which involved 3,996 offspring of parents who have congenital heart disease. They found the risk for all defects was markedly higher if the affected parent was the mother rather than the father (table).

The risk ratio ranged from a high of 6.39 for aortic stenosis to a low of 1.48 for patent ductus arteriosus, and the ratio was statistically significant in aortic stenosis and ventricular septal defect. Unfortunately, despite the relatively large number of cases, there were too few patients to

SUGGESTED RECURRENCE RISK IN OFFSPRING FOR EIGHT CONGENITAL HEART DEFECTS WHEN ONE PARENT IS AFFECTED (%)*

Defect	Father Affected	Mother Affected
AS	3	13–18
ASD	1.5	4–4.5
AV	1	14
Coarc.	2	4
PDA	2.5	3.5–4
PS	2	4–6.5
TOF	1.5	2.5
VSD	2	6–10

**AS*, aortic stenosis; *ASD*, atrial septal defect; *AV*, atrioventricular canal; *Coarc.*, coarctation of aorta; *PDA*, patent ductus arteriosus; *PS*, pulmonary stenosis; *TOF*, tetralogy of Fallot; *VSD*, ventricular septal defect.

(Courtesy of Nora, J.J., and Nora, A.H.: Am. J. Cardiol. 59:459–463, February 1987.)

reveal a statistical significance for a malformation such as atrioventricular canal, in which there were 5 affected offspring among 36 children of mothers who had atrioventricular canal and no affected children among 16 offspring of affected fathers.

Although many familial cases of congenital heart disease are compatible with multifactorial inheritance and vulnerability to teratogens, an important subset of cases, particularly in some high-risk families, may be better explained by cytoplasmic inheritance. The authors recommend that genetic counseling should take into account the differences in risk to offspring of affected mothers while further investigation and confirmation proceed.

▶ As more and more people with congenital heart disease (CHD) are enabled to become adults, through good luck of having a minor abnormality or the good fortune of survival through medical/surgical treatment, cardiologists will increasingly be asked by these patients about the risk of a cardiac problem in their babies. This review and "rethink" by the Noras, with their well-known interest and expertise in genetics and in pediatric cardiology, addresses this question. After reviewing their own collection of data on parents with CHD having babies with CHD, and reports of some other well-studied series, they conclude that not all cases are due to multifactorial causes but that some could be better explained by cytoplasmic inheritance. They analyzed eight common malformations and found that the risk to offspring was greater if the affected parent were the mother than if it were the father. They tabulated estimated risk rates from guidance in genetic counseling, a table reproduced herein.—M.A. Engle, M.D.

Malformation Patterns in Children With Congenital Heart Disease

Hans-Heiner Kramer, Frank Majewski, Hans Joachim Trampisch, Spiros Rammos, and Maurice Bourgeois (Univ. of Düsseldorf, West Germany)

Am. J. Dis. Child. 141:789–795, July 1987 2–4

Patterns of extracardiac malformations were examined in a prospective series of 1,016 infants and children aged 16 years and younger with cardiovascular malformations. In 881 cases within this group, the congenital cardiac malformation was isolated or was accompanied by a major extracardiac malformation (Table 1). In the other 135 cases the congenital heart disease was part of a malformation syndrome, embryopathy, association of anomalies, or complex.

Fifty-four percent of the 881 patients (479) had no extracardiac malformation. Eight percent (68) of other children had a major extracardiac malformation. (Patients with inguinal hernias or undescended testes were excluded.) Children with tetralogy of Fallot had major extracardiac malformations more often than the others, and these usually were more serious (Table 2). Most major extracardiac anomalies involved the musculoskeletal system, and most were not very serious.

Malformation syndromes of chromosomal origin were diagnosed in

TABLE 1.—PREVALENCE OF CONGENITAL HEART DEFECTS*

Type of CHD	Present Study (n = 1016) No. (%) of Patients	Present Study 95% CL	Hospital for Sick Children, Toronto, Study[16] (n = 15 104), % of Patients	Baltimore-Washington Infant Study[15] (n = 664) % of Patients	Baltimore-Washington 95% CL
VSD	285 (28.1)	25.3-31.0	28.3	23.3	20.5-26.8
ASD II	82 (8.0)	6.3-9.8	7.0	8.6	6.6-10.9
PDA	63 (6.2)	4.8-7.9	9.8	2.4	1.4-3.9
ECD	52 (5.1)	3.8-6.6	3.4	9.8	7.8-12.4
PS	79 (7.7)	6.1-9.5	9.9	5.1	3.7-7.1
AOS	59 (5.8)	4.6-7.6	7.1	3.0	2.0-4.7
CoA	77 (7.6)	6.0-9.4	5.1	6.5	4.9-8.7
Fallot	106 (10.4)	8.6-12.5	9.7	7.1	5.4-9.4
D-TGA	64 (6.3)	4.9-8.0	4.4	5.7	3.9-7.3
Other	149 (14.8)	12.8-17.3	15.3	28.5	24.9-32.0

*VSD, ventricular septal defect; ASD II, atrial septal defect (secundum type); PDA, persistent ductus arteriosus; ECD, endocardial cushion defect; PS, pulmonary stenosis; AOS, aortic stenosis; CoA, coarctation of aorta; Fallot, tetralogy of Fallot; D-TGA, D-transpositon of great arteries; and CL, confidence limits.

(Courtesy of Kramer, H.-H., et al.: Am. J. Dis. Child. 141:789–795, July 1987.)

TABLE 2.—FREQUENCY OF EXTRACARDIAC MALFORMATIONS (ECMS) IN CHILDREN WITH TETRALOGY OF FALLOT COMPARED WITH MOST COMMON CONGENITAL HEART DEFECTS (CHDS)

Type of CHD*	No. of Patients	No. (%) of Patients With ECMs	P†
Fallot	88	14 (15.7)	. . .
D-TGA‡	61	4 (6.6)	NS
PDA	50	2 (4.0)	.03
VSD	249	17 (6.8)	.01
ASD II	74	5 (6.8)	NS
ECD	36	3 (8.3)	NS
PS	58	2 (3.4)	.01
AoS	46	3 (6.5)	NS
CoA	71	4 (5.6)	.03
Other	148	14 (9.5)	NS
Total, excepting Fallot	793	54 (6.8)	.01
Total	**881**	**68** (7.7)	. . .

*See Table 1 for explanation of abbreviations.

†Fisher's exact test was used to compare tetralogy of Fallot with other CHDs; NS, not significant.

‡Frequency of ECMS in children with D-TGA was not significantly reduced, compared with other diagnoses listed below it.

(Courtesy of Kramer, H.-H., et al.: Am. J. Dis. Child. 141:789–795, July 1987.)

5.5% of the overall series. Thirty patients had malformation syndromes of nonchromosomal origin. Findings of embryopathy were present in 27 cases; rubella embryopathy and alcohol embryopathy were most frequent. Seventeen patients had malformation associations such as hypoplasia of the depressor anguli oris muscle. Malformation complexes were diagnosed in 5 patients.

One of 8 children in this series had a malformation syndrome, embryopathy, malformation association, or complex. This emphasizes the need to carefully examine all children with congenital heart disease for extracardiac malformations.

▶ When it comes to congenital heart disease (CHD), isn't it remarkable how much we've learned yet how little we know! How often have you been asked by parents, "Why did this happen to my baby?" or "Is there anything else wrong besides the heart?"

Kramer and colleagues in Dusseldorf decided to take a new look at the question of malformation patterns by personally examining in a prospective manner, 1,016 German infants through adolescents referred over a 12-month period because of their heart disease.

They divided the patients according to (1) those 881 patients with CHD with or without a major extracardiac malformation and (2) those whose cardiac defect was part of a malformation syndrome, embryopathy, or complex. The largest subgroup in (1) consisted of 479 children without an extracardiac malformation (ECM): 54.4%. Only 7.7% had a major ECM. Of these, patients with tetralogy of Fallot were more often afflicted than those with other malformations. Most major ECMs were muskuloskeletal in nature and not very serious. With a minor ECM (41.9%) there was no association with a specific cardiac anomaly.

It was not surprising that in group (2) chromosomal abnormalities were chiefly in children with Down's syndrome. Rubella embryopathy in 1.3% was followed closely by alcohol embryopathy in 1%.

If we agree that rubella and alcohol embryopathies should be preventable, we are still left with about 98% of the people with congenital heart disease from other causes that at this time are probably not preventable.—M.A. Engle, M.D.

Life Expectancy in Down Syndrome

Patricia A. Baird and Adele D. Sadovnick (Univ. of British Columbia, Vancouver, and Health Surveillance Registry, Ministry of Health, British Columbia, Canada)
J. Pediatr. 110:849–854, June 1987 2–5

Although the use of prenatal diagnosis of Down's syndrome (DS) in older women has increased, it is not expected that the total population incidence of DS will decrease significantly in the future. This study was part of a collaborative effort between the Ministry of Health and the University of British Columbia. The purpose of the study was to calculate the life expectancy for children born with DS, using vital and health data comprising more than 1 million consecutive live births recorded in the province of British Columbia.

A total of 1,341 children, 703 boys and 638 girls, were born with DS in British Columbia between 1952 and 1981. Congenital heart disease (CHD) was recorded in 388 children (28.9%) born with DS, including 176 boys (25.0%) and 212 girls (33.2%). Thus, the incidence of CHD was significantly higher in girls than in boys. IQ levels, which were recorded for 434 subjects (32.4%) in the DS cohort, ranged from 35 to 49.

For patients with DS and CHD, survival to age 1 year was 76.3%; to age 5, 61.8%; to age 10, 57.1%; to age 20, 53.1%; and to age 30, 49.9%. For patients with DS without CHD, survival to the same ages was 90.7%, 87.2%, 84.9%, 81.9%, and 79.2%, respectively.

Overall, 70.96% of the total DS cohort survived to age 30 years. When all DS patients born with CHD were excluded, 79.19% of the remaining DS patients survived to age 30, which is still lower than the percentage of the general population living to age 30 (96.66%), or that of the mentally retarded population (92.20%).

Accurate survival data for DS are essential to those who counsel the families involved as to the prognosis of their affected children, and to those who need to plan facilities to care for patients who survive until adulthood.

▶ Accurate survival data for patients with Down's syndrome (DS) are important for counseling of families and in planning for programs of education and care. The population-based Health Surveillance Registry of British Columbia provides an opportunity to obtain these data from an entire community, not just from hospitals or institutions.

This report concerns 1,341 patients from more than 1 million live births between 1952 and 1981. The incidence of DS was 1 in 795 live births. Of the patients with DS, 28.9% had congenital heart disease (CHD). The greatest risk for dying was in the first year of life, with or without CHD. Survival to age 30 was less for the group with DS (70.9%) than for the general population (96.66%) and for the population of mentally retarded from other causes (92.2%). Those with DS and CHD had a lower survival (less than 50%) than those without CHD (79.19%). Surprising to me, there was not much evidence of improvement in survival during each of the last three decades, despite changes in medical and surgical care for those with congenital heart disease.—M.A. Engle, M.D.

Subaortic Fibrous Ridge and Ventricular Septal Defect: Role of Septal Malalignment

Paulo Zielinsky, Marinez Rossi, José Carlos Haertel, Domingos Vitola, Fernando Antonio Lucchese, and Rubem Rodrigues (Inst. of Cardiology of Rio Grande do Sul, Porto Alegre, Rio Grande do Sul, Brazil)

Circulation 75:1124–1129, June 1987 2–6

It is now possible to recognize and characterize a "discrete" or fixed subaortic ridge by two-dimensional echocardiography. Because of this investigators can prospectively study the coexistence of ventricular septal defects (VSDs) and subaortic shelf. The present study was carried out to test the hypothesis that the presence of a subaortic ridge associated with a VSD is related to a malaligned ventricular septum caused by anterior or posterior deviation of the infundibular septum with or without obstructive lesions of the aortic arch.

The study group consisted of 32 of 295 patients in whom a diagnosis of VSD was made by two-dimensional echocardiography and who presented with a subaortic shelf (Fig 2–1). Every patient had a malalignment type of defect; the defect resulted from anterior deviation of the

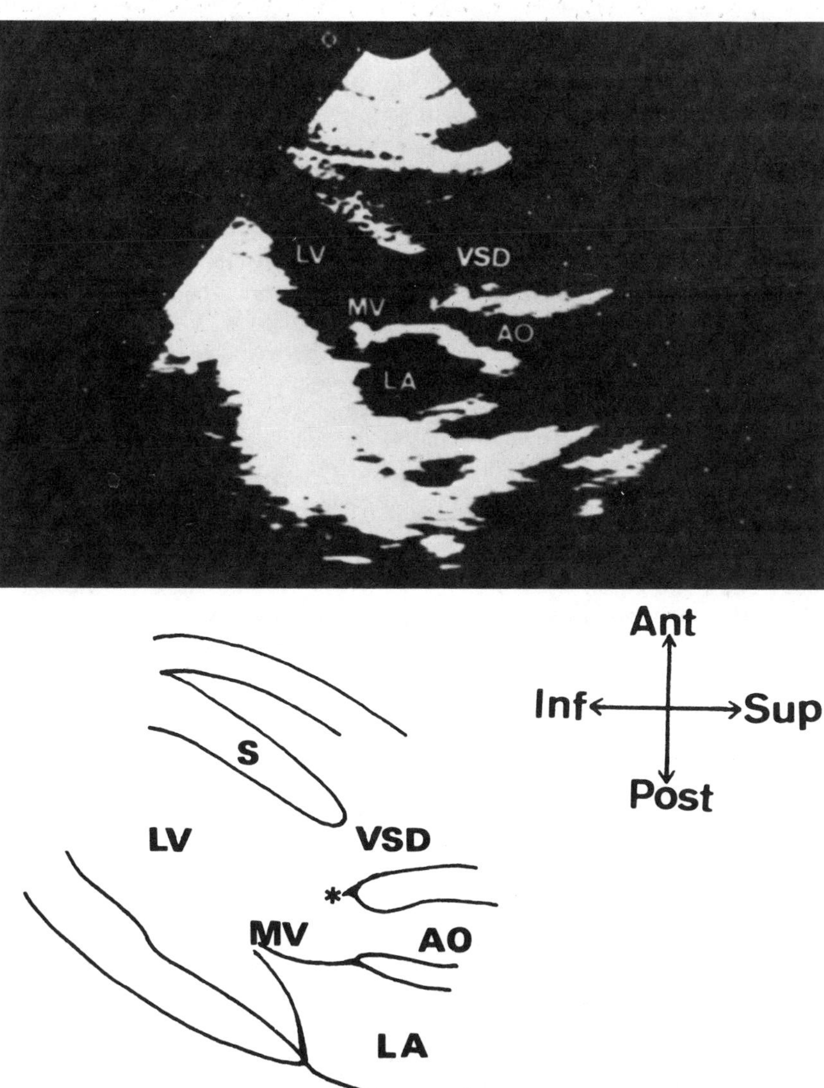

Fig 2–1.—VSD with subaortic shelf. Apical long-axis view. Notice the septal malalignment produced by posterior deviation of the infundibular septum. LF, left ventricle; MV, mitral valve; LA, left atrium; AO, aorta; S, trabecular septum. *Subaortic shelf. (Courtesy of Zielinsky, P., et al.: Circulation 75:1124–1129, June 1987.)

outlet septum in 28 and by posterior deviation of the infundibular septum in 4. The authors noted that the prevalence of a subaortic shelf in the malalignment VSD group was 82% (32 of 39 patients). Among 28 patients with a subaortic ridge and anterior deviation of the outlet septum, only 3 had aortic coarctation, but all 4 patients with subaortic stenosis and posterior infundibular malalignment had obstructive lesions of the aortic arch. Of these 4 patients, 3 had coarctation, and 1 had interruption of the aortic arch.

A malalignment type of VSD may be a consistent feature in patients with VSD and associated discrete subaortic stenosis. Because they also noted a high prevalence of subaortic ridge in the presence of a malalignment VSD, the authors speculate that there may be a common morphogenesis for malalignment VSD, subaortic shelf, and obstructive lesions of the aortic arch.

▶ Not only is ventricular septal defect (VSD) the most common kind of congenital heart disease but it is also one of the most fascinating because of its spontaneous changes and its association with other anomalies that may change as well. This prospective study in children with VSD, well characterized echocardiographically, demonstrates that a subaortic shelf, which may progress to discrete subaortic stenosis, is related to malalignment of the ventricular septum. Either anterior or posterior deviation of the septum results in the malalignment, and this can occur in VSD with or without obstruction to aortic flow.—M.A. Engle, M.D.

Coarctation and Other Obstructive Aortic Arch Anomalies: Their Relationship to the Ductus Arteriosus

Nynke J. Elzenga, Adriana C. Gittenberger-de Groot, and Arentje Oppenheimer-Dekker (Erasmus Univ., Rotterdam, The Netherlands)

Int. J. Cardiol. 13:289–308, December 1987 2–7

Coarctation and other aortic arch abnormalities that interfere with normal flow through the aortic arch are frequently part of a complex congenital heart defect. The authors studied the relationship between coarctation and other arch anomalies, reappraised the relationship of the arterial duct and anomalies of the aortic arch.

The authors studied 43 specimens with an intracardiac anomaly and also with an obstructive aortic arch. These were obtained from infants who had died younger than the age of 1 year. They examined all of the specimens morphologically, and 20 histologically. The morphological aspect of the investigation included measurements of all the segments of the aortic arch and establishment of the localization of any associated coarctation. They divided the specimens according to the appearance of the isthmus, which was not present in 4, was atretic in 2, hypoplastic in 19, and of normal diameter in 18 cases. All cases, except 5 (2 with atresia and 3 with hypoplasia of the isthmus) showed an associated coarctation.

Most of the coarctations (28) were located preductally. All such preductal coarctations had ductal tissue in the obstructing ridge. Of the 5 paraductal coarctations; 2 also had ductal tissue in the obstructing ridge. The distribution of the ductal tissue among the two types of coarctation suggested a spectrum of anomalies, rather than two completely different entities. The patterns of the aortic arches appeared to be predictive for the type of coarctation present. The arches that tapered normally toward the isthmus either presented with a preductal coarctation (20 cases) or without a coarctation (3 cases). All of the specimens in which the isthmus was lacking (4 cases) also had a preductal coarctation. The 5 paraductal coarctations were found in arches that showed a reverse pattern, tapering toward the brachiocephalic arches. Abnormal extension of ductal tissue far into the descending aorta was present in each of the 28 preductal coarctations but not in 3 of the 5 juxtaductal coarctations. All the preductal coarctations contained ductal tissue, whereas only 2 of the 5 paraductal coarctations had ductal tissue in the obstructing ridge.

Careful evaluation of all the segments of the aortic arch may be helpful in the clinical evaluation of infants with an obstructive aortic arch anomaly.

▶ Among many controversies and confusions concerning coarctation of the aorta have been variations in nomenclature and in the relation of ductal tissue to the obstruction. This study from The Netherlands focuses on specimens from infants dying in the first year of life, usually by 3 months of age. All 43 specimens had other associated anomalies, principally ventricular septal defect (29), hypoplastic left ventricle (5), and univentricular heart (3). Interestingly, and in contrast to some other earlier studies, malformations of the mitral valve were not mentioned and bicuspid aortic valve was rare.

The authors studied about half of the specimens histologically. While there was considerable variation, they found that the majority of these coarctations were preductal and that all such had ductal tissue in the obstructing ridge, which was not always circumferential, and often far into the descending aorta. Two of 5 paraductal coarctations had ductal tissue in the ridge. Ductal tissue sometimes extended into or around the origin of the left subclavian artery if it arose below the coarctation.

This detailed analysis has surgical implications, as well as material of interest to those who have been concerned with the question of contractile ductal tissue and its role in development of coarctation pre- or postnatally.—M.A. Engle, M.D.

Hemodynamic and Hormonal Abnormalities in Canine Aortic Coarctation at Rest and During Exercise

Richard J. Declusin, Lawrence E. Boerboom, Gordon N. Olinger, Anthony B. Gustafson, and Lawrence I. Bonchek (Med. College of Wisconsin, Milwaukee)

J. Am. Coll. Cardiol. 9:903–909, April 1987 2–8

The neurohumoral adaptations and the pressure and flow dynamics at rest and during exercise accompanying aortic coarctation are incompletely understood. The authors determined the hemodynamic and hormonal consequences of induced aortic coarctation at rest and during treadmill exercise.

They studied 12 normal adult dogs as controls, and 8 dogs with coarctation, created within 1 week of birth by banding the aorta just proximal to the ductus ligament, thereby fixing the luminal diameter at 1–2 mm. Eighteen months after the operation, the authors monitored vascular pressures proximal and distal to the coarctation; evaluated cardiac output and regional blood flow using radioactive microspheres; and collected blood samples for determination of hormone levels and blood gas volumes. At rest, systolic pressure in the proximal aorta was 130 ± 12 mm Hg in the control group and 167 ± 16 mm Hg in dogs with coarctation. During exercise at a level that doubled heart rate and cardiac index, mean aortic pressure increased by 11% in the control dogs, and by 31% in the coarctation group. Mean distal aortic pressure increased by 8% during exercise in control dogs, but decreased by 29% in dogs with coarctation. Exercise decreased flow to the kidneys and the large intestine in the coarctation group. Plasma norepinephrine concentrations were greater in the coarctation group than in control dogs at rest; during exercise, plasma norepinephrine, epinephrine, and renin activity increased in both groups, but to a greater degree in the group with coarctation.

They concluded that there is an abnormality in renal and gut perfusion in experimental coarctation that may be related to a decline in perfusion pressure. They demonstrated that cardiac performance was well preserved in this model with hypertension of long duration, and that sympathoadrenal activity was increased.

▶ This elegant study provides answers in a canine model of coarctation of the aorta, created at 4–7 days of life and studied at adult size (18 months) by hemodynamic and hormonal studies during rest and exercise. When compared with control animals, the 8 dogs with coarctation had forearm limb hypertension at rest that increased markedly after 10 minutes of running on a treadmill while hind limb pressure decreased and blood flow to the kidneys and gut decreased. Left ventricular subendocardial to subepicardial blood flow remained unchanged. At rest their norepinephrine levels were greater, and on exercise, epinephrine, norepinephrine and plasma renin activity increased more.

Since distal pressure with coarctation decreased on exercise, decreased vascular resistance distally was more important than the sum effect of increased proximal aortic pressure plus vasodilation or recruitment from chest wall vessels. With coarctation, cardiac output increased on exercise due to an increase in heart rate and stroke volume, rather than in heart rate alone as in the controls. This could relate to enhanced sympathetic activity. The rise in plasma renin activity on exercise in coarctation correlated with decrease in renal blood flow, implicating the renin-angiotensin system in the hypertension.—M.A. Engle, M.D.

Diagnostic Techniques

First-Pass Anger Camera Radiocardiography: Biventricular Ejection Fraction, Flow, and Volume Measurements

Martin L. Nusynowitz, Anthony R. Benedetto, Richard A. Walsh, and Mark R. Starling (Univ. of Texas, Galveston, Univ. of Texas Health Science Ctr., San Antonio)

J. Nucl. Med. 28:950–959, June 1987 2–9

To accomplish the difficult task of assessing the dimensions and function of the right ventricle at the same time as the left ventricle, these authors conducted a study in which first-pass right and left ventricular ejection fraction results were compared with equilibrium radiocardiographic measurements and first-pass left ventricular ejection fraction (LVEF) values obtained with biplane contrast angiographic measurements.

Thirteen patients with and seven patients without regurgitant valvular disease were studied. Regurgitant fractions were determined from the differences between the first-pass right and left ventricular stroke volumes. The mean LVEF by first pass and equilibrium radiocardiographic measurements were essentially identical; both were lower than biplane contrast angiographic measurements. First-pass LVEF was found to correlate with LVEF by equilibrium radiocardiography and biplane contrast angiography. Mean RVEF by first pass and equilibrium radiocardiography were also found to be correlated. Correlation was also found between corrected first pass and contrast angiography left ventricular stroke, end-diastolic, and end-systolic volumes, but underestimation was noted when uncorrected flows were used. The first pass regurgitant fraction measurements separated the patients with and without regurgitant disease and correlated well with contrast angiographic grading of regurgitation.

Studies of ejection fraction, flow, and volume information were done for both ventricles in a modified left anterior-oblique view that separated the two ventricles. Reasonable correlations were demonstrated among the methods used—equilibrium radiographic measurements, biplane contrast angiographic measurements, and first-pass left ventricular ejection fraction. First-pass Anger camera studies distinguished patients with and without regurgitant valve disease.

► Many methods exist for evaluating dimensions and function of the left ventricle. The right ventricle, on the other hand, because of its geometry is difficult to assess. Several techniques have been proposed, but no "gold standard" exists for validation.

These authors performed studies of ejection fraction, flow, and volume information for both ventricles in a modified left anterior-oblique view that separated the two ventricles. They sought to estimate regurgitant valvular disease after comparing Anger counter results with those from equilibrium radiographic measurements for both ventricles, biplane cineangiographic measurements and first-pass left ventricular ejection fraction.

They demonstrated quite reasonable correlation between the different methods, and that first-pass Anger camera studies distinguished patients with regurgitant valve disease from those without. This might become a useful technique for study of patients with congenital heart disease especially when the right ventricle supplies the systemic circulation, as it does after venous-switch operations for transposition of the great arteries—M.A. Engle, M.D.

Angiography for Delineation of Systemic-to-Pulmonary Shunts in Congenital Pulmonary Atresia: Evaluation With the Dynamic Spatial Reconstructor

Yun-He Liu, Douglas D. Mair, Donald J. Hagler, James B. Seward, Paul R. Julsrud, and Erik L. Ritman (Mayo Clinic)

Mayo Clin. Proc. 61:932–941, December 1986 2–10

It is difficult to diagnose and formulate medical and surgical plans in many types of congenital heart disease. In recent years new diagnostic modalities such as two-dimensional echocardiography have provided additional noninvasive information about the central pulmonary artery, but the standard diagnostic modality is angiography.

The authors believe that potential advantages are offered through the use of high-temporal-resolution synchronous volumetric scanning computed tomography, and they use the dynamic spatial reconstructor (DSR), a high-speed three-dimensional computed tomography system. They present results from two patients with congenital pulmonary atresia who have undergone scanning with the DSR.

When information that was obtained from conventional diagnostic angiography was compared with information which was obtained from the DSR, it was found to be equivalent. However, the quality of the DSR images (in terms of spatial and density resolution) was not as good as that provided by conventional angiography. With the use of DSR it was possible to demonstrate numerous shunts, stenoses, and systemic collateral arteries. This procedure involved only one or two nonselective injections of a contrast agent and less exposure to radiation than that which is normally necessitated by angiographic study.

This study demonstrates the feasibility of acquiring data on dynamic volume imaging from pediatric patients by the use of DSR scanning. The authors recommend that the quality of DSR images should be upgraded before a more definitive study is conducted, i.e., a prospective comparison of DSR and routine angiographic techniques.

▶ This report from the Mayo Clinic is a clear exposition of the potential uses and present drawbacks of a new imaging system: dynamic spatial reconstruction. This equipment is available only to a few at this time, and it needs improvements in quality of images before it will be more than an investigational tool. Yet the two cases selected, with their multiple vessels of collateral circulation from aorta to pulmonary tree, illustrate the future potential of a powerful new tool to display complex vascular arrangements and anatomy.—M.A. Engle, M.D.

Doppler Echocardiographic Evaluation of the Normal Human Fetal Heart

Lindsey D. Allan, Sunder K. Chita, Widad Al-Ghazali, Diane C. Crawford, and Michael Tynan (Guy's Hosp., London)

Br. Heart J. 57:528–533, June 1987 2–11

From as early as 16 weeks' gestation, the anatomy of the fetal heart can be studied by echocardiography and blood flow velocity can be estimated by Doppler examination. Previous studies have focused principally on the lamb; the authors report on Doppler evaluation of blood flow in a series of normal human fetuses.

In 120 normal fetuses Doppler velocity measurements were obtained across the mitral, tricuspid, aortic, and pulmonary valves. Measurements were taken at all four sites in 36 fetuses. Maximum and mean velocities were calculated for each valve and values were related to gestational age. Cross-sectional echocardiography was used to measure the size of the openings in the valves. Blood flow values were calculated from the product of the mean velocity and the valve orifice dimensions.

The pulmonary orifice was larger than the aortic at all ages, and the tricuspid orifice was larger than the mitral. In most cases, the output of the right ventricle was greater than that of the left ventricle. At 18 weeks, the combined ventricular output was approximately 50 ml per minute; by term, it had increased to 1,200 ml per minute.

It is difficult to be certain that the fetus is in a resting state when Doppler tracings are obtained. Movement would alter the results. However, these data demonstrate that Doppler echocardiography can be used to evaluate human fetal cardiac function. Normal values provide a basis for interpretation in fetuses with abnormal Doppler findings.

▶ Use of two-dimensional echocardiography to analyze the fetal heart for structural defects and arrhythmias has been possible since 1980. Addition of Doppler methodology enhances the diagnostic value of these studies. This report by Dr. Lindsey Allan and her colleagues provides a basis for comparison of those suspected to be abnormal with normal fetuses of a gestational age from 16 to 36 weeks. Orifice dimensions, blood flow velocity, and ventricular output increased steadily, with right-sided structures and output greater than left.—M.A. Engle, M.D.

Measurement of Cardiac Output and Exercise Factor by Pulsed Doppler Echocardiography During Supine Bicycle Ergometry in Normal Young Adolescent Boys

Gerald R. Marx, Richard W. Hicks, and Hugh D. Allen with the technical assistance of Scott M. Kinzer (Univ. of Arizona, Tucson)

J. Am. Coll. Cardiol. 10:430–434, August 1987 2–12

Doppler echocardiographic estimates of resting cardiac output have compared well with the results when invasive methods are used. The usefulness of this technique in measuring cardiac output during exercise was studied in 34 healthy young adolescent boys with a mean age of 13 years who underwent pulsed Doppler echocardiography during supine bicycle exercise at varying intensities at four different sessions. The CO_2 rebreathing method was used for comparison.

Successful rest and exercise studies were carried out by the Doppler method in 52 of 64 attempts. As measured by this method cardiac output at rest and during submaximal exercise correlated well with simultaneous oxygen consumption values. The mean exercise factor in 20 subjects, as determined on two occasions 3 months apart, was 6.2 on both occasions. This mean exercise factor was similar to that determined by the CO_2 rebreathing method.

The pulsed Doppler echocardiographic technique can be used to estimate both cardiac output and the exercise factor in adolescents. It remains to be determined whether Doppler studies are valid in more heterogeneous populations and whether the exercise factor, as measured during submaximal exercise, will help distinguish persons with cardiovascular disease from normal subjects.

▶ Simple, straightforward, illuminating are terms that can appropriately be applied to this study in 34 healthy adolescent boys to determine whether pulsed Doppler echocardiography can consistently and accurately measure cardiac output on exercise as well as at rest. The answer is equally simple. It can.—M.A. Engle, M.D.

Cross-Sectional Echocardiography With Pulsed and Continuous Wave Doppler in the Management of Ventricular Septal Defects

Andrea Magherini, Lia Simonetti, Carlo R. Tomassini, Carlo Moggi, Francesco Ragazzini, and Giorgio Bartolozzi (Univ. of Florence, Italy)

Int. J. Cardiol. 15:317–328, June 1987 2–13

The recent increase in resolution with cross-sectional echocardiography and the introduction of subcostal projections have made it possible to determine the site and size of ventricular septal defects (VSDs). Previous studies in patients with large VSDs have provided ample data, since surgical and autopsy findings were often available to confirm anatomical and echocardiographic findings. However, small-to-moderate VSDs have not been documented extensively, because cardiac catheterization or operation are often not required in these cases. This study compared data obtained from cross-sectional echocardiography with those obtained from Doppler echocardiography and determined which cross-sectional projections were most valuable in the diagnosis of VSDs.

The authors studied 71 patients, aged 10 days to 18 years, with confirmed small-to-moderate VSDs. Cross-sectional echocardiography imaged the VSD in 49 patients (group 1), but not in the other 22 patients (group 2). Pulsed Doppler detected a left-to-right shunt at the ventricular level in group 1, and a positive signal but no defect in the ventricles in group 2. Pulsed Doppler provided supplemental information to that detectable from cross-sectional echocardiography in small defects. Thus, pulsed Doppler diagnosed those defects that were not imaged by cross-sectional echocardiography because of their site, size, or both.

Of the five subcostal projections evaluated in this study, the right oblique subcostal view and the four-chamber view were the most useful projections. The right oblique subcostal view passes simultaneously through both the inlet and outlet of the right ventricle. The appearance of a hole in the four-chamber view indicates that it opens between the inlets of the two ventricles.

Cross-sectional echocardiographic imaging will contribute greatly to the study of congenital heart disease.

▶ Still the most common congenital cardiac anomaly in clinical practice, the ventricular septal defect (VSD) continues to intrigue us with its variation in size, location, complexity, and association with other congenital and acquired anomalies. To image the defect is difficult when it is small, as was true in 22 patients in this study, but to detect its presence by pulsed Doppler identification of the left-to-right shunt overcomes this problem. The continuous-wave Doppler helps in judging pressures on either side of the defect, but not always reliably when there is a problem of aligning the jet when the signal is poor. This occurs, for instance, when other pathologic conditions exist in the right heart. In their study of 71 infants and children with VSD, the authors found that the right oblique subcostal view is one of the most useful and important views for identifying and classifying the various types of VSD.

This article is replete with examples of various echocardiographically demonstrated defects and is accompanied by an editorial by Dr. Edward J. Baker of Guy's Hospital. He points out the significance of identifying the precise location of the defect and using the four-chamber view and the right subcostal view as especially valuable imaging planes.—M.A. Engle, M.D.

Noninvasive Doppler Echocardiographic Evaluation of Shunt Flow Dynamics of the Ductus Arteriosus

Satoshi Hiraishi, Yasunori Horiguchi, Hitoshi Misawa, Kohki Oguchi, Nobuaki Kadoi, Nobuyuki Fujino, and Kimio Yashiro (Kitasato Univ., Sagamihara, Kanagawa, Japan)

Circulation 75:1146–1153, June 1987 2–14

Previous studies have shown that two-dimensional/Doppler echocardiography is a highly sensitive technique for detecting ductal patency in patients with patent ductus arteriosus (PDA). Because few studies have been done to assess shunt flow within the ductus, the authors designed a study to assess whether two-dimensional/Doppler echocardiography can determine the direction of shunt flow in the ductus arteriosus.

The study was done with 26 patients, aged 1 day to 3.5 years, with either isolated or complicated PDA as confirmed by cardiac catheterization and surgery, and with 42 patients, aged 1 day to 6 years, who did not have PDA as confirmed by cardiac catheterization and angiography. Diagnoses in the latter group included ventricular septal defect (n = 12), Kawasaki disease (n = 10), valvar pulmonary stenosis (n = 8), atrial septal defect (n = 7), valvar aortic stenosis (n = 2), tetralogy of Fallot (n = 2), and transposition of great arteries (n = 1). All study subjects were examined by two-dimensional and Doppler echocardiography.

Abnormal Doppler signals, indicating left-to-right (L-R) or right-to-left (R-L) shunt flow, or both, could be obtained at the site of the ductus arteriosus in all 26 patients with PDA, while no Doppler signals of shunt flow were noted in any of the 42 control subjects. The peak, mean, and diastolic velocities of the L-R shunt flow within the ductus could be measured from the obtained ductal flow velocity profiles. Using these measurements, patients with normal pulmonary arterial pressure could then be distinguished from those with pulmonary hypertension.

Two-dimensional/Doppler echocardiography cannot only assess the presence of PDA accurately, but can also determine shunt dynamics in infants and children.

▶ Increasing application of two-dimensional echocardiography with Doppler evaluation brings heightened validity of the method in detecting anomalies and quantifying shunts in patients with congenital heart disease. The study by Hiraishi and colleagues adds to this capability in the study of patients with simple (16) or complicated (10) patent ductus arteriosus (PDA) in comparison with 42 children with acquired or congenital heart disease and without a ductus. Confirmation of the presence or absence of the ductus was by cardiac catheterization and, in the former, by surgery. Direction of flow in those with PDA was verified by contrast echocardiography. Pulmonary-to-systemic pressure (Pp/Ps) was measured at catheterization in 23 patients with PDA and was estimated by Doppler peak flow velocity.

The authors found they could visualize the ductus in all patients with a PDA, could evaluate patency sensitivity by pulsed Doppler, and could correctly distinguish between normal and elevated pulmonary pressure through analysis of mean and diastolic flow velocities.

This study provides much useful information concerning the noninvasive assessment by echo-Doppler, not only of the presence of the common anomaly of PDA, but also of the shunt dynamics.—M.A. Engle, M.D.

Preoperative Two-Dimensional Echocardiographic Prediction of Prosthetic Aortic and Mitral Valve Size in Children

Randall L. Caldwell, Donald A. Girod, Roger A. Hurwitz, Lynn Mahony, Harold King, and John Brown (Indiana Univ., Indianapolis)

Am. Heart J. 113:873–878, April 1987 2–15

Cardiovascular surgeons have perceived a need for an accurate means of predicting potential size of prosthetic valves in patients who are undergoing valve replacement. The techniques used for this purpose include the aortic root angiogram and the two-dimensional echocardiographic (2D-ECHO) prediction.

The authors describe a 2D-ECHO technique for predicting the size of mitral and aortic valve prostheses in children who have valve replacement, and they have also evaluated intraobserver variability. The study group included 18 consecutive pediatric patients with a mean age of 11.5 years (range, 2 to 17 years) who underwent preoperative 2D-ECHO study. Fourteen patients subsequently underwent primary valve replacement and 4 had repeat valve replacement.

The 2D-ECHO–measured mitral or aortic valve anulus was compared with the external diameter of the largest prosthetic valve that could be inserted. A strong correlation was found between the 2D-ECHO measurements and the size of the prosthetic valve in patients who underwent primary valve replacement. However, the correlation was poor for those who had repeat valve replacement.

It is concluded that 2D-ECHO prediction of the size of prosthetic mitral and aortic valves is accurate in children who undergo primary valve replacement but is poor in those who have repeat valve replacement.

▶ Pediatric cardiologists strive to make as accurate and precise a preoperative diagnosis as possible. This saves minutes in the operating room, benefits the patient, and reinforces the teamwork of cardiologist and surgeon. In the child undergoing valve replacement, the cardiologist was able reproducibly to predict valve prosthesis size for primary replacement. However, not unexpectedly, this preoperative assessment was not helpful for reoperations. In that situation, the surgeon expects to find that the size of the anulus has been fixed by prior valve placement and that the second valve will be about the same size as the original artificial valve.—M.A. Engle, M.D.

Catheter Therapy

Anatomic Features of Congenital Pulmonary Valvar Stenosis

Betty Muthoni Gikonyo, Russell V. Lucas, and Jesse E. Edwards (Univ. of Minnesota and United Hosps., St. Paul)

Pediatr. Cardiol. 8:109–116, 1987 2–16

A good understanding of the pathologic anatomy of congenital pulmonary valvar stenosis helps to select the best candidates for balloon valvuloplasty of the pulmonary valve. The authors examined 31 hearts with congenital pulmonary valve stenosis and 210 specimens having a normal pulmonary valve.

They found five types of stenosis: the domed type (most frequent), followed by unicommissural, bicuspid, tricuspid, dysplastic, and hypoplastic anulus types. The valve leaflets were thickened in all of these types along the entire length of the leaflet. Microscopy showed that increased myxomatous tissue usually accounted for the increase in thickness. The valve anulus commonly was abnormal, due to partial or complete absence, or to replacement of the fibrous backbone by myxomatous tissue.

The changes in the hypoplastic pulmonary valve and anulus may preclude successful valvuloplasty.

▶ Now that pediatric cardiologists tend increasingly to perform balloon valvoplasty for moderate and severe forms of pulmonary valvar stenosis (PVS), rather than to refer the children to a cardiac surgeon for valvotomy under direct vision, it is timely for the doctors at University of Minnesota to remind us of the anatomy of the congenitally stenosed valve.

From their extensive collection of heart specimens, they reviewed 31 with VPS and compared them with 210 specimens with normal valves. They divided the stenotic specimens into five groups, based on number of leaflets (one to three), size of anulus, and dysplastic tissue. They also commented on the 14 specimens that had been treated by open surgical valvotomy and on 2 specimens following closed (Brock) valvotomy. When the lines of fusion were opened, the results were evident relief of obstruction, but if the incision of the fused commissures was incomplete or leaflets were incised, relief was incomplete or the leaflet was flail.

They concluded that the valve is thickened along the entire leaflet due to an increase in myxomatous tissue and that the valve anulus in most instances is abnormal due to lack of all or part of the fibrous backbone.

Surely these variations are important in considering balloon valvoplasty versus surgery under direct vision and in weighing potential complications and judging results.—M.A. Engle, M.D.

The Morphology of the Right Ventricular Outflow Tract After Percutaneous Pulmonary Valvotomy: Long Term Follow Up

M. Robertson, L.N. Benson, J.S. Smallhorn, N. Musewe, R.M. Freedom, C.A.F. Moes, P. Burrows, A.. Johnston, F.A. Burrows, and R.D. Rowe (Hosp. for Sick Children, Toronto)

Br. Heart J. 58:239–244, September 1987 2–17

Certain patients have hemodynamically significant obstruction of the right ventricular outflow tract after percutaneous balloon pulmonary valvotomy despite an apparent tear in the valve. This obstruction was studied by echocardiography in 29 patients undergoing pulmonary valvotomy for moderate to severe isolated valvular stenosis. Seven cases with valve dysplasia were excluded. Echocardiography was done immediately prior to and 24 hours after balloon dilatation of the valve and after a mean follow-up of 10 months.

All but two patients had commissural fusion of a tricuspid pulmonary valve as the cause of the stenosis. None had pulmonary regurgitation. After valvoplasty, the valve gradient declined significantly (by 47%), whereas the cardiac index did not change in the short term. The infundibular ratio also did not change after the procedure. The valve commissure was torn in 27 patients after dilation. Two patients with bicuspid valves had flail leaflets. All patients had evidence of mild pulmonary insufficiency at follow-up. After 10 months, the mean valve gradient was

31 mm Hg, compared with 37 mm Hg immediately after the procedure. Two patients had a second valvotomy.

Dynamic obstruction of the subpulmonary outflow tract appears frequently to be a component of pulmonary valve stenosis, and it may persist after balloon dilation of the valve. If an adequate commissural tear is accomplished, the gradient may be expected to decline in time as infundibular hypertrophy regresses. Further dilations with larger balloons are usually not necessary.

▶ This sampling of 29 patients treated by pulmonary balloon valvoplasty provided an opportunity for pre- and postprocedure analysis of valve anatomy, the gradient across the valve, and the morphology of the right ventricular (RV) outflow tract.

The good news is that the reduction in peak systolic pressure gradient measured immediately after the procedure still held at postprocedure study almost 1 year later. The infundibular ratio (ratio of systolic to diastolic endocardial dimensions) was unchanged by the procedure. Dynamic RV outflow tract obstruction relaxes, just as it does after open valvotomy with incision along the lines of commissural fusion.

The bad news was that mild pulmonic regurgitation developed in all and that 2 with bicuspid valves were left with flail valves.

Commissural tears appear to be the primary mechanism of valve disruption.—M.A. Engle, M.D.

Balloon Dilation of the Aortic Valve: Studies in Normal Lambs and in Children With Aortic Stenosis

Hrodmar Helgason, John F. Keane, Kenneth E. Fellows, Thomas J. Kulik, and James E. Lock (The Children's Hosp. and Harvard Univ., Boston)

J. Am. Coll. Cardiol. 9:816–822, April 1987 2–18

Static balloon dilation has been used to treat valvular pulmonary stenosis, as well as other valvular obstructive lesions such as aortic and mitral stenosis. The authors evaluated the effects of balloons of various sizes on the aortic valve and paravalvular structures of 16 normal live newborn lambs and described their initial experience with balloon dilation in 15 patients with valvular aortic stenosis.

In the lambs, ratio of the diameters of the inflated balloon to aortic anulus ranged from 0.9 to 1.5. Immediately after the procedure, the authors found that ratios of 0.9 to 1.1 did not cause significant damage to the left ventricular outflow tract, whereas those of 1.2 to 1.5 caused tears or hematomas, or both, of the aortic valve leaflets (n = 3), mitral valve leaflets (n = 4), and interventricular septum (n = 4).

The 15 patients, aged 10 days to 15 years, underwent 16 balloon aortic valvulotomy procedures with the balloon anulus diameter ratios ranging from 0.67 to 1.1. The average pressure gradient decreased 69% and, overall, the peak systolic gradient decreased from 86 ± 21 to 28 ± 14 mm Hg and the aortic valve area increased from 0.44 ± 0.11 to 0.73 ±

0.22 sq cm/sq m. An increase in aortic regurgitation was observed immediately after the procedure in 8 (57%) of 14 patients. However, the regurgitation was greater than 3+ and it was well tolerated in short-term followup. The other early complications included transient left bundle-branch block in 2 patients, temporary femoral artery occlusion in 3 patients, and femoral artery rupture requiring operative management in 1 infant.

Balloon valvotomy can reduce the transvalvular gradient in selected patients with valvular aortic stenosis when a balloon less than 1.1 times the aortic root diameter is used. Although an increase in aortic regurgitation occurred in more than half the patients, it appears to have been well tolerated thus far in 6 weeks' to 6 months' follow-up.

▶ As pulmonary balloon valvoplasty has gained wide acceptance as a safe and effective way to relieve most instances of moderate or severe congenital pulmonic stenosis, some investigators have explored possible extension to other obstructions to blood flow. This article provides information from an experimental model in lambs and from clinical application in 15 infants and children with congenital valvar aortic stenosis. The predilation systolic pressure gradient ranged from 58 to 130 mm Hg and immediately afterward, from 10 to about 55 mm. At follow-up catheterization, 5 patients had the same level of reduction but 3 had a greater gradient. Aortic regurgitation appeared after dilation in 4 of 8 patients who had none prior to dilation.

This report serves as a useful, forthright analysis of the problems encountered in choice of balloon size, in maintaining placement during inflation, and in complications, as well as in short-term outcome. The patients were carefully selected after prior experience in animals and the results were reported helpfully. The authors plan to continue aortic balloon dilation as an investigational procedure.—M.A. Engle, M.D.

Aortic Valve Damage Caused by Operative Balloon Dilatation of Critical Aortic Valve Stenosis

Rachel R. Phillips, Leon M. Gerlis, Neil Wilson, and Duncan R. Walker (Killingbeck Hosp., Leeds, England)

Br. Heart J. 57:168–170, February 1987 2–19

Percutaneous balloon dilation of the pulmonary or aortic valve is used to relieve critical valvular stenosis in children and in adults. Experimental and necropsy findings following this procedure have shown linear tears of the valve or transverse tears in the aortic wall. The authors describe 7 patients with operative balloon dilatation of the aortic valve that in 4 cases damaged the valve leaflets and caused severe aortic regurgitation.

Girl, age 4 days, presented with cardiac failure. Echocardiography and angiocardiography demonstrated a ventricular septal defect, severe aortic stenosis, patent ductus arteriosus, and preductal coarctation. She underwent surgical repair of the coarctation with a Goretex gusset and ligation of the ductus arteriosus at age 18 days. After the surgery, she developed episodes of acute left ventricular failure that were unresponsive to medical treatment, and she required mechanical ventilation. These episodes were due to massive left-to-right shunting through the ventricular septal defect. The shunt was worsened by the critical obstruction of the left ventricular outflow tract. The diameter of the valve seen on echocardiography was 6 mm. The ventricular septal defect was closed surgically on day 47, and at the same time, balloon dilation of the aortic valve was performed through an apical left ventricular stab incision with an 8-mm diameter balloon catheter. Although there was some improvement immediately after the operation, the infant died the next day with severe aortic regurgitation.

In three patients, necropsy demonstrated partial detachment of the right coronary cusp of the aortic valve. Damage to the valve leaflet due to balloon dilatation was probably the result of using a balloon with a diameter that was too large in relation to the aortic ring diameter and of shearing forces created in the aortic wall by the contracting ventricle. If this procedure is undertaken, the authors recommend that the diameter of the inflated balloon should not be larger than the diameter of the aortic valve ring.

▶ When new procedures are developing, it is essential that we analyze failures as well as successes. Probably there are fewer conditions in congenital heart disease that are more imminently life-threatening in newborns than critically severe aortic stenosis, which causes cardiac failure in the first two days of life. It would appear highly desirable to confirm the diagnosis and to relieve the condition immediately. Aortic balloon valvoplasty seems a reasonable possibility as palliation in this situation.

Balloon dilation was carried out in the operating room in seven babies. The outcome in four infants was highly unsatisfactory due to the development of severe aortic regurgitation. Postmortem examination in three showed dysplastic aortic valves with tears and partial detachment of the cusp, especially the right coronary cusp.

The authors advised that in order to avoid damage to the aortic wall and to the leaflets, while effecting relief of the severe obstruction, a balloon size somewhat less than that of the aortic ring should be used. Clearly, we do not yet have the best solution for this problem.—M.A. Engle, M.D.

Transluminal Balloon Dilatation for Discrete Subaortic Stenosis

Zuhdi Lababidi, Larry Weinhaus, Harry Stoeckle, Jr., and Joseph T. Walls (Univ. of Missouri)

Am. J. Cardiol. 59:423–425, Feb. 15, 1987 2–20

Recently successful transluminal balloon angioplasty and valvuloplasty have been reported in left-sided cardiac obstructive lesions such as coarctation of the aorta and valvular aortic stenosis. The authors describe their experience with 10 children with discrete subaortic stenosis (DSS) who underwent transluminal balloon dilatation to alleviate the obstruction.

The DSS was visualized by two-dimensional echocardiography and cineangiography. Six patients had a thin discrete "membrane" immediately below the aortic valve (group I) and 4 had a thicker fibromuscular ring about 1 cm below the aortic valve (group II). In group I the mean gradient decreased from 82 mm Hg to 22 mm Hg; in group II it decreased from a mean of 155 mm Hg to 85 mm Hg.

One year later three patients underwent follow-up cardiac catheterization. Mean gradient soon after the procedure was 37 mm Hg and on follow-up it was still 37 mm Hg, indicating persistence of relief from the obstruction. In group II the patients had a high residual gradient and three of them had surgical relief of the obstruction.

The extent of aortic regurgitation that was present before the dilatation in all ten patients did not change after the procedure. Relief of the obstruction was provided by tearing the subaortic membrane.

These data suggest that relief of subaortic obstruction is more favorable in the thin, membranous DSS.

▶ Discrete subaortic stenosis comes in several forms, none of them simple to manage because the obstruction tends to worsen as time goes by, to be associated with the development of aortic regurgitation, and to recur after surgery. Therefore, it is appropriate in an investigational and controlled manner to see whether balloon dilation has something to offer. Based on short-term experience in a small number of children, the group at Columbia, Mo., which is experienced in balloon dilation techniques, reported that in six patients with a discrete membrane, the mean systolic pressure gradient dropped from 82 ± 19 to 22 ± 15 mm Hg and remained at that level in three who were restudied 1 year later. However, in four patients with a thicker, fibromuscular ring, the residual gradient was 85 ± 44 mm Hg compared with 155 ± 18 before the dilation. Aortic regurgitation in five of the ten children was said to be the same after the procedure.

Clearly this malformation is still a lesion in search of a cure.—M.A. Engle, M.D.

Balloon Angioplasty for Coarctation of the Aorta in Infancy

P. Syamasundar Rao (King Faisal Specialist Hosp., Riyadh, Saudi Arabia)
J. Pediatr. 110:713–718, May 1987 2–21

Percutaneous balloon angioplasty was used to treat six infants with coarctation of the aorta. These infants had associated aortic stenosis, ventricular septal defect, and patent ductus arteriosus. Balloon dilation was repeated at least three times in each patient, 5 minutes apart.

No significant complications were encountered. The systolic pressure proximal to the coarctation decreased significantly from 122.2 ± 11.5 to 104.4 ± 15.4 mm Hg. The systolic pressure distal to the coarctation increased significantly from 78.0 ± 12.9 to 99.7 ± 9.2 mm Hg. The systolic pressure gradient across the coarctation decreased significantly from 44.2 ± 14.7 to 11.7 ± 9.4 mm Hg. The coarcted segment significantly increased in diameter from 2.9 ± 0.7 mm to 5.3 ± 1.2 mm. The mean

Doppler flow velocity decreased from 3.5 m per second to 2.1 m per second. A follow-up of 10–16 months revealed excellent results in four infants and the need for additional treatment in two infants. Aneurysm was not seen in any of these patients.

Balloon angioplasty is recommended as the procedure of choice for severe unoperated coarctation of the aorta in infants. The size of the balloon should be limited by the size of the aorta proximal to the coarcted segment or to the diameter of the descending aorta at diaphragm level.

▶ Dr. Rao has had excellent results in Saudi Arabia with balloon dilation of valvular pulmonic stenosis. While the balloon dilation of native coarctation of the aorta offers the possibility of relatively safe immediate relief of obstruction, it has also the possibility of an unfavorable outcome a year or so later, either because of restenosis or of aneurysm formation. This report of six babies, aged 1–18 months, with coarctation and all with associated cardiac anomalies can add to the data base of immediate and of short-term (up to 16 months) results. All six survived the dilation and had relief of the systolic pressure gradient, which decreased from a mean of 44 to a mean of 17 mm Hg. Two infants had restenosis relieved in one by surgery and in the other by repeat dilation.—M.A. Engle, M.D.

Angioplasty for Coarctation of the Aorta: Long-Term Results

Rubin S. Cooper, Samuel B. Ritter, William B. Rothe, C.K. Chen, Randall Griepp, and Richard J. Golinko (Brookdale Hosp. Med. Ctr. and State Univ. of New York, Brooklyn)

Circulation 75:600–604, March 1987 2–22

For the past 5 years, clinicians have used percutaneous balloon angioplasty to treat patients with various congenital and acquired heart lesions. The initial and long-term results of a study of seven patients exhibiting discrete coarctation are reviewed.

The patients were five boys and two girls, aged 18 months to 18 years, with isolated discrete unoperated coarctation of the aorta. For surgery a No. 8F or 9F catheter was employed with balloon lengths of 30 mm or 40 mm and maximum inflation diameters of 1 mm less than the smallest measured aortic diameter determined 1 cm proximal to the site of coarctation. A 10-second inflation-deflation cycle of 6–8 atmospheres, 90–120 psi, was performed. Before balloon coarctation angioplasty, the peak systolic pressure gradient ranged from 35–70 mm Hg, with a mean of 58 mm Hg. Immediately after balloon coarctation angioplasty, it dropped to 0–20 mm Hg, with a mean of 7 mm Hg. At follow-up 1–2 years later, the peak systolic pressure gradient was 10–30 mm Hg, with a mean of 19 mm Hg. Angiography was repeated immediately proximal to the coarctation site. Three patients (43%) showed evidence of aneurysm formation at or just distal to the balloon dilatation site. One patient demonstrated coarctation restenosis.

As in previous studies, these early observations with balloon angioplasty for unoperated coarctation of the aorta appeared encouraging. Nevertheless, the follow-up data raise serious concern about the long-term safety and efficacy of this procedure.

▶ Long-term follow-up of this newly introduced form of treatment is not yet very long: 1–2 years with a mean of 14 months. The authors initially were encouraged by the immediate drop in peak systolic pressure from a range of 35–70 mm Hg down to 0–20 mm Hg. Later their enthusiasm dampened because although the gradient was only 10 mm more after 1–2 years, three of the seven patients (43%) had evidence of aneurysm formation in the area of original coarctation. The long-term effects of that complication are unkonwn, but I join the authors in urging cautious consideration of the long-term safety, efficacy, and ill effects of this new modality.—M.A. Engle, M.D.

Double Balloon Technique for Dilation of Valvular or Vessel Stenosis in Congenital and Acquired Heart Disease

Charles E. Mullins, Michael R. Nihill, G. Wesley Vick III, Achi Ludomirsky, Martin P. O'Laughlin, J. Timothy Bricker, and Victoria E. Judd (Baylor College and Texas Children's Hosp., Houston)

J. Am. Coll. Cardiol. 10:107–114, July 1987 2–23

Although balloon dilation for the stenotic lesions of congenital and acquired heart disease generally yields excellent results, technical difficulties can prevent good results. Such difficulties include a large diameter of the anulus of the stenotic lesion, compared with available balloon diameter; difficulty inserting or removing larger balloon catheters; and permanent damage to or obstruction of the femoral vessels by redundant deflated balloon material of large balloons. A double balloon technique developed to resolve these difficulties, is described.

With this method, the surgeon inserts percutaneous balloon angioplasty catheters in right and left femoral vessels (so that they are side by side across the stenotic lesion) and inflates them simultaneously. Dilatation procedures were performed using this technique in 41 patients: 18 with pulmonary valve stenosis, 14 with aortic valve stenosis, 5 with mitral valve stenosis, 3 with vena caval obstruction after the Mustard or Senning procedure, and 1 with tricuspid valve stenosis (Fig 2–2). Patients ranged in age from 1 to 75 years (mean, 17.8 years) and in weight from 8.9 to 89 kg (mean, 42.3 kg). Balloon catheters were 10–20 mm in diameter. The average maximal pressure gradient before dilation in mm Hg was 61 in pulmonary stenosis, 68 in aortic stenosis, 21 in mitral stenosis, 12 in tricuspid stenosis, and 25 in vena caval stenosis. After dilatation, the average maximal valvular pressure gradient was 13 in pulmonary stenosis, 24 in aortic stenosis, 4 in mitral stenosis, 0 in tricuspid stenosis, and 1 in vena caval stenosis. There were no major complications.

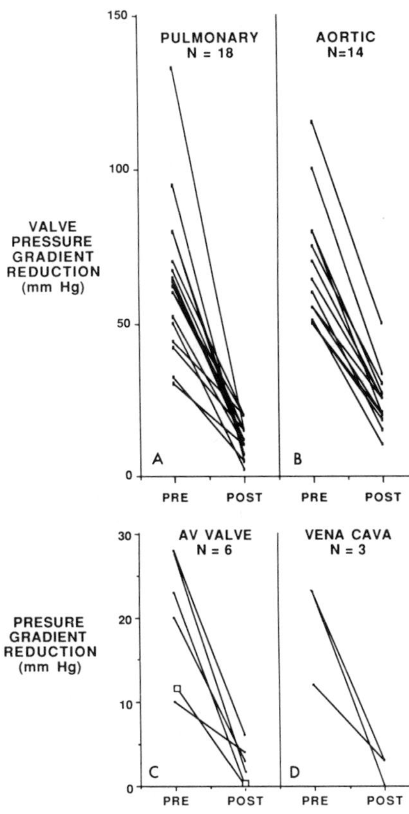

Fig 2–2.—Simultaneously inflated balloons positioned across the pulmonary valve. (Courtesy of Mullins, C.E., et al.: J. Am. Coll. Cardiol. 10:107–114, July 1987.)

The two-balloon technique of percutaneous balloon dilation appears effective and safe and in selected cases, has substantial advantages over techniques that use a single large angioplasty balloon.

▶ The authors describe the reasons for and the technique of using two balloons rather than a single one for dilation of stenotic lesions. They found no problems that were different from those with a single balloon. However, an obvious drawback in infants and small children is that venous cannulation is necessary from both groins. Occasionally there are residua, with edema of the extremity and with difficulty in entering the vein again, should a repeated study or dilation be necessary. The advantages are that, with two balloons, there is still an opening for blood to continue to pass through the stenosis during the actual dilatation. In contrast, a single balloon completely occludes the area of stenosis. The authors state that the double balloon technique extends the range of conditions that can be dilated.

The immediate results of this procedure are impressive, as the figure indicates.—M.A. Engle, M.D.

Acute Complications of Catheter Therapy for Congenital Heart Disease

Kenneth E. Fellows, Wolfgang Radtke, John F. Keane, and James E. Lock
(Children's Hosp. and Harvard Univ., Boston)

Am. J. Cardiol. 60:679–683, Sept. 15, 1987 2–24

Dilation of peripheral pulmonic stenosis (PS) is often done and evaluated because few or no surgical options exist. Dilation of valvular PS and coil embolization of systemic-pulmonary collaterals are reasonable alternatives to surgery, and newer therapies are being explored. At this stage, the literature emphasizes the success rates of the various procedures and does not provide extensive reviews of complications. A review was made of the acute complications resulting from 417 therapeutic catheter procedures from one institution to better define the risks and to identify risk factors.

The patients, aged 1 day to 51 years, underwent catheter procedures between 1984 and 1987. The procedures consisted mainly of vascular dilatations and embolizations. Dilatations were of peripheral pulmonic stenosis in 97, valvular pulmonic stenosis in 67, valvular aortic stenosis in 62, and recurrent coarctation in 49. Embolizations involved double umbrella devices in 36 and steel coils in 45 cases. Acute complications were considered to be adverse effects recognized clinically within 1 week of the procedure. They did not include late complications in this study. Overall, 50 acute complications occurred, yielding an incidence of 12%. Twenty-four (6%) were major, and 26 (8%) were minor. The mortality was 0.7%. Complication rates varied from 4% for dilation of recurrent coarctation to 40% for dilation of aortic stenosis. A strong age dependency was noted for the incidence of vascular access complications, usually persistent pulse loss or venous occlusion. Eight of ten such events occurred in patients younger than 6 months. Also, 3 of 4 patients who had cardiac arrest or ventricular fibrillation were younger than 6 months. No statistically significant trend toward diminishing overall complication rates was found during the 37 months of the study.

Based on these findings, it appears that serious arrhythmias and complications of vascular access are more common in patients younger than 6 months old and that pulmonary artery rupture represents a life-threatening risk in dilation of peripheral PS.

▶ This is a most important article by the group at Boston Children's Hospital, who analyzed their extensive experience with 417 such procedures in a recent 3-year period. Carefully they reported on the acute complications within the week following the procedure and they offered responsible words of caution to teams of experienced cardiologists who undertake this new type of therapy.

They pointed out the high-risk procedures such as in dilating valvular aortic stenosis, with a 40% complication rate. This includes postprocedure aortic regurgitation, which was at least moderate in 8% and severe in 2%. Although they stated that "Aortic regurgitation to some degree is expected after surgical valvotomy," that has not been my experience since our cardiac surgeons learned to accept less complete relief of stenosis without regurgitation rather than to make incisions all the way out to the anulus, thereby inviting valvular incompetence. I am not in favor, at the present time, of aortic balloon valvuloplasty.

Long-term complications, such as edema of the leg, are not the subject of this analysis. Nor is fluoroscopy time reported. This can be lengthy.

The authors are to be commended for a forthright sharing with us the wisdom of their great experience with catheter therapy of congenital heart disease.—M.A. Engle, M.D.

Cardiac Surgery

Correlates of Resting and Maximal Exercise Systolic Blood Pressure After Repair of Coarctation of the Aorta: A Multivariable Analysis

Stephen R. Daniels, Frederick W. James, Jennifer M.H. Loggie, and Samuel Kaplan (Children's Hosp. Med. Ctr., Cincinnati)
Am. Heart J. 113:349–353, February 1987 2–25

It has been shown that corrective surgery for coarctation of the aorta may not prevent subsequent late development of elevated systemic blood pressure and the associated premature morbidity and mortality as these patients grow into adulthood. In addition, the systolic blood pressure response to exercise may also be abnormal in patients who have had corrective surgery for coarctation.

The authors have conducted a retrospective investigation to test a number of potential correlates of systolic blood pressure in patients who have undergone repair of coarctation of the aorta. The study group included 42 patients who had graded exercise tests after correction of coarctation of the aorta.

The independent variables that were tested included height, weight, body surface area, age at surgery, age at exercise testing, time between surgery and exercise testing, highest systolic blood pressure prior to surgery, gradient across the coarctation at preoperative catheterization, and residual postoperative gradient across the coarctation.

The same combination of independent variables provided the best regression model for explanation of the variance of both postoperative resting and maximal exercise systolic blood pressure. The models included height, highest preoperative systolic blood pressure, and residual gradient; none of the other variables added significant explanatory ability to either model.

The preoperative level of systolic blood pressure may be the best determinant of timing corrective surgery. The authors believe that as long as blood pressure remains normal, the operation can probably be delayed until an age when repair is less likely to lead to recurrent coarctation.

▶ The authors provide a retrospective, multivariate analysis of 42 children with simple coarctation, operated on 9 months to 18 years earlier when they were aged 2 months to 18 years. The article merits careful study because of the long-standing interest and expertise of the authors in hypertension, exercise testing, and congenital heart disease at their well-known medical center. After analyzing many potentially informative variables, they found that the following were the most important for predicting postoperative outcome: height, highest preoperative systolic blood pressure (BP), and residual gradient. Of these, the height of the systolic BP "may be the best determinant of timing" of surgical repair. This implies that a recent trend to rush the asymptomatic, nonhypertensive child with coarctation to the operating room in order to protect him from late postoperative hypertension may not be necessary.—M.A. Engle, M.D.

Survival After Balloon Atrial Septostomy for Complete Transposition of Great Arteries

Q. Mok, F. Darvell, S. Mattos, T. Smith, P. Fayers, M.L. Rigby, and E.A. Shinebourne (Brompton Hosp., London)

Arch. Dis. Child. 62:549–553, June 1987 2–26

The authors describe the mortality rate in 102 infants with transposition of the great arteries who underwent balloon atrial septostomy between December 1984 and January 1985. The outcome was considered unsuccessful if the patient died of any cause between the septostomy and the subsequent repair by Mustard's operation or the arterial switch operation.

Death occurred in 18% of these patients prior to surgery. All deaths occurred within 6 weeks of septostomy. Of the 102 patients, 53 had complete transposition and an intact ventricular septum. Death occurred in 19% of these cases. The presence of low weight, persistent arterial duct, and coarctation were significant risk factors. In 3 patients, balloon atrial septostomy was insufficient. Atrial septectomy was performed, but the patients died in the perioperative period.

The introduction of balloon atrial septostomy has greatly increased survival of infants with transposition of the great arteries. However, significant death still occurs before surgical repair. This must be considered in the assessment of overall outcome.

▶ One of the most remarkable accomplishments in the field of cyanotic congenital heart disease in the past quarter century was the introduction by the late Dr. William Rashkind of the balloon atrial septostomy (BAS) procedure for newborns with completely transposed great arteries (TGA). This event of interventional cardiac catheterization, applied worldwide soon after its introduction, converted a mortality rate of about 95% for babies with TGA to a salvage of about 95%.

The procedure was palliative but was effective for the next 4–6 months, at which time a Mustard operation was performed. This is a venous switch to conform physiologically to the anatomically transposed great arteries. It was performed with a mortality rate of about 5%.

Two recent changes in surgical care have come about. One is the use of the Senning operation for venous switch at about the same low mortality rate. The other is the use of the arterial switch operation in the first 2 weeks of life to accomplish an anatomical repair but with higher mortality.

The "right choice" is not yet clear. However, this article from London provided some data to help decision-making. It analyzes the outcome after balloon septostomy and before reparative surgery in 102 infants over a 10-year period, 1975–1984.

The article points out an attrition rate that totaled 18% in the 6 weeks after BAS. Risk factors were low weight and the presence of two associated defects: persistent patent ductus and coarctation of the aorta.—M.A. Engle, M.D.

Results of the Senning Procedure in Infants With Simple and Complex Transposition of the Great Arteries

Barbara L. George, Hillel Laks, Thomas S. Klintzner, William F. Friedman, and Roberta G. Williams (Univ. of Calif., Los Angeles)

Am. J. Cardiol. 59:426–430, February 1987 2–27

Over the past 10 years surgical management of patients with simple and complex d-transposition of the great arteries (TGA) has improved markedly because of venous switch procedures, Mustard and Senning operations, or an arterial switch procedure. The authors have examined recent experience with the Senning operation in patients with simple as well as complex TGA and compared early and late mortality with published results of the arterial switch procedure.

The study group included 35 patients with simple TGA (group I) and 10 patients with complex TGA (group II) who underwent a Senning operation. Mean duration of follow-up was 14 months for group I and 24 months for group II. One patient in group I died early, and no patient had a late death, in addition, there was infrequent occurrence of right ventricular dysfunction, tricuspid regurgitation, baffle obstruction, or arrhythmias. In group II no patients died early, and 3 patients had a late death; in addition, many patients required prolonged digoxin therapy.

Because the arterial switch operation has a high early mortality risk and an undetermined long-term morbidity and mortality risk, the Senning operation is considered the preferred surgical approach for simple TGA. The authors recommend further studies to compare the early and late morbidity and mortality of the arterial versus the venous switch operations in order to select the appropriate surgical approach to complex TGA.

▶ The pediatric and surgical cardiologists at UCLA review in a thoughtful manner the options available today for surgical relief of transposition of the great arteries (TGA), simple and complex. They present their recent experience in one of the two most frequently used venous switch operations, in which systemic and pulmonary venous return is rerouted to match physiologically the transposed aorta and pulmonary artery. They conclude that for simple TGA, a venous switch operation (Senning or Mustard) is the preferred surgical approach. This preference is based on the low early and late mortality and morbidity of venous switch versus the higher early mortality and undetermined late morbidity and mortality of the arterial switch.

Based on our experience since 1972, I agree with their view for this point in time, that rerouting of venous return is preferable to reconnecting the arterial trunks.—M.A. Engle, M.D.

Replacement of Obstructed Extracardiac Conduits With Autogenous Tissue Reconstructions

Gordon K. Danielson, T. Peter Downing, Hartzell V. Schaff, Francisco J. Puga, Roberto M. DiDonato, and Donald G. Ritter (Mayo Clinic and Found.)

J. Thorac. Cardiovasc. Surg. 93:555–559, April 1987 2–28

The failure rate of tissue-valved prosthetic extracardiac conduits within 5 years of implantation is 6% to 30%. Failure is caused by both valve degeneration and conduit peel formation. This article reviews a technique that allows replacement of the obstructed extracardiac valved conduit with a new conduit by using the previous conduit bed as the posterior wall and an onlay patch as the anterior wall or roof of the conduit.

During a 2.5-year period, 16 patients, aged 10–23 years, underwent autogenous tissue reconstruction of an obstructed right-sided valved conduit. The initial operation had been performed at a younger age for transposition of the great arteries (n = 8); truncus arteriosus (n = 3); pulmonary atresia (n = 3); complicated tetralogy of Fallot (n = 1); or isolated dextrocardia with atrioventricular discordance, double-outlet right ventricle, and pulmonary atresia (n = 1). All patients developed obstruction of a previously inserted Hancock porcine bioprosthesis.

The roof of the conduit was fashioned from a patch of xenograft pericardium in 10 patients, from homograft dura mater in 5 patients, and from Dacron in 1 patient. One patient with pulmonary hypertension required insertion of a Björk-Shiley pulmonary valve, but the other 15 patients did not need a new valve. Intraoperative pressure measured after completion of repair in the right ventricle (n = 14) ranged from 31–65 mm Hg, and that in the pulmonary artery (n = 12) ranged from 30–55 mm Hg. Right ventricular pressure in all patients was less than one half of systemic pressure. No early deaths occurred. Hospital stays ranged from 6–26 days. No late deaths occurred during follow-up for up to 17 months.

It appears that this technique simplifies conduit replacement. Moreover, this repair allows for a generous-sized outflow tract that may grow as the patient grows, and it uses material that is not likely to become obstructed.

▶ Sometimes dramatic, innovative surgery for complex congenital heart disease has late effects not anticipated when the procedure was introduced. Such is the case when an external conduit of synthetic material with porcine valve is used to establish continuity between the pulmonary pumping ventricle—usually the right ventricle (RV)—and the main pulmonary artery (PA) or its branches. Valve deterioration and/or obstruction by conduit "peel" occur within 5 years in about one fourth of these children, who then need replacement of the conduit. In England, where homografts consisting of aortic leaflet of the mitral valve, aortic valve, and ascending aorta are used, this problem occurs less frequently.

It is no fun for anyone when reoperation is needed for conduit obstruction—not for the patient, parents, pediatric cardiologist, or cardiac surgeon. This report from the Mayo Clinic describes one method currently in use to simplify the replacement somewhat. They simply leave the sides and posterior wall and replace the ventral aspect with tissue, such as xenograft pericardium or dura mater or with Dacron. If there is no obstruction distal to the main pulmonary artery, the valve can be omitted.

They caution that great care must be taken on reentry through the sternum. They reduced the right ventricular hypertension to 50% of systemic systolic pressure or less by the repair. All patients survived reoperation and continued well up to 17 months of follow-up. Unfortunately, conduit obstruction can recur. I have observed one such instance 11 months after the replacement of the obstructed conduit in this manner.

One should not deny a child with truncus arteriosus or pulmonary atresia in tetralogy of Fallot the benefits that accrue to most of them through closure of the ventricular septal defect and establishment of RV to PA flow via an external conduit. At the same time it behooves surgeons to continue to seek a longer-lasting conduit. One cannot expect it to grow in a baby or young child, but one can hope that it will not become blocked and that the valve will not deteriorate.—M.A. Engle, M.D.

Flow Dynamics in the Main Pulmonary Artery After the Fontan Procedure in Patients With Tricuspid Atresia or Single Ventricle

Makoto Nakazawa, Keiko Nojima, Hirofumi Okuda, Yasuharu Imai, Toshio Nakanishi, Hiromi Kurosawa, and Atsuyoshi Takao (The Heart Inst. of Japan, Tokyo Women's Med. College)

Circulation 75:1117–1123, June 1987 2–29

The authors have observed that patients with a large pulmonary artery do better after the Fontan procedure than patients with a small pulmonary artery. Similarly, patients with tricuspid atresia do better than those with single ventricle after the operation. The authors hypothesize that these differences influence the postoperative hemodynamics. To test this theory, they analyzed the flow velocity pattern in the main pulmonary artery after Fontan operation in patients with tricuspid atresia ($n = 10$) or with single ventricle ($n = 10$).

The authors used a catheter-mounted velocity probe and integrated the area underneath the velocity signal of the forward flow, and then calculated ratios of the portions during atrial systole (Fa) and during the diastolic phase (Fd) to the total area. The Fa was 0.54 ± 0.09 in patients with tricuspid atresia and 0.45 ± 0.05 in those with single ventricle. Car-

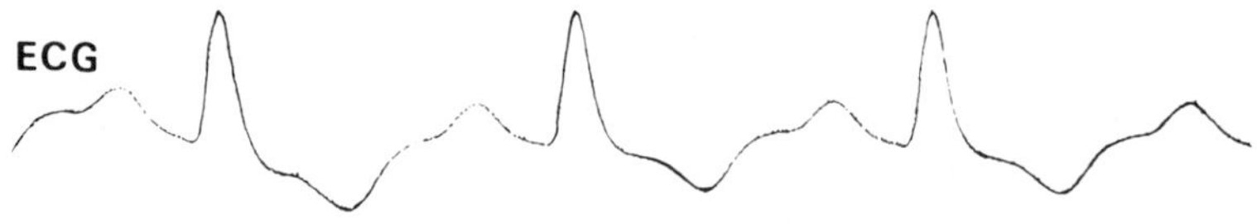

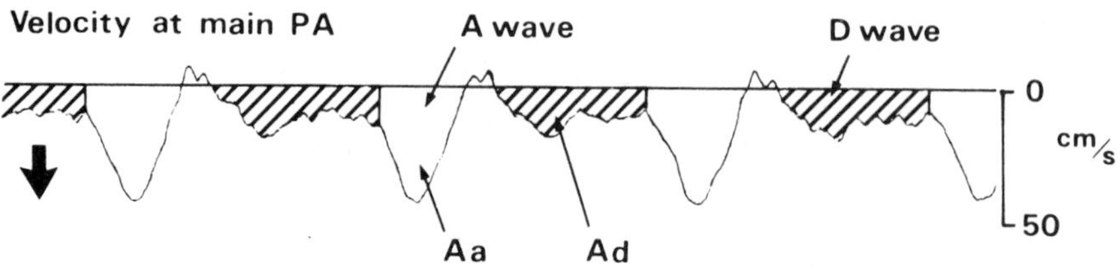

$$Fa = Aa/(Aa + Ad)$$

Fig 2–3.—The area underneath the forward flow of the velocity signal recorded at the main pulmonary artery (PA) was integrated. The areas underneath the A wave (Aa) and the diastolic flow (Ad) were separated by drawing a vertical line to the zero line at the beginning of upstroke of the A wave. Then a fraction (Fa) of atrial systolic flow to the total flow was calculated by dividing Aa by (Aa + Ad). Fd was obtained by dividing Ad by (Aa + Ad). The *heavy arrow* indicates the direction of forward flow. (Courtesy of Nakazawa, M., et al.: Circulation 75:1117–1123, June 1987.)

diac output was shown to be 2.45 ± 0.48 L/min/sq m in patients with tricuspid atresia and 2.75 ± 0.72 L/min/sq m in patients with single ventricle. The forward flow during atrial contraction was observed to be 1.32 ± 0.35 L/min/sq m in patients with tricuspid atresia and 1.23 ± 0.33 L/min/s m in those with single ventricle. The diastolic forward flow, was observed to be 0.99 ± 0.25 L/min/sq m in patients with tricuspid atresia and 1.52 ± 0.45 L/min/sq m in those with single ventricle.

When the authors normalized the sum of cross-sectional areas of the right and left pulmonary arteries by body surface area (PA index), they obtained values of 282 ± 85 sq cm/sq m in patients with tricuspid atresia and 462 ± 65 sq cm/sq m in patients with single ventricle. In the whole group the Fa was inversely correlated with the PA index and was also inversely correlated with the PA index in the tricuspid atresia group alone. The postoperative right atrial and pulmonary atrial pressures were 16 ± 3 and 16 ± 4 mm Hg in patients with tricuspid atresia and 15 ± 3 and 13 ± 3 mm Hg in those with single ventricle. Finally, the right atrial maximum volume, determined angiographically, was 169 ± 87% of normal in patients with tricuspid atresia and 105 ± 32% of normal in patients with single ventricle; however, the ejection fraction was the same in the two groups (Fig 2–3).

The relative role of right atrial contraction may become more important in patients with a smaller PA index. Furthermore right atrial output is constant regardless of the PA index or the type of anomalies, and the amount of diastolic forward flow is influenced by the PA index. The preoperative PA index appears to be an important determinant of postoperative hemodynamics.

▶ To determine why patients did better after the Fontan operation if they had a large rather than a small pulmonary artery and when they had tricuspid atresia rather than a single ventricle, the authors at the Heart Institute of Japan in Tokyo analyzed flow dynamics in the main pulmonary artery. They found that the relative role of atrial contraction became more important in those with smaller pulmonary arteries. Diastolic forward flow was higher in the 10 postoperative patients with single ventricle than it was in the 10 with tricuspid atresia. Atrial systolic output was the same in both groups.

They reaffirmed as key in their selection criteria for the Fontan operation the condition of the pulmonary circulation. Large arteries were more favorable than small vessels.—M.A. Engle, M.D.

Tricuspid Atresia in Adolescents and Adults: Current State and Late Complications

Carole A. Warnes and Jane Somerville (Natl. Heart Hosp., London)

Br. Heart J. 56:535–543, December 1986 2–30

As a result of early palliative and reparative operations, increasing numbers of patients with tricuspid atresia are surviving to adolescence and adult life. However, information about late results is scarce and little is known about the medical and social problems that these patients encounter in adulthood.

In the present study data were reviewed on all patients with tricuspid atresia and normally related great arteries who were treated at the National Heart Hospital since 1965 and survived past age 14 years. These 29 patients were aged 15 to 35 years, and 20 were alive at the time of this investigation. Ten patients who had had a Fontan operation (group 1) were compared with 9 patients with palliative shunts and 1 patient with no surgery (group 2). The patients were given an ability index based on their ability to lead a normal life (Fig 2–4).

Patients in group 1 tended to have a better ability index, a greater exercise capacity, and fewer social and extracardiac problems, compared to the patients in group 2. Mean left ventricular ejection fraction as measured by radionuclide angiography was the same in both groups. Ar-

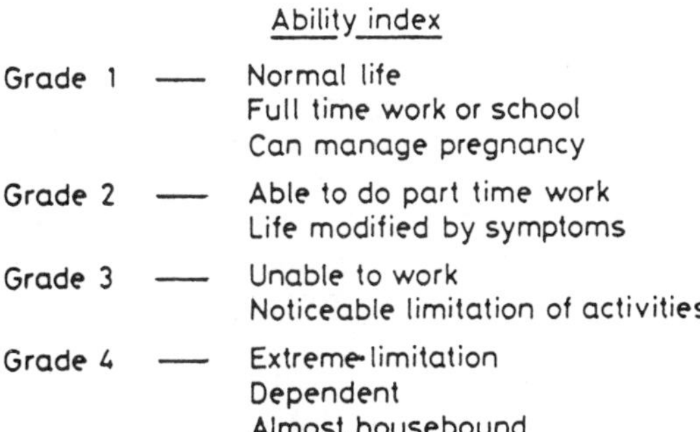

Fig 2–4.—Ability index classification. (Courtesy of Warnes, C.A., and Somerville, J.: Br. Heart J. 56:535–543, December 1986.)

rhythmias were equally common and appeared to be age-related and to occur independently of left ventricular function.

It is concluded that the status of patients who had a Fontan procedure is slightly better than the status of those who had palliative procedures. The authors recommend the Fontan procedure if ideal criteria can be fulfilled. If these criteria cannot be fulfilled, then they believe that the Blalock-Taussing shunt is the shunt of choice.

▶ What are the chances of an infant's reaching the age of 14 years or older if he is born with tricuspid atresia with normally related great arteries? That question is not answered in this article, but the question of how he does function if he makes it is addressed in a comparison of 10 survivors who had been treated by a variety of shunt procedures to increase pulmonary blood flow and another 10 who in addition had a different palliation, the Fontan procedure. Remarkably, both groups functioned about equally well, in a quietly active life, and had comparable exercise capacity and RNCA-measured ejection fraction. Arrhythmias tended to appear in about 50% of both groups around 20 years of age.

One aspect not discussed is a difference in the two groups: the freedom from cyanosis, polycythemia, and the complications of right-to-left shunting that those survivors with the Fontan procedure enjoy.—M.A. Engle, M.D.

The Long-Term Risk of Warfarin Sodium Therapy and the Incidence of Thromboembolism in Children After Prosthetic Cardiac Valve Replacement

Scott Stewart, Diane Cianciotta, Chlor Alexson, and James Manning (Univ. of Rochester, N.Y.)

J. Thorac. Cardiovasc. Surg. 93:551–554, April 1987 2–31

To determine the effectiveness of warfarin therapy, 30 children, aged 6–17 years, who underwent cardiac valve replacement with a prosthetic valve were followed for 1–17 years. All patients began warfarin therapy before leaving the hospital.

In the 211 total patient years of therapy, there were five bleeding episodes, with an incidence of 2.3 per 100 patient-years. However, three of these episodes were preventable, since the children were either receiving excess anticoagulation or were participating in inappropriate activities. There were five thromboembolic events in 211 total patient-years, with an incidence of 2.3 per 100 patient-years. Three of these patients had halted therapy. Eight teenaged patients were noncompliant, and the incidence of thromboembolic events in this group was 5.5 per 100 patient-years. In the group of 22 compliant patients, the incidence was 1.3 thromboembolic events per 100 patient-years.

There is no greater risk of bleeding from warfarin therapy in pediatric patients than there is in adults. The incidence of thromboembolism in this series was lower than that reported for adults. Discontinuation or noncompliance increased the risk of thromboembolism. Therefore, continuous warfarin therapy is recommended for children after prosthetic valve replacement.

▶ Since there may sometimes be no surgical alternative for a child with serious heart disease than valve replacement, this analysis of an experience that covers 211 patient-years of warfarin therapy in 30 children aged 6–17 years when they were operated on should be useful. The good news is that, in comparison with reports on adults taking warfarin for the same reason, there was no greater risk of bleeding and even less risk of embolism than in adults. Furthermore, most of the episodes of either bleeding or clotting were preventable. Of 22 compliant patients, the incidence of thromboembolism was only 1.3 per 100 patient-years.—M.A. Engle, M.D.

Aspirin Anticoagulation in Children With Mechanical Aortic Valves

Edward D. Verrier, Robert F. Tranbaugh, Scott J. Soifer, Edward S. Yee, Kevin Turley, and Paul A. Ebert (Univ. of California, San Francisco, and State Univ. of New York, Brooklyn)

J. Thorac. Cardiovasc. Surg. 92:1013–1020, December 1986 2–32

The best means of anticoagulating children with mechanical heart valves remains uncertain. Aspirin, alone or combined with dipyridamole, was used in 51 such children (mean age, 13 years), who were followed up for a mean of 36.5 months after heart valve insertion. Forty-five patients received aspirin alone in a dose of 6 mg/kg daily, up to 600 mg daily. Six patients also received dipyridamole in a dose of 25 or 50 mg daily. Fifty Björk-Shiley tilting spherical disc valves and a St. Jude bileaflet valve were placed.

There were few early complications, and the late mortality was 8%. No late deaths were related to thrombosis or embolism. There were no postoperative thromboembolic events. Eleven asymptomatic patients who underwent brain computed tomography (CT) or magnetic resonance (MR) imaging had no evidence of silent cerebral thromboembolism. Minor hemorrhagic complications occurred in 6% of patients.

Therapy for 5 patients was changed to warfarin. No mechanical valve failures occurred. All patients have remained in normal sinus or paced rhythm.

It appears that children with mechanical valve prostheses in normal sinus rhythm can safely be given aspirin, alone or with dipyridamole. Hemorrhagic complications of aspirin are not serious and are easily managed. Antiplatelet drugs are relatively inexpensive, easily administered, and do not require laboratory monitoring.

▶ Most of us are reluctant to recommend valve replacement in children until it is absolutely necessary. Our concerns are due not only to the problems of the valve itself, which cannot grow and in time will malfunction, but are also related to the long-term use of anticoagulants in active children. This study from the University of California in San Francisco offers an alternative for children with artificial aortic valves in normal sinus rhythm. The 45 children treated with aspirin alone and 6 others given aspirin and dipyridamole had little risk of thromboembolic events, valve thrombosis, or valve failure, and only minor risk of hemorrhage in a mean follow-up period of 36.5 months.—M.A. Engle, M.D.

Arrhythmias

Cardiac Arrhythmias in Healthy Children Revealed by 24-Hour Ambulatory ECG Monitoring

Masami Nagashima, Masaki Matsushima, Akimasa Ogawa, Akiko Ohsuga, Tetsuichi Kaneko, Takehiko Yazaki, and Mitsuharu Okajima (Nagoya Univ. and Chukyo Hosp., Nagoya, and Fujita-Gakuen Health Univ., Toyoake, Japan)
Pediatr. Cardiol. 8:103–108, 1987 2–33

Cardiac arrhythmias are presumed to be rare in children, but resting surface ECGs usually are recorded only for short periods. The authors performed ambulatory ECG monitoring in 360 healthy children, including 63 neonates, 50 infants aged 1–11 months, 53 children aged 4–6 years, 97 primary school children aged 9–12 years, and 97 junior high school students aged 13–15 years.

Both peak and minimum heart rates were significantly greater in infants than in older children. Sinus arrhythmia was a universal finding. One older child had an episode of sinus arrest unaccompanied by symptoms. First-degree atrioventricular (AV) block and Wenckebach type second-degree AV block occurred only in children older than 1 year, and were most frequent in the oldest group and during sleep. The most frequent type of arrhythmias were supraventricular premature contractions, present in more than half of the children. Many newborns and many older children had frequent ventricular as well as supraventricular premature beats. Ventricular tachycardia occurred only in a newborn infant who had no associated symptoms.

This ambulatory ECG study demonstrated an increasing incidence of arrhythmia with advancing age in children, except in the neonatal period. Arrhythmias are much more frequent in children than is apparent from resting ECG studies.

▶ It is very helpful to have the results of this study as guidelines when we encounter healthy children with an arrhythmia, and we must decide whether that is benign or serious, within the normal range or a real problem. This is especially so when we evaluate children in long-term postoperative follow-up and find an arrhythmia.

It is interesting that the incidence of arrhythmias increased with rising age, that more than half of the children had supraventricular premature beats, and that newborns and adolescents tended more to have ventricular premature contractions than the older children. Older children during sleep also had Wenckebach and first-degree heart block.—M.A. Engle, M.D.

Familial Occurrence of Accessory Atrioventricular Pathways (Preexcitation Syndrome)

Humberto J. Vidaillet, Jr., Joyce C. Pressley, Elizabeth Henke, Frank E. Harrall, Jr., and Lawrence D. German (Duke Univ.)
N. Engl. J. Med. 317:65–69, July 9, 1987 2–34

The cause of the preexcitation syndrome, which is considered to be a congenital but sporadic entity, is unknown. It has been theorized that accessory conduction pathways are the result of an unpredictable developmental failure to eradicate the remnants of the atrioventricular conections present during cardiogenesis. Although a genetic factor in the formation of accessory pathways has not been confirmed, there have been isolated reports of familial preexcitation. This study was done to determine whether preexcitation syndromes could also be transmitted genetically.

The records of 456 consecutive patients with electrophysiologically confirmed accessory pathways were reviewed. Of 456 patients, 383 (84%) could be contacted and were able to give a complete family his-

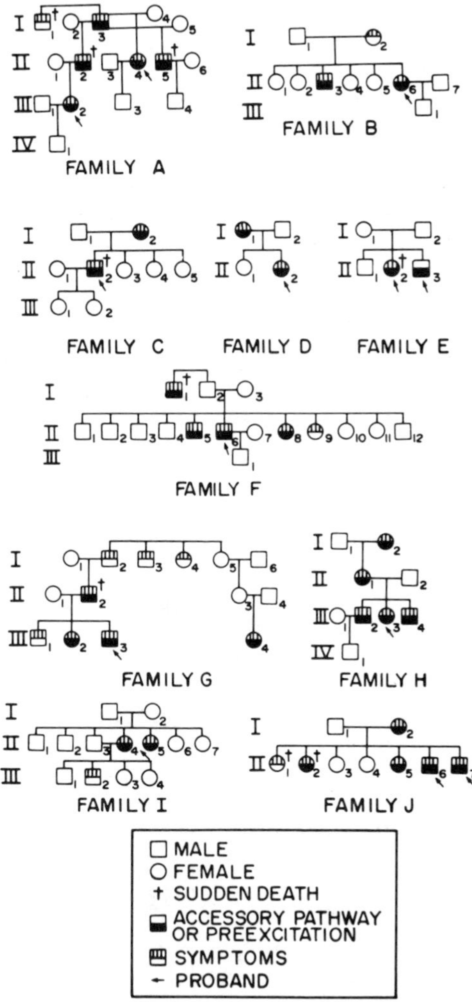

Fig 2–5.—Family trees of ten kindreds with the familial preexcitation syndrome. (Courtesy of Vidaillet, H.J., Jr., et al.: N. Engl. J. Med. 317:65–69, July 9, 1987.)

tory. The total study population comprised 2,343 first-degree relatives. The observed frequency of preexcitation in this cohort was compared with a prevalence of accessory pathways in the general population.

Thirteen (3.4%) of the 383 contacted patients had one or more first-degree relatives with documented accessory pathways (Fig 2–5). The 13 probands came from ten families. Preexcitation was confirmed in 15 of the 2,343 first-degree relatives, including 2 who had pathways that conducted only in the retrograde direction, and 13 (0.55%) who had the Wolff-Parkinson-White syndrome with anterograde preexcitation. This 0.55% prevalence was significantly higher than the 0.15% prevalence found in a general population sample. Because clinical information was obtained only about symptomatic relatives, identification of affected relatives may have been incomplete. Patients with familial preexcitation had a higher incidence of multiple accessory pathways and possibly an increased risk of sudden cardiac death.

These findings suggest a hereditary contribution to the development of accessory pathways. The pattern of inheritance appears to be autosomal dominant.

▶ The cardiologists and cardiac surgeons at Duke University continue to study preexcitation syndromes and to expand our knowledge concerning this interesting congenital anomaly. It was at Duke that mapping techniques made possible the surgical approach Dr. Will Sealy introduced to interrupt the accessory pathway that had led to intractable arrhythmias that defied medical management.

This study pooled results from 14 reports in the literature to estimate the incidence of preexcitation syndrome in the general population (0.15%). They contacted first-degree relatives of 383 of their 456 patients and compared the frequency of the syndrome among 2,343 such relatives with that found in the general population. They documented the condition in 1 or more first-degree relatives in 13 (3.4%) of the index patients. At least 13 of 2,343 relatives (0.55%) had pre-excitation; none had other forms of congenital heart disease.

Their data suggest a hereditary contribution to the development of accessory pathways in human beings. The pattern of inheritance in 10 kindreds (see Fig 2–5) suggests autosomal dominance as the mechanism.—M.A. Engle, M.D.

Lorcainide Treatment of Wolff-Parkinson-White Syndrome in Children and Adolescents

Milan Šamánek, Věra Hroboňová, and Helena Bartáková (Univ. of Prague, Czechoslovakia)

Pediatr. Cardiol 8:3–9, 1987 2–35

Serious supraventricular tachyarrhythmias may occur in children with Wolff-Parkinson-White (WPW) syndrome. Lorcainide is an antiarrhythmic agent with local anesthetic properties; it is effective when used during attacks of supraventricular tachycardia. The authors used lorcainide in an attempt to block conduction via the accessory pathway in 17 children and adolescents with a WPW pattern but no previous episodes of supraventricular tachycardia. Patients received age-related doses of lorcainide ranging from 10–100 mg.

Lorcainide controlled attacks of supraventricular tachycardia in 8 of 11 patients with tachyarrhythmias. Long-term administration prevented new attacks of tachyarrhythmia for an average of 9 months in all 7 patients who tolerated the drug. The WPW pattern normalized in 9 of 11 children with tachyarrhythmias, and in 3 of 6 others. The ECG effects of lorcainide usually appeared 2 hours after oral administration. Dizziness was an occasional problem, but no hematologic or biochemical effects occurred.

Lorcainide blocks antegrade conduction through the accessory pathway in WPW syndrome and also increases the effective refractory period of retrograde conduction. Toxicity from the drug is relatively low. Dosage should be adjusted individually for pediatric patients.

▶ Dr. Šamánek and colleagues have provided us with yet another drug for treatment of children with WPW syndrome and symptomatic tachycardia that is unresponsive to the usual drug regimens. Quite remarkably, they noted disappearance of the WPW pattern on ECG during therapy. They attributed this to antegrade blockage down the accessory pathway. They suggested that this change in ECG could be used to titrate drug dosage. Even more remarkable to me was the suggestion that the drug be used in asymptomatic children with WPW to prevent attacks of tachycardia in the future. They tried this in 6 such children, and in 3 the ECG normalized.

Even though the drug complications in short-term usage were low, I would be reluctant to begin using lifelong antiarrhythmic therapy for an asymptomatic child with a variant ECG of WPW type, who might never have an arrhythmia during many long and healthy years. The risk of arrhythmia in those with incidentally discovered WPW is not known, but from my experience, I would say it is small.—M.A. Engle, M.D.

Rapid and Safe Termination of Supraventricular Tachycardia in Children by Adenosine

B. Clarke, E. Rowland, P.J. Barnes, J. Till, D.E. Ward, and E.A. Shinebourne
(Brompton Hosp. and St. George's Hosp., London)

Lancet 1:299–300, Feb. 7, 1987 2–36

Adenosine is a potent antiarrhythmic agent that impairs atrioventricular (AV) nodal conduction and thereby terminates reentrant supraventricular tachycardias (SVT) that involve the AV node. Because most episodes of SVT in children are caused by AV reentry, adenosine should be appropriate for the treatment of such tachycardias. The authors report their experience with adenosine in the treatment of SVT in children.

Three seriously ill newborn infants with recurrent SVT that was unresponsive to other agents, and who were in cardiac failure resulting from long-term spontaneously occurring SVT, and a 10-year-old child with AV nodal reentrant tachycardia who had been admitted for an elective electrophysiologic study were treated with adenosine. None of the children was receiving theophylline, which is a known adenosine antagonist. Adenosine was administered through an intravenous catheter. All children were monitored by ECG throughout adenosine administration.

Adenosine successfully terminated SVT within 20 seconds of injection by a sudden slowing of AV conduction. No fall in blood pressure was observed. One child had atrial echo beats, and another child had anterograde conduction down an accessory pathway. Because the first patient treated with adenosine developed sinus bradycardia for a few seconds as the tachycardia terminated, the dose schedule was subsequently revised.

The authors conclude that adenosine is a safe and effective first-line agent for the acute termination of SVT in children. However, it is of no value in prophylaxis against recurrent SVT.

▶ This report from London presents information on an interesting new drug, already used intravenously in adults for termination of supraventricular tachycardia. Adenosine, an endogenous purine nucleoside, acts to impair atrioventricular nodal conduction by prolonging A-H but not H-V intervals. It breaks down to inosine, which is inactive. It has a very short half-life and it can be titrated, even in very sick newborns.

The authors successfully treated three newborns and one 10-year old child. The tachyrhythmia ended within 20 seconds of intravenous injection. The patients experienced no ill effects from the drug.

The agent cannot be used as prophylaxis against recurrence of arrhythmia, but this report is impressive for its benefits in rapid termination of supraventricular tachycardia.—M.A. Engle, M.D.

Arrhythmias Before and After Anatomic Correction of Transposition of the Great Arteries

Robin P. Martin, Rosemary Radley-Smith, and Magdi H. Yacoub (Harefield Hosp., Harefield, Middlesex, England)

J. Am. Coll. Cardiol. 10:200–204, July 1987 2–37

Cardiac arrhythmias are a problem after intra-atrial repair of transposition, and sudden deaths have resulted. It is not clear whether the arrhythmias result from operative injury or are an inherent feature of transposition of the great arteries. Ambulatory ECG monitoring of 92 survivors of anatomical repair was carried out to determine the rate of arrhythmia. In more recently treated patients pulmonary artery banding was combined with placement of a modified Blalock-Taussig shunt.

Only 1 of 41 patients evaluated had supraventricular premature beats preoperatively, and 1 had paroxysmal atrial fibrillation. Six patients had ventricular arrhythmias, usually modified Lown grade 1 ventricular premature beats. First-stage surgery did not alter the incidence of arrhythmias. No deaths from arrhythmia occurred during a mean 3-year follow-up, and no patient required treatment for symptomatic arrhythmia. Infrequent supraventricular premature beats occurred in 23% of the patients, but the rate of ventricular arrhythmias was unchanged. One patient acquired complete heart block.

Significant arrhythmias are infrequent after anatomical correction of transposition, at least in the medium term, but longer follow-up is necessary. Significant arrhythmias do not seem to be inherent to patients with transposition of the great arteries.

▶ As normal children age, they are more prone to develop supraventricular and ventricular premature beats and first- as well as second-degree heart block. In long-term postoperative follow-up, therefore, the patient is more likely to have arrhythmias than when he was younger and preoperative. This should be borne in mind in any analysis of postoperative arrhythmias in children.

In the present report of 41 children studied with 24-hour ECG monitoring, 17% had arrhythmias before operation. Postoperatively, over a 3-year period in which there were no symptomatic arrhythmias or arrhythmia deaths, 38% had some kind of arrhythmia, especially with supraventricular premature beats.

The group from Middlesex, who have a large number of survivors of anatomical correction (specifically, 92 in this study), concluded that in medium-term follow-up the incidence of important arrhythmias is low and is similar to that in normal children.—M.A. Engle, M.D.

Atrial Tracking (Synchronous) Pacing in a Pediatric and Young Adult Population

Paul C. Gillette, Alex Zinner, John Kratz, Cathleen Shannon, Deborah Wampler, and David Ott (South Carolina Children's Heart Ctr., Med. Univ. of South Carolina, and Texas Children's Hosp., Baylor College of Medicine)

J. Am. Coll. Cardiol. 9:811–815, April 1987 2–38

It has been proposed that pediatric and young adult patients should benefit more than other groups from the use of atrial tracking pacemakers because they are more likely to have a nearly normal myocardium and a nearly normal sinus node response to exercise. Despite the theoretical advantages of the use of atrial tracking pacemakers in children, several potential technical drawbacks have prevented their use in large numbers of these patients. The authors have investigated whether recent improvements in pulse generators and leads make atrial track pacing feasible in pediatric and young adult patients.

The study group included 100 pediatric and young adult patients who underwent implantation of an atrial tracking pacemaker. Seventy-four pacemakers paced in an atrioventricular (AV) sequential mode at the lower rate limit and 26 paced in a ventricular demand mode at the lower rate limit.

Five patients required reoperation during follow-up of 1 month to 2.5 years. Six other patients required programming to ventricular demand (3) or AV sequential pacing (3) because of sinus bradycardia (2), atrial sensing problems (1), or pacemaker-mediated tachycardia (3). Pulse generators that could sense atrial signals of less than 1.0 mV and had a programmable atrial refractory period did not require reprogramming out of the atrial tracking mode. No patient developed atrial flutter or fibrillation.

There were sensing problems during exercise in 37% of the first 60 pacemakers but in none in the last 40, which had improved electronic components. Atrial tracking pacing may be feasible in pediatric and young adult patients.

▶ A worthy goal for children who need pacemakers is for the unit to resemble as much as possible the normal state of sinus-node acceleration or deceleration on exercise and at rest, transmission to the junctional region with an appropriate delay and then to the ventricles. The generator should be small and long-lived, and the transvenous or epicardial leads should be secure.

Dr. Gillette has been a pioneer in pacemakers for children—indications, selection of the appropriate unit, monitoring for problems. This article serves as a progress report on the odyssey of continuing pursuit of the goal. An experience in 100 children and young adults is sizable, and the experience accumulated is worthy of report. Along with the problems recited, Dr. Gillette and colleagues report that the wearers felt better and had better exercise tolerance with atrial tracking pacemakers than with ventricular demand units.—M.A. Engle, M.D.

Incessant Ventricular Tachycardia in Infants: Myocardial Hamartomas and Surgical Cure

Arthur Garson, Jr., Richard T. Smith, Jr., Jeffrey P. Moak, Debra L. Kearney, Edith P. Hawkins, Jack L. Titus, Denton A. Cooley, and David A. Ott (Baylor College, Texas Children's Hosp., St. Luke's Episcopal, and Texas Heart Inst., Houston)

J. Am. Coll. Cardiol. 10:619–626, September 1987 2–39

Pathologic studies have described infants with incessant ventricular tachycardia—ventricular tachycardia that persists for more than 10% of the day. The cases of 21 infants with incessant ventricular tachycardia present for more than 90% of the day and night are described.

The patients ranged in age from birth to 30 months, with a mean of 10.5 months. Cardiac arrest, occurring in 11 babies, was the most common presenting symptom. Another 6 babies had congestive heart failure, and 4 were asymptomatic. Three patients had Wolff-Parkinson-White syndrome as well. The rates of incessant ventricular tachycardia ranged from 167–440 beats per minute, and the QRS duration ranged from 0.06–0.11 second. In 10 patients, the predominant ECG pattern was right bundle branch block with left axis deviation; other right and left bundle branch block patterns also occurred (Fig 2–6). Nine patients received amiodarone. Conventional and investigational antiar-

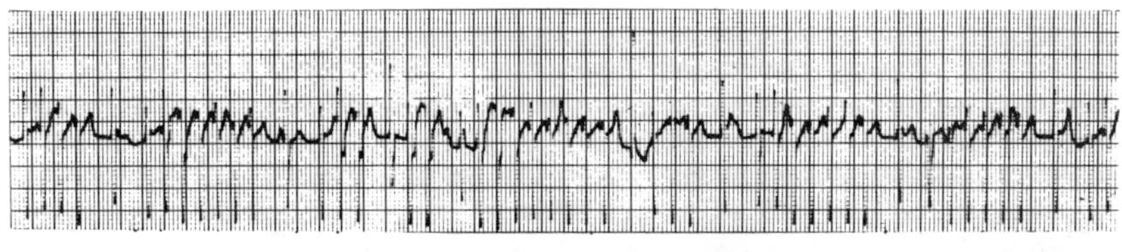

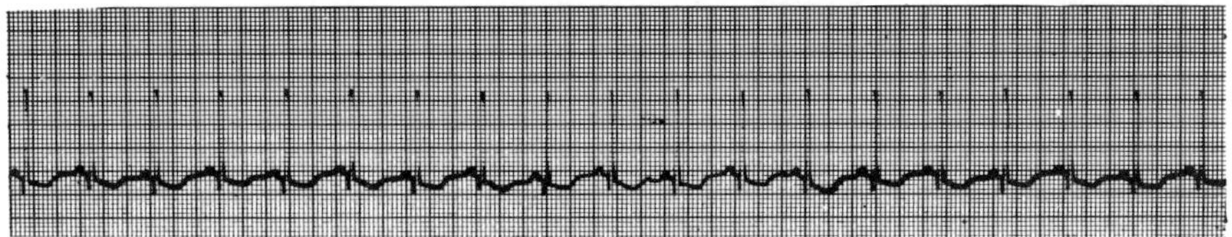

Fig 2–6.—Top, electrocardiogram (lead II) of incessant ventricular tachycardia. A sinus capture beat is shown. Also evident are fusion beats and AV dissociation. **Bottom,** lead II after surgical tumor excision. The sinus rhythm QRS has a similar configuration and capture beat in ventricular tachycardia. (Courtesy of Garson, A., Jr., et al.: J. Am. Coll. Cardiol. 10:619–626, September 1987.)

rhythmic agents did not eliminate incessant ventricular tachycardia in all.

With electrophysiologic studies, it was possible to localize the disorder to the left ventricle in 17 babies—to the apex in 2, the free wall in 9, and the septum in 6—and to the right ventricular septum in 4. No structural abnormalities were discovered on echocardiogram or angiocardiogram. All patients underwent surgery at 3.5–31 months. Fifteen patients had a tumor: 13 had myocardial hamartomas, and 2 had rhabdomyomas. Nine of the myocardial harmartomas were discrete, and 4 were diffuse throughout both ventricles. One rhabdomyoma was multiple. The oldest patient had myocarditis. Four patients had only myocardial fibrosis, 1 with normal biopsy results. Two patients died in the immediate postoperative period, and 1 died later from congestive heart failure. Nine months to 7 years later, the remaining 18 patients are asymptomatic, and only 1 takes medication.

Incessant ventricular tachycardia in infants is distinct from paroxysmal ventricular tachycardia. It is most commonly associated with a tumor, despite "normal" echocardiogram and angiocardiogram results. Because medical management usually fails, operation is recommended early in the disease course in infants younger than 24 months.

▶ It is unusual for a child to have ventricular tachycardia that persists through 90% of the day and night. That was the situation in 21 patients, aged 3½ to 31 months, who were referred to the cardiologists at Baylor because of the excellence of their program of diagnosis and treatment of arrhythmias. After evaluation, 15 were found at surgery to have a tumor. One had myocarditis and 4 had myocardial fibrosis. Eighteen patients are now asymptomatic after removal of the tumor; only 1 requires treatment to suppress ventricular arrhythmia.

Since medical management of this condition usually does not succeed, one should consider a resectable lesion and have a good expectation of helping.—M.A. Engle, M.D.

Congestive Heart Failure

Plasma Norepinephrine Levels in Infants and Children With Congestive Heart Failure

Robert D. Ross, Stephen R. Daniels, David C. Schwartz, David W. Hannon, Rakesh Shukla, and Samuel Kaplan (Children's Hosp. Med. Ctr. and Univ. of Cincinnati)

Am. J. Cardiol. 59:911–914, April 1, 1987 2–40

No objective laboratory measurements have been established to assess the degree of congestive heart failure (CHF) in children. It was hypothesized that plasma norepinephrine levels would reflect the presence and degree of CHF in children with congenital defects producing a large left-to-right shunt and in those with cardiomyopathy or obstructive left-sided lesions. To characterize catecholamine levels in children with CHF and to evaluate its relation to the severity of CHF, measurements were made of plasma norepinephrine, epinephrine, and hemodynamic values in 102 children undergoing routine cardiac catheterization.

The patients ranged from 0.1–14.7 years old, with a mean of 3.3 years. Sixty-one had left-to-right shunts. The mean plasma norepinephrine level in 41 children with signs or symptoms of CHF was 694 ± 384 pg/ml, significantly higher than that in the 61 patients without CHF, whose mean value was 277 ± 138 pg/ml. A highly significant association was noted between the level of plasma norepinephrine and the severity of the CHF symptoms. This relationship was present for CHF secondary to lesions producing a left-to-right shunt and CHF resulting from primary myocardial dysfunction. In children with congenital lesions with a left-to-right shunt, plasma norepinephrine levels correlated strongly with size of shunt and degree of pulmonary arterial hypertension.

It appears that the plasma norepinephrine level is an indicator of the presence and severity of CHF in infants and children. Increases in plasma norepinephrine concentrations were associated with severe CHF, regardless of its origin.

▶ This study from Cincinnati of plasma norepinephrine of children undergoing indicated cardiac catheterization for heart disease provides a hormonal basis for use of vasodilator therapy for infants and children in cardiac failure. Among 102 children who were catheterized, 1% were considered to have grade III or IV (on a scale of I to IV) signs of cardiac failure, and 24 were classed II. Plasma norepinephrine levels were significantly higher in those with cardiac failure and the height of that measurement correlated with severity of failure. The norepinephrine levels also correlated with size of a left-to-right shunt and level of pulmonary hypertension. Both are aspects of cardiac failure due to a large left-to-right shunting malformation.—M.A. Engle, M.D.

Guidelines for Vasodilator Therapy of Congestive Heart Failure in Infants and Children

Michael Artman and Thomas P. Graham, Jr. (Univ. of South Alabama and Vanderbilt Univ.)
Am. Heart J. 113:994–1005, April 1987 2–41

Recently investigators have begun to apply vasodilator therapy to infants and children with inadequate systemic output. The authors have attempted to provide a rational approach to vasodilator therapy in infants and children by combining physiologic and pharmacologic principles with available clinical experience.

The vasodilator drugs that are used most commonly in pediatric patients include those with a venous site of action such as nitroglycerin; drugs with an arteriolar site of action such as hydralazine or nifedipine; and drugs with a mixed site of action such as nitroprusside, phentolamine, captopril, enalapril, or prazosin.

Nitroglycerin and nitroprusside act by causing direct vasodilation that is mediated by changes in intracellular cyclic guanosine 3′,5′-monophosphate. Nifedipine blocks calcium channels, and hydralazine causes direct vasodilation by an unknown mechanism. Phentolamine competitively blocks α_1- and α_2-adrenergic receptors, prazosin competitively blocks α_1-adrenergic receptors, and captopril and enalapril competitively inhibit angiotensin-converting enzyme.

The authors recommend that nitroglycerin and nitroprusside be used to treat postoperative low-cardiac output syndrome and pulmonary hypertension or systemic venous congestion, or both. Phentolamine can also be used to treat postoperative low-cardiac output syndrome. Hydralazine, captopril, or enalapril is suggested for treatment of chronic ventricular dysfunction; aortic or mitral regurgitation, or both; and systemic to pulmonary shunts. Prazosin can also be used for chronic ventricular dysfunction and aortic or mitral regurgitation, or both; nifedipine can be used for aortic and or mitral regurgitation, or both, and for systemic to pulmonary shunts.

The authors point out that they rarely use a vasodilator as sole therapy and that almost all their patients are treated concomitantly with a diuretic. They emphasize that many of the recommendations and guidelines that are outlined in this article are based on experience that has been published regarding the pharmacology of these drugs in adult patients. Additional clinical studies are recommended to clarify the clinical pharmacology and consequences of long-term vasodilator therapy in infants and children with inadequate systemic output.

▶ This article provides a useful review of the pharmacology of selected vasodilators and the rationale for choosing venous dilators, arteriolar dilators, and mixed-type vasodilators when children have inadequate systemic output. Desired, as well as adverse, effects are described and clinical settings in which these agents might be useful are mentioned, together with suggested dosage regimens.

Since much of the information on these drugs is derived from studies in adults, it is important for investigations and report of clinical experience in infants and children to be extended and updated from time to time, as in this report.—M.A. Engle, M.D.

Acquired Heart Disease

Acute Rheumatic Fever in Western Pennsylvania and the Tristate Area

Ellen R. Wald, Barry Dashefsky, Cindy Feidt, Darleen Chiponis, and Carol Byers
(Children's Hosp. of Pittsburgh and Univ. of Pittsburgh)
Pediatrics 80:371–374, September 1987 2–42

The marked decline in the incidence and severity of rheumatic fever in the past 20 years has prompted some clinicians to propose "a more relaxed policy" toward the diagnosis and treatment of pharyngitis. Prompted by a recent occurrence of 17 cases of acute rheumatic fever in an 18-month period, the authors reviewed their experience with this disease to determine whether such a policy would be wise.

The records of 243 children with acute rheumatic fever, who were cared for at two institutions from 1965–1986, were reviewed. The diagnoses were made using the modified Jones criteria. The cases were classified using major criteria such as arthritis, arthritis and carditis, carditis alone, carditis and chorea, chorea alone, and arthritis and chorea. Of the 17 patients presenting most recently—between 1985 and 1986—59% had carditis, 30% had chorea, and 24% had arthritis alone. Proportions of children with particular major manifestations were similar over the last 20 years and from 1985 to 1986. The most recently presenting patients were aged 6–13 years, with a median age of 10 years. There were 16 white children and 1 Asian child. Only 4 lived in an urban area.

The demographic features of the most recent patients were compared with those of patients in the past 20 years; a decrease was noted in the proportion of children who lived in urban settings and were black. Four of the recently seen children had a history of preceding sore throat, although only 3 sought medical care; 9 had no memorable illness; and 4 had either a nonrespiratory illness or a respiratory illness with no sore throat.

It appears that a diligent approach to diagnosing and treating streptococcal infections is still of prime importance.

Outbreak of Acute Rheumatic Fever in Northeast Ohio

Blaise Congeni, Christopher Rizzo, Joseph Congeni, and V.V. Sreenivasan
(Northeastern Ohio Univs., and Children's Medical Center of Akron)
J. Pediatr. 111:176–179, August 1987 2–43

Recent outbreaks of acute rheumatic fever (ARF), the leading cause of acquired heart disease, have occurred in Utah and Ohio; clinicians in northeastern Ohio faced an outbreak in 1986. A study was conducted to determine whether an actual increase in ARF was occurring, to assess the nature of the disease in hospitalized patients, and to examine the epidemiologic features of the latest outbreak.

Twenty-three children, aged 3–16 years, had new diagnoses of ARF in 1986. Fourteen of these were inpatients. Seventy-eight percent had polyarthritis, and 30% had carditis. All children with carditis had new mitral valve insufficiency murmurs. Clinicians found evidence of chamber enlargement or effusion on echocardiograms in five patients and on chest films in two. Parents of all the children completed questionnaires that indicated the children were generally not indigent, had good access to medical care, and were from a nonurban setting. A review of the records of inpatients with ARF from 1976 to 1985 indicated that the clinical manifestations in these former patients were not significantly different from those of the current inpatients.

Outbreaks of ARF have occurred in different parts of the United States. Physicians should be aware of a possible resurgence of classic ARF and ensure compliance with an appropriate treatment course for patients with streptococcal pharyngitis.

▶ The disconcerting resurgence of acute rheumatic fever in children is attested to by descriptions of two more outbreaks, one in the western Pennsylvania area (Abstract 2–42) and the other in northeastern Ohio in 1985–1986 (Abstract 2–43). Those of us who had long grown used to seeing only a sporadic case of rheumatic fever were shocked last year with the report of the outbreak in Utah.

Particularly alarming in these recent epidemics is the paucity of a history of sore throat; although most of these children were not socioeconomically deprived or living in crowded urban communities and most had access to medical care, they felt no illness that called for a visit to the doctor.

Another unusual feature is the high incidence of chorea (30%) in the children in Pennsylvania and in those reported previously from Utah.

Certainly, rheumatic fever is not a vanishing problem. Perplexing now are these questions: Why the resurgence? Why so few antecedent strep throats? Has the *Streptococcus* changed? How can we prevent the rheumatic fever if children are not ill enough to visit a doctor and to be cultured for β-hemolytic *Streptococcus* and treated for 10 days with therapeutic doses of penicillin?—M.A. Engle, M.D.

Coronary Artery Caliber in Normal Children and Patients With Kawasaki Disease but Without Aneurysms: An Echocardiographic and Angiographic Study

Kalavathy Arjunan, Stephen R. Daniels, Richard A. Meyer, David C. Schwartz, Hal Barron, and Samuel Kaplan (Children's Hosp. Med. Ctr., Cincinnati)

J. Am. Coll. Cardiol. 8:1119–1124, November 1986 2–44

In the United States the first description of mucocutaneous lymph node syndrome (Kawasaki disease) was published in 1974. Since that time the incidence has steadily increased, and it has been shown that coronary artery aneurysms with thrombosis constitute a major complication of this disease. Although these aneurysms can be detected accurately by using

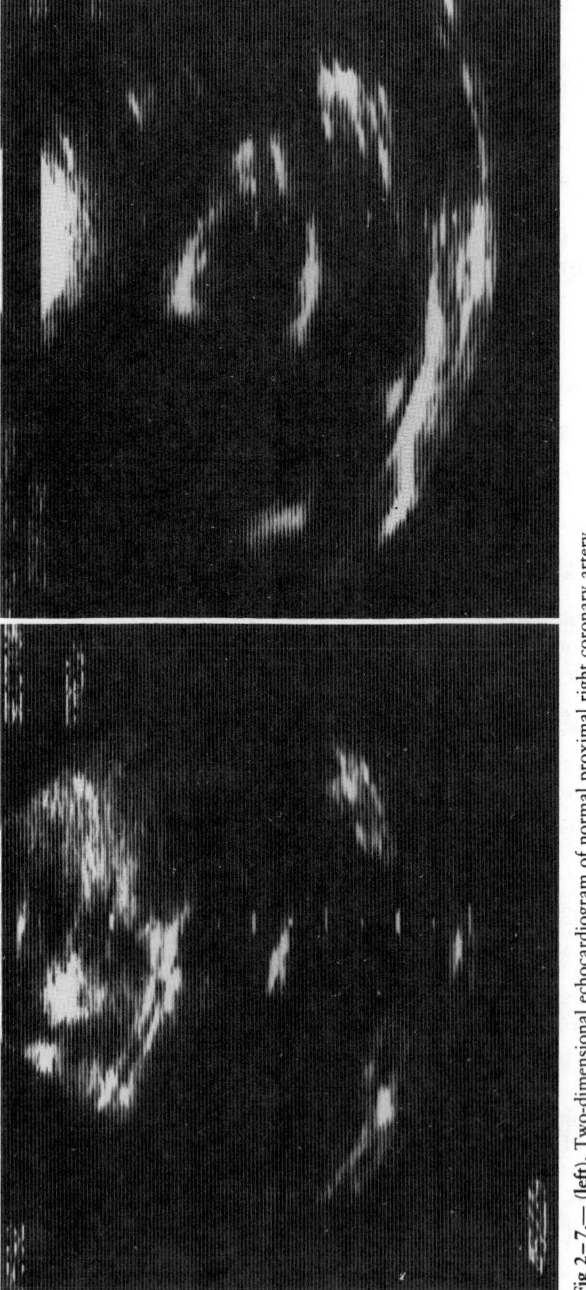

Fig 2–7.— (left). Two-dimensional echocardiogram of normal proximal right coronary artery.
Fig 2–8.—(right). Two-dimensional echocardiogram of normal left main coronary artery.
(Courtesy of Arjunan, K., et al.: J. Am. Coll. Cardiol. 8:1119–1124, November 1986.)

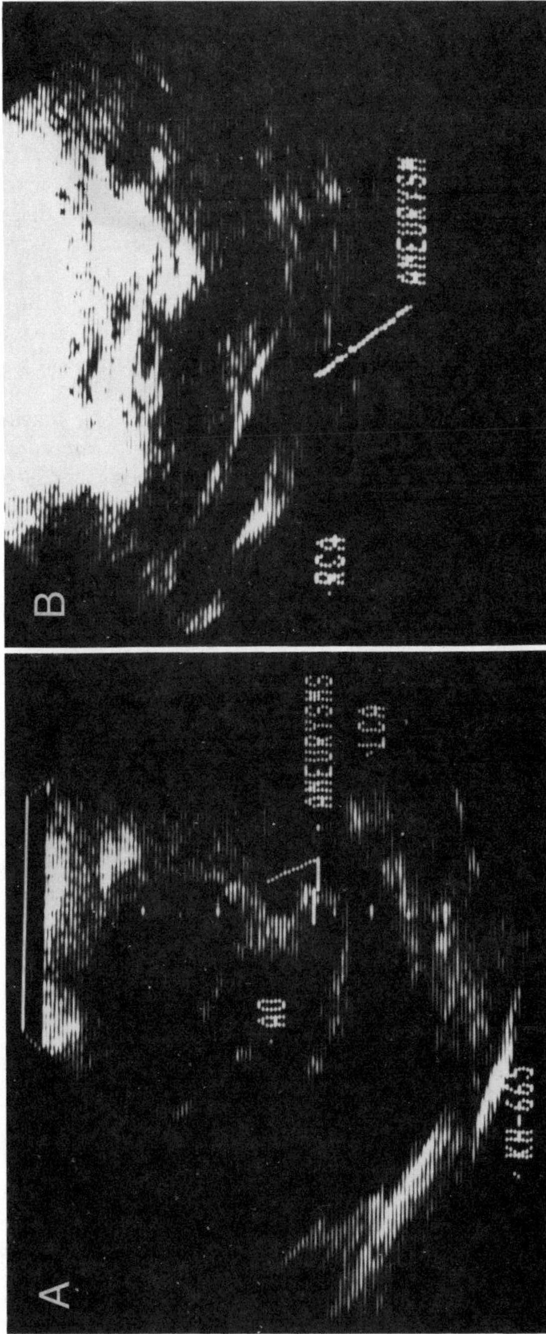

Fig 2–9.—Patient with saccular aneurysms of the proximal left coronary artery (LCA) (A) and of the right coronary artery (RCA) (B). There is tapering of the right coronary artery beyond the aneurysm. (Courtesy of Arjunan, K., et al.: J. Am. Coll. Cardiol. 8:1119–1124, November 1986.)

two-dimensional echocardiography, only preliminary data that characterize normal coronary arteries in children are available.

The authors carried out an echocardiographic and angiographic study of the caliber of coronary arteries in normal children and in patients with Kawasaki disease but without aneurysms. The study group included 110 children aged 3 months to 16 years who underwent two-dimensional echocardiography with special attention to the coronary arteries. There were 42 normal children and 68 patients with Kawasaki disease. All the patients with Kawasaki disease also underwent selective coronary arteriography.

It was found that in both the normal subjects (Figs 2–7 and 2–8) and in the patients with Kawasaki disease the caliber of the coronary arteries exhibited little variability from the ostium to 10 mm distally and ranged in size from 2 mm in infants to 5 mm in teenagers. There was no significant difference between male and female subjects. The feature that distinguished the large but normal coronary artery without aneurysm from one with an aneurysm was its uniformity of caliber (Fig 2–9). Furthermore, the caliber of the opposite coronary artery was generally at the lower limits of normal.

The proximal coronary arteries in infants and children can be assessed accurately by using high-resolution two-dimensional echocardiography, and sequential evaluation of subtle changes over time may be carried out.

▶ Since Kawasaki syndrome is now the most common cause of pancarditis and vasculitis, not only in Japan but also in the United States, and since abnormality of the coronary arteries is the chief risk factor in that illness, this article from Cincinnati is most timely and important. Two-dimensional echocardiography has become the chief laboratory tool to identify aneurysms and dilatation of the coronary arteries in this illness.

The authors studied coronary arteries in 42 normal children to determine normal size and pattern. They carefully evaluated coronary arteries by echocardiography and angiocardiography in 68 children with Kawasaki syndrome, to characterize abnormalities and to compare with normal children.

They verify that two-dimensional echocardiography is accurate, reliable, and sensitive in recognizing coronary abnormality. The chief feature that distinguishes the large coronary artery without an aneurysm from one with an aneurysm is the uniform caliber of the artery from ostium to distal extent. Aneurysms narrow abruptly or taper gradually.—M.A. Engle, M.D.

Incomplete Kawasaki Disease With Coronary Artery Involvement

Anne H. Rowley, Frank Gonzalez-Crussi, Samuel S. Gidding, C. Elise Duffy, and Stanford T. Shulman (Northwestern Univ. and Children's Mem. Hosp., Chicago)
J. Pediatr. 110:409–413, March 1987 2–45

Kawasaki disease is diagnosed on clinical grounds because the cause of Kawasaki disease is not known and no specific diagnostic test is available. Although the diagnostic guidelines are useful, they may result in failure to recognize incomplete forms of illness. The authors describe four children in whom significant coronary artery abnormalities developed after an illness that included some of the clinical features of Kawasaki disease but that did not fulfill the classic diagnostic criteria, and a fifth child with severe multiple vessel coronary artery disease of several months' duration in whom no antecedent illness other than desquamation of the hands several months before presentation could be recalled by the parents.

Boy, 7 months, had a 5-day history of fever and irritability. Laboratory test results showed evidence of bacterial or viral infection. He exhibited left posterior cervical adenopathy and red fissured lips. There was no history or finding of conjunctival injection, rash, or swelling or erythema of the hands or feet. Laboratory data included leukocytes, 19,900/cu mm, with 35% polymorphonuclear neutrophils, 19% band cells, 9% eosinophils, 36% lymphocytes, and 1% monocytes; erythrocyte sedimentation rate, 65 mm/hr; platelets, 761,000/cu mm; and serum glutamic oxaloacetic transaminase, 50 IU/L. Because of the suspicion that the illness might be Kawasaki disease despite incomplete diagnostic criteria, aspirin therapy was begun. Several days later, desquamation of the fingers and toes developed. Echocardiograms beginning on day 20 after onset of illness revealed a fusiform aneurysm of the left main coronary artery extending into the proximal left anterior descending and left circumflex coronary arteries, and a saccular aneurysm of the right coronary artery at its origin.

The authors reported on four other patients, one of whom died of cardiac failure. Autoplasty showed severe myocardial abnormalities with involvement of the mitral and aortic valves and of the coronary arteries. Fever, present in four of the five patients, lasted in three of them from 7 to 14 days. Although these patients did not manifest classic acute clinical features of Kawasaki disease, 3 of 4 patients showed desquamation of the fingers and toes 10–14 days after onset of illness, and the fifth patient, who died, had shown desquamation several months earlier.

Strict adherence to currently accepted criteria for diagnosis of Kawasaki disease may lead to failure to recognize incomplete forms of the disease, with potential sequelae of myocardial infarction or sudden death. Children with prolonged unexplained febrile illnesses, especially when associated with subsequent peripheral desquamation, should undergo echocardiography 3–4 weeks after onset of the illness. This practice may help to identify those patients with illnesses characterized by incomplete diagnostic criteria, but in whom significant coronary abnormalities develop.

▶ Although we still do not know the etiology of this syndrome, at least we continue to learn more about its clinical aspects. One problem with this syndrome, as in many others, is that there is no specific diagnostic test. Instead, we physicians must rely on a constellation of findings that characterize the febrile illness with pan-vasculitis and with potential pancarditis that is the mucocutaneous lymph node syndrome. Most of us have used criteria developed in Japan and regularly updated there by their research group.

This article presents five children who did not fulfill all of those criteria, yet who developed significant coronary artery abnormalities. This really should not be surprising, since in many illnesses and infections, for every apparent case, there may be other milder or even inapparent ones.

We must be careful not to overdiagnose the condition but also not to overlook incomplete forms of the illness.—M.A. Engle, M.D.

Cardiac Performance in Children With Homozygous Sickle Cell Disease

Edward E. Chung, Sinda B. Dianzumba, Priscilla Morais, and Graham R. Serjeant (Univ. of the West Indies, Kingston, Jamaica)

J. Am. Coll. Cardiol. 9:1038–1042, May 1987 2–46

Adults with homozygous sickle cell anemia generally have cardiomegaly, flow murmurs, and evidence of increased cardiac output. Recent studies have shown that hemoglobin levels in children with sickle cell disease will have decreased by the time they are 1 year old to levels seen in adults with the disease. It is not known at what age cardiac changes begin to occur. Left ventricular function was evaluated in an unbiased asymptomatic group of children with sickle cell disease.

The study was done in 10 asymptomatic children (six boys) with sickle cell disease and 14 control children (8 boys) who had a normal hemoglobin genotype. The children, part of a Jamaican sickle cell cohort study, were examined within 2 months of their 8th birthday by M-mode echocardiography.

The children with sickle cell disease had significantly lower hemoglobin levels, height, weight, and body surface area than the control children. They also showed a significant increase in left ventricular dimension index, diastolic, diastolic volume, left ventricular mass index, and cardiac index in comparison with those in the control subjects. Nevertheless, there was no significant difference between the two groups in ejection fraction, velocity of circumferential fiber shortening, percent fractional shortening, systolic time intervals, wall stress, and ratio of wall stress-systolic volume.

It appears that despite a finding of increased cardiac dimensions and cardiac output, left ventricular function in sickle cell disease remains normal during the first 8 years of life.

▶ In an attempt to determine at what age the cardiovascular effects of sickle cell anemia began in a cohort identified from birth and not just in a hospitalized setting, these doctors from Jamaica studied patients born with sickle cell anemia (SCA) and an age- and sex-matched control group. At age 8 years, they found that ECG studies in the 10 with SCA and the 14 controls showed increased chamber dimension but normal left ventricular contractile function in the former. The children with SCA were asymptomatic though they had significantly lower hemoglobin levels, as well as height and weight, in comparison with the controls.—M.A. Engle, M.D.

Cardiovascular Findings in Adolescent Inpatients With Anorexia Nervosa

G. William Dec, Joseph Biederman, and Thomas J. Hougen (Massachusetts Gen. Hosp., Children's Hosp., and Harvard Univ., Boston)

Psychosom. Med. 49:285–290, May–June 1987 2–47

Anorexia nervosa has the highest mortality rate of all the major psychiatric disorders, with many deaths occurring suddenly. Left ventricular function, resting ECG, and Holter recordings were assessed in 25 hospitalized patients with anorexia nervosa.

No serious arrythmias, abnormal prolongation of the QT interval, conduction abnormalities, or depression of left ventricular systolic function was observed. Mitral valve prolapse was seen in 9 patients.

No evidence of cardiac dysfunction was obtained with ECG, 24-hour Holter monitoring, and M-mode echocardiography in 25 adolescents hospitalized with anorexia nervosa.

▶ Self-inflicted illness is difficult to comprehend and to cure. This group from Boston studied 25 seriously ill, emaciated adolescents and found, to my surprise, preservation of good left ventricular function and freedom from serious arrhythmias and from QT prolongation. This is a rare piece of good news in a problem that has afflicted many adolescent girls for more than 100 years and has often been the cause of their sudden death.—M.A. Engle, M.D.

Report of the Second Task Force on Blood Pressure Control in Children—1987

Michael J. Horan, Bonita Falkner, Sue Y.S. Kimm, Jennifer M.H. Loggie, Ronald J. Prineas, Bernard Rosner, Janice Hutchinson, Shirley Mueller, Donald A. Riopel, Alan Sinaiko, and William H. Weidman (Natl. Heart, Lung, and Blood Inst., Bethesda, Md., and various U.S. universities, hospitals, and clinics)

Pediatrics 79:1–25, January 1987 2–48

There is ample evidence to support the concept that roots of essential hypertension extend back into childhood, although the prevalence of clinical hypertension is of a far less magnitude in children than adults. This article revises the 1977 report and includes normative blood pressure (BP) data from more than 70,000 children.

Pathophysiologic causes of secondary hypertension in children are well-described, but in most cases the etiology is not understood. These individuals thus fall into a category characterized as primary, essential hypertension. These children should be identified early so that surveillance and possible prevention or intervention can be undertaken. If fixed hypertension should occur, treatment is required. All physicians who care for children from age 3 years through adolescence should be encouraged to measure BP once a year when the child is well. Blood pressure is a physiologic parameter that when elevated, becomes a risk factor either for developing hypertension or premature cardiovascular morbidity, if not during childhood, then during adulthood.

The curves describing age-specific distributions of systolic and diastolic BPs are intended to replace those of the 1977 curves. Variations in BP readings may occur without the presence of sustained hypertension or other detectable disease; consequently, BP readings on a single occasion are insufficient for identifying subjects with hypertension. Measurements above the 90th percentile should be repeated during subsequent visits. If the patient has an average BP value greater than the 90th percentile for age but is not unusually tall or heavy, there is greater probability that the elevation results from some pathologic process, and that the patient needs special consideration.

If the average BP measurement is at the 95th percentile or higher, a diagnostic evaluation should be made and therapy considered unless there is obesity, in which case weight control may be attempted first. Diagnostic evaluation should be tailored to each hypertensive child or adolescent and an attempt should be made to determine whether there is a family history of essential hypertension and to identify secondary causes of hypertension that may be amenable to specific therapy.

One of the most important aspects of the diagnostic evaluation of hypertension is an extensive family history emphasizing age of onset of hypertension and age of occurrence of complications such as stroke, heart failure, and renal failure. Hypertension should be approached with emphasis on general counseling about cardiovascular risk factors. The initial treatment can be nonpharmacologic. Patients with severe hypertension can receive traditional forms of antihypertensive drug therapy. Optimal treatment for childhood elevated BP is the least amount of intervention required to reduce the BP successfully.

▶ Ten years ago a group of experts in childhood hypertension compiled the best data available on normal ranges for blood pressure in infants and children. Although the data were useful, a drawback was that they came from a variety of reports, which were not always standardized and rarely longitudinal.

The present report recommends the proper technique for measuring blood pressure in the pediatric age range and encourages all physicians caring for children to measure the pressure once a year. A manometer, a cuff of appropriate size, and a cooperative, seated child are necessary. The Task Force recommends use of the Korotkoff fourth sound in children and fifth sound in adolescents as the diastolic pressure.

The article presents distribution curves by age and denotes normal, high normal, and hypertensive. Furthermore, it recommends follow-up of those with borderline hypertension, workup of those with sustained hypertension, and treatment strategies.

This Task Force Report is a helpful update.—M.A. Engle, M.D.

Adult Heart Disease Prevention in Childhood: A National Survey of Pediatricians' Practices and Attitudes

Philip R. Nader, Howard L. Taras, James F. Sallis, and Thomas L. Patterson (Univ. of California, San Diego)
Pediatrics 79:843–850, June 1987 2–49

There are many apparent reasons to start primary preventive efforts against atherosclerotic disease in children, but it has not been directly shown that risk factor reduction in children lessens morbidity and mortality later in life. The attitudes and practices of 2,000 randomly selected primary care pediatricians were sought, and 1,165 responses were reviewed. The final sample included 779 board-certified pediatricians.

Blood pressure measurement after infancy was the most commonly reported practice. Lipid estimates were least frequent. Smoking was considered the most important topic for discussion at child and/or parent visits. Exercise was considered more important than diet for children older than 6 years. Obesity was the topic most often selected for continuing medical education. Few respondents reported feeling confident about altering patient life-styles. Pediatricians older than 45 years were more likely than others to assess cardiovascular disease risk, provide health counseling, and feel confident about their ability to promote life-style changes.

Pediatricians generally are aware of the need to detect risk factors for cardiovascular disease and to counsel intervention. It is likely that much premature heart disease can be prevented by intervention in childhood, without creating any risk of other disorders. It is especially important to measure serum cholesterol in high-risk groups, provide dietary advice, and discuss smoking. Further efforts are needed to increase physicians' skills in altering patient behavior when that seems indicated.

Should the Primary Prevention of Coronary Heart Disease Commence in Childhood?

Michael D. Gliksman, Terence Dwyer, and T. John C. Boulton (Univ. of Tasmania, Hobart, Royal Newcastle Hosp., Newcastle, and Newcastle Mater Hosp., Weratch, New South Wales, Australia)
Med. J. Aust. 146:360–362, April 6, 1987 2–50

Atherosclerosis is the end-stage of a process that begins in childhood. There now is evidence that elevations of serum lipoprotein cholesterol levels and systolic blood pressure in childhood are closely related to later atherosclerosis in the aorta and/or coronary vessels. Several randomized risk factor intervention trials in adults have shown that life-style-based interventions prevent or reverse elevations in risk factors and are safe, and that progression to coronary heart disease is countered. The benefit seems to be proportionate to the extent of risk factor reduction. Significant changes in life-style are necessary. It may well be that interventions in childhood will yield similar or greater benefit. Daily activity limits body fatness in children, and reductions in saturated fat intake influence serum lipid levels favorably.

Both a "whole population" approach and intervention with children who have significant risk factors may be worthwhile. High-risk subjects could be detected by screening children with a family history of hypercholesterolemia or coronary heart disease in a parent before age 60 years. In the United States, dietary interventions intended to lower fat and cholesterol intake are coupled with longitudinal assessments of response for children having triglyceride and low-density lipoprotein-cholesterol levels above the 75th percentile. In addition, overweight should be eliminated and cigarette smoking should actively be discouraged. Exercise-based interventions also are worthwhile. In the future, socioeconomic and ethnic variables may be of value in identifying at-risk groups to which screening efforts may be directed.

▶ About 20 years ago, when the late Dr. Helen B. Taussig was president of the American Heart Association, she began to encourage pediatric cardiologists, pediatricians, and epidemiologists to direct their attention to children when they contemplated the epidemic of coronary artery disease and problems of arteriosclerosis in adults. She encouraged all of us to look into exercise, diet, correction of obesity, recognition early of hypertension, and prevention of smoking. These risk factors were already being identified for their role in disability and premature death in adults. She reasoned that the disease process had its beginnings in childhood and that if prevention were ever to be effective, alertness to the problem and efforts to control risk factors should begin then.

Some progress has been made, and recommendations continue to be promulgated, but there is still some controversy, particularly when it comes to nationwide modifications of diet.

The special article from Australia (Abstract 2–50) on this question presents the problem and concludes that current evidence favors strongly a combination of dietary, antismoking, and exercise-induced interventions to commence in childhood.

The article from the Child and Family Health Studies Division of General Pediatrics at the University of California in San Diego (Abstract 2–49) reports a survey by mail of 2,000 pediatricians to determine their knowledge, attitudes, and practices regarding risk factors. It is comforting to know that the majority of pediatricians do take a family history for hypertension and death from heart disease, assess blood pressure, recommend exercise, and advise against smoking.—M.A. Engle, M.D.

3 Heart Disease in Adults

Introduction

The 8 articles dealing with valvular heart disease review the normal nonplanar orientation of the mitral valve in normal individuals (which may explain some false positive echocardiographic diagnoses of mitral valve prolapse); the current status of balloon catheter valvuloplasty for mitral and aortic stenosis; the occurrence of calcific aortic stenosis in patients with chronic renal failure or on chronic hemodialysis; the possible importance of idiopathic dilatation of the ascending aorta as a cause of chronic aortic regurgitation; and the difficulty of determining the cause (such as endocarditis) of fever early in patients who use intravenous drugs and develop fever.

The 17 articles on myocardial disease deal with selenium deficiency in dilated cardiomyopathy in China; the immunology of Chagas' disease; the use of postextrasystolic potentiation to evaluate ventricular function in dilated cardiomyopathy; the pathophysiology of Friedreich's cardiomyopathy; the value of verapamil in preventing alcoholic cardiomyopathy in the Syrian hamster; two excellent reviews of hypertrophic cardiomyopathy, including the pathophysiology of the outflow tract "obstruction" when present, the coronary circulation, including the smaller, intramyocardial vessels, the occasional development of dilated cardiomyopathy, and its treatment with verapamil; the echocardiographic characteristics of amyloid heart disease; the diagnosis of hemochromatosis with cardiac involvement; and the use of myocardial biopsy to distinguish restrictive cardiomyopathy from constrictive pericarditis.

The two articles in the section on diseases of the pericardium deal with management of tuberculous pericarditis and of malignant pericordial effusions.

There are 18 articles abstracted in the section on disturbances of cardiac rhythm and conduction. These deal with the prognosis of idiopathic sinus bradycardia; the usefulness of anticoagulant therapy in patients with atrial fibrillation; the value of acebutolol in preventing atrial fibrillation or flutter after coronary bypass grafting; the importance of magnesium deficiency in the genesis of cardiac arrhythmias; the relationship of ventricular arrhythmias to sudden cardiac death; the proarrhythmic effects of class IA antiarrhythmic drugs; the negative inotropic effect of flecainide; the possible relationship between nitrous oxide and episodes of atrioventricular junctional rhythm; the clinical pharmacology of amiodarone; the clinical value of signal-averaged electrocardiography; clinical experiences with the automatic implantable cardioverter-defibrillator; the diagnosis and management of the preexcitation syndromes including the localization of bypass tracts from the conventional 12-lead cardiogram and the use of sotalol to manage associated supraventricular tachycardia; the value of electrophysiologic testing to guide therapy in patients with aborted sudden death; and the limitations of ambulatory ECG recordings in predicting patients likely to have ventricular tachycardia induced during programmed electrical stimulation.

Five articles on miscellaneous topics describe characteristics of subjects most likely to experience sudden death in Framingham; the hypothesis that individuals with more lateralized frontal lobe activity may be at increased risk of having fatal cardiac arrhythmias; the value of the pill electrode and esophageal electrocardiography in the diagnosis of many tachyarrhythmias; the increased survival of patients with heart failure who have enalapril added to their therapeutic regimen of digoxin and diuretics; and the effects of different types of exercise on the development of different patterns of cardiac hypertrophy and systolic function.

Robert C. Schlant, M.D.

Valvular Heart Disease

The Relationship of Mitral Annular Shape to the Diagnosis of Mitral Valve Prolapse

Robert A. Levine, Marco O. Triulzi, Pamela Harrigan, and Arthur E. Weyman (Massachusetts Gen. Hosp. and Harvard Univ.)
Circulation 75:756–767, April 1987 3–1

The geometric or anatomical diagnosis of mitral valve prolapse is based on the relationship of the mitral leaflets to the surrounding anulus. Current echocardiographic criteria for making this diagnosis involve displacement above the anular hinge points in any two-dimensional view. This equivalent use of intersecting views assumes that the mitral anulus is a euclidean plane. Using these criteria, prolapse is found in a surprisingly large proportion of the general population. However, in most affected individuals, prolapse is present in the apical four-chamber view and absent in roughly orthogonal long-axis views of the left ventricle. This discrepancy between leaflet-anular relationships in intersecting views suggests an underlying geometric property of the mitral apparatus that would produce the appearance of prolapse in one view without actual leaflet distortion.

To address this possibility, a model of the mitral valve and anulus was developed (Fig 3–1). Clinical observations were reproduced when the model anulus was given a nonplanar, saddle-shaped configuration. The leaflets appeared to lie above the low points of the anulus in one plane and below its high points in a perpendicular plane. The appearance of mitral valve prolapse can, therefore, occur without actual leaflet displacement above the most superior points of the mitral anulus if the anulus is nonplanar. Twenty patients without evident anular or rheumatic valvular

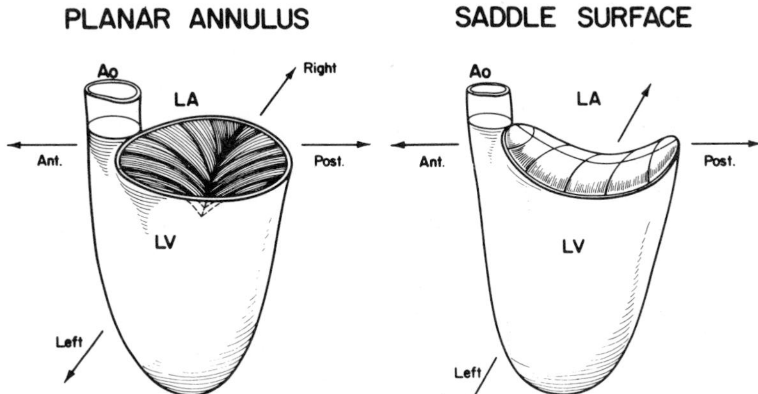

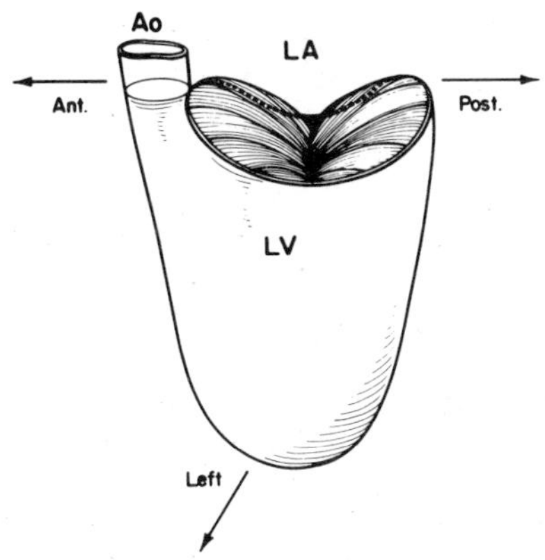

Fig 3–1.—Models of mitral valve and anulus. Adjacent cardiac structures are also diagrammed. *Ant.* indicates anterior; *Ao,* aorta; *LA,* left atrium; *LV,* left ventricle; *Post.,* posterior. **Top left,** model with a planar anulus and leaflets curving downward toward zone of coaptation. **Top right,** model with leaflets and anulus shaped to lie on a saddle-shaped surface. **Bottom,** model restructured with leaflets concave toward left ventricle, reflecting systolic pressure but not protruding above anterior and posterior high points of saddle-shaped anulus. (Courtesy of Levine, R.A., et al.: Circulation 75:756–767, April 1987.)

disease were examined to determine whether this pattern is reflected in the human mitral anulus. Two-dimensional echocardiographic views of the mitral apparatus were obtained by rotation around the cardiac apex. In all cases, the mitral anulus had a nonplanar systolic configuration, with high points located anteriorly and posteriorly. This finding is consistent with findings in other animals and favors the appearance of prolapse in the four-chamber view and its absence in long-axis views oriented anteroposteriorly.

This model explains the often observed discrepancy between

leaflet-anular relationships in roughly orthogonal views. It challenges the assumption that the mitral anulus is planar and calls into question the diagnosis of prolapse in many otherwise normal persons.

▶ This important article, which documents that the mitral valve is nonplanar in a group of 20 normal persons, should be studied by all who are in a position to diagnose mitral valve prolapse on the basis of the echocardiogram or any other planar or tomographic imaging technique. The findings, which help explain many false positive echocardiographic diagnoses of mitral valve prolapse, emphasize the relative accuracy of the parenteral long-axis views as compared to the four-chamber view.

The relation between clinical features of the mitral valve prolapse syndrome and echocardiographically documented mitral valve prolapse were also recently studied by Devereaux et al. (*J. Am. Coll. Cardiol.* 8:763–772, 1986), and the clinical and epidemiologic issues in mitral valve prolapse have been well reviewed in a symposium (*Am. Heart J.* 113:1265–1332, 1987). The history of mitral valve prolapse was reviewed by Wooley (*Am. J. Cardiol.* 59:1183–1186, 1987), and the history of DaCosta's Syndrome was reviewed by Paul (*Br. Heart J.* 58:306–315, 1987).—R.C. Schlant, M.D.

Balloon Dilation of Mitral Stenosis in Adult Patients: Postmortem and Percutaneous Mitral Valvuloplasty Studies

Raymond G. McKay, James E. Lock, Robert D. Safian, Patricia C. Come, Daniel J. Diver, Donald S. Baim, Aaron D. Berman, Sanford E. Warren, Valerie E. Mandell, Henry D. Royal, and William Grossman (Beth Israel Hosp. and Children's Hosp., Harvard Med. School)

J. Am. Coll. Cardiol. 9:723–731, April 1987 3–2

Although preliminary reports have shown the utility of percutaneous balloon valvuloplasty of the mitral valve in adult patients with mitral stenosis, the mechanism of successful dilatation of the valve and the effect of mitral valvuloplasty on cardiac performance is not known.

The authors performed mitral valvuloplasty in 5 postmorten specimens and in 18 adult patients with rheumatic mitral stenosis by using either one (25 mm) or two (18 and 20 mm) dilation balloons.

Postmortem balloon dilation resulted in increased area of the valve orifice in all 5 postmortem specimens, secondary to separation of fused commissure and fracture of nodular calcium within the mitral leaflets. The balloon dilation did not tear the valve leaflets, disrupt the mitral ring, or liberate potentially embolic debris.

In the 18 patients with severe mitral stenosis, percutaneous mitral valvuloplasty resulted in increased cardiac output and mitral valve area and in a decrease in mean mitral pressure gradient, pulmonary capillary wedge pressure, and mean pulmonary artery pressure. None of the patients experienced embolic phenomena. Left ventriculography before and after valvuloplasy in 14 of the 18 patients revealed a mild increase in mitral regurgitation in 5 and no change in the others.

When serial radionuclide ventriculography was carried out, there was an increase in left ventricular peak filling rate. In addition, serial echocardiography-phonocardiography demonstrated an improvement in mitral valve excursion, mitral EF slope, left atrial diameter, S_2-opening snap interval, and mitral valve area. All patients were discharged from the hospital with decreased symptoms after valvuloplasty.

Percutaneous mitral valvuloplasty can be performed in adult patients with mitral stenosis, including patients with calcific disease and can lead to significant improvement in valvular function. It is likely that the mechanisms of successful dilation include commissural separation and fracture of nodular calcium.

► As noted by Beckman in his accompanying editorial (*J. Am. Coll. Cardiol.* 9:732–733, 1987), balloon mitral and aortic valvuloplasty are exciting new techniques but, at present, they should be used only in the context of investigative protocols. There is now a need for larger, controlled clinical trials to determine the ultimate role of these techniques and to answer many questions: Which patients are most likely to benefit? How long does the benefit last? How often will embolic events, valvular regurgitation, or significant atrial septal defects occur? What are the short- and long-term advantages and disadvantages compared with surgical therapy? Hopefully, such trials will be performed in the near future. The following abstract (3–3) deals with catheter balloon valvuloplasty of the aortic valve.—R.C. Schlant, M.D.

Percutaneous Transluminal Balloon Valvuloplasty of Adult Aortic Stenosis: Report of 92 Cases

Alsin Cribier, Thierry Savin, Jacques Barland, Paulo Rocha, Rachid Mechmeche, Nadir Saoudi, Patrick Behar, and Brice Letac (Hôpital Charles-Nicolle, Centre Hospitalier at Universitaire de Rouen, France)

J. Am. Coll. Cardiol. 9:381–386, February 1987 3–3

Surgical valve replacement is a well-established effective treatment of aortic stenosis; nevertheless, mortality increases in high-risk surgical patients, particularly elderly patients. Percutaneous transluminal balloon valvuloplasty was attempted in 92 adult patients with severe calcific aortic stenosis. Mean age was 75 ± 11 years (range, 38–91), and 35 patients were more than 80 years old. Most of the patients were severely disabled; 66 were in New York Heart Association functional class III or IV, 27 had syncopal attacks, and 17 had severe angina pectoris. Altogether, considering these risks, 42 patients could not be considered for valve replacement. The femoral route was used in 82 patients and the brachial route in 10.

After valvuloplasty, mean systolic gradient fell significantly; the final gradient was less than 40 mm Hg in 78 patients, and mean calculated aortic valve area was grossly doubled. Ejection fraction increased significantly immediately after dilatation. Valvuloplasty resulted in moderately severe aortic regurgitation in 2 patients, although it generally resulted in a minor increase in aortic insufficiency in the other patients. There was no clinical evidence of embolic phenomena. Mean hospital stay was 6 days.

A dramatic rapid clinical improvement was evident in all severely disabled patients during the first few days after dilatation. This clinical improvement was sustained and marked in 73 of 81 patients after a mean follow-up of 18 ± 9 weeks (range, 8–44). This was confirmed by stable hemodynamic improvement noted during repeat catheterizations performed an average of 14 weeks postoperatively in 12 patients.

Three in-hospital deaths occurred; two resulted from complications of arterial catheterization, and one was related to insufficient valve dilatation. Eight patients died 4–12 weeks after the procedure; all but 1 were more than 80 years old and were in functional class III or IV before valvuloplasty.

Aortic valvuloplasty can become a relatively simple and safe possible therapeutic procedure in patients considered at high risk for valve replacement, particularly the elderly. The procedure requires only standard cardiac catheterization, low-cost materials, and 5 or 6 days of hospital stay, with immediate resumption of a normal life.

▶ The group at Rouen now has the largest experience with this procedure in the world. Their results appear to have improved significantly since they treated their initial cases. In the present study, the mean calculated aortic valve area increased approximately 0.4 sq cm. Not all other groups have had such satisfactory results, and additional studies are needed to determine which patients are best treated by this technique. Long-term studies will be especially important. Isner et al. (*Am. J. Cardiol.* 59:313–317, 1987) reported their experiences in 9 patients, and Safian et al (*J. Am. Coll. Cardiol.* 9:655–660, 1987) studied the mechanisms of successful balloon dilation.—R.C. Schlant, M.D.

Valvular Aortic Stenosis: A Clinical and Hemodynamic Profile of Patients

J. Timothy Lombard and Arthur Selzer (Pacific Presbyterian Med. Ctr., San Francisco)

Ann. Intern. Med. 106:292–298, February 1987 3–4

In the past few decades in developed countries, there has been a dramatic fall in the prevalence of acute rheumatic fever, which has significantly altered the prevalence and nature of valvular heart disease. Valvular aortic stenosis has surpassed mitral stenosis as the principal significant lesion. The authors established a profile of patients with valvular aortic stenosis seen over a 20-year period.

The clinical and hemodynamic findings in 397 patients with valvular aortic stenosis at their first hemodynamic evaluation were reviewed. This series was considered to be representative of aortic stenosis because it was heavily weighted toward older patients and severe aortic stenosis. Two categories of symptoms were identified: angina and syncope, which develop during a fully compensated stage of aortic stenosis (prefailure symptoms); and dyspnea or congestive failure, which signifies various degrees of left ventricular malfunction.

The preponderance of soft or medium intensity systolic murmur and normal or widened pulse pressure emphasizes the changing clinical picture of aortic stenosis in an aging population. Although coexisting coronary artery disease was found in 60% of patients, those with and without coronary disease did not differ significantly, even in the presence of angina.

▶ As noted by the authors, the clinical picture of patients seen with severe aortic stenosis has gradually changed over the last three or four decades. Their data support the significance of any of the classic triad: congestive heart failure (dyspnea), angina pectoris, or syncope. A major clinical problem, however, exists in determining whether or not dyspnea on exertion is truly heart failure or is merely the manifestation either of aging and deconditioning or of an hypertrophied left ventricle without severe or critical aortic stenosis. Actually, virtually everyone has dyspnea on sufficient exertion. Thus, unless there is evidence of pulmonary congestion on physical examination or chest roentgenogram, it is necessary to document a quantitative decrease in exercise tolerance or habits by a careful history, which is often better obtained in the presence of the spouse.

The ability to obtain regular Doppler echocardiograms is a major advance in the management of patients with basal systolic murmurs or known mild aortic stenosis, which can progress over a few years. Hofmann et al. (*Am. J. Cardiol.* 59:330–335, 1987) reported very good results estimating the aortic valve orifice area using two-dimensional transesophageal echocardiography. Selzer has also reviewed the changing natural history of aortic stenosis (*N. Engl. J. Med.* 317:91–98, 1987). The progression of aortic stenosis in adult men was further documented by Nitta, et al. (*Chest* 92:40–43, 1987).—R.C. Schlant, M.D.

Calcific Aortic Stenosis: A Complication of Chronic Uraemia

E.R. Maher, M. Pazianas, and J.R. Curtis (Charing Cross Hosp., London)

Nephron 47:119–122, October 1987 3–5

Chronic renal failure is associated with increased occurrence of calcified mitral valve annulus, and mitral stenosis or regurgitation may result. The incidence of aortic stenosis due to premature calcification of the valve was studied in a series of 174 consecutive patients who began maintenance hemodialysis before age 55 years. Sixty-one patients were alive at the time of study; 28 were undergoing dialysis and 33 had a functioning renal transplant.

Six patients developed severe isolated aortic stenosis about 10 years on average after the start of hemodialysis. (The incidence was significantly higher than expected.) All 6 had a long history of uremia, and 4 had been dialyzed for longer than 8 years. Five patients with a tricuspid aortic valve had severe calcification that caused stenosis. Two patients had successful valve replacement and another is awaiting surgery. Two patients who refused surgery died, 1 with infective endocarditis. Three patients had had parathyroidectomy at the time of diagnosis; 1 had severe hyperparathyroidism.

Autopsy showed aortic valve calcification in 9 of 32 cases. In 2 instances it was severe and caused stenosis. Patients with calcified valves were older at the start of dialysis and had been dialyzed longer than the others.

Two-dimensional echocardiography will facilitate the diagnosis of aortic stenosis in patients on long-term hemodialysis. Untreated severe aortic stenosis in this setting carries a poor prognosis. Replacement with a mechanical prosthesis is indicated in patients in chronic renal failure who have severe aortic stenosis.

▶ This report emphasizes the increased calcification of apparently normal tricuspid aortic valves in patients undergoing long-term hemodialysis for chronic renal failure (CRF). As more and more patients with CRF are sustained, it is important for the physicians caring for them to be aware of the increased likelihood of cardiac calcification, which may occur in the mitral valve leaflet, mitral annulus or aortic valve. Premature fibrocalcification of bioprosthetic heart valves also occurs in patients in chronic renal failure on hemodialysis, as well as in younger patients.—R.C. Schlant, M.D.

Aortic Root Dilatation as a Cause of Isolated, Severe Aortic Regurgitation: Prevalence, Clinical and Echocardiographic Patterns, and Relation to Left Ventricular Hypertrophy and Function

Mary J. Roman, Richard B. Devereux, Nathaniel W. Niles, Clare Hochreiter, Paul Kligfield, Nina Sato, Mariane C. Spitzer, and Jeffrey S. Borer (New York Hosp.-Cornell Med. Ctr., New York)

Ann. Intern. Med. 106:800–807, June 1987 3–6

Dilatation of the aortic root has been recognized as a significant cause of aortic regurgitation, and recent pathologic studies suggest it may be the most frequent cause in industrialized societies. The clinical, echocardiographic, and radionuclide cineangiographic findings were reviewed in 102 patients with severe isolated aortic regurgitation who were followed up for 6 months or longer. In all cases there was hemodynamically severe regurgitation, and left heart catheterization confirmed 4+ regurgitation in all 56 patients studied.

In 31 patients (30%) aortic root dilatation was the only apparent cause of aortic regurgitation. It was independently associated only with older age. Dilatation was localized to the sinuses of Valsalva in some cases and generalized in others. The latter patients had more abnormal left ventricular size and more functional impairment. Nine of 15 patients with generalized dilatation and 2 of 15 with localized dilatation underwent valve replacement during a mean follow-up of 28 months. There was no consistent independent relation between aortic size and blood pressure in this series.

These findings confirm the high prevalence of idiopathic root dilatation as a cause of aortic regurgitation. Generalized aortic root dilatation is associated with marked ventricular dilatation, hypertrophy, and dysfunction.

▶ I still think that systemic hypertension is probably the most common cause of aortic regurgitation in the entire world, even though only a small fraction of patients with hypertension develop aortic regurgitation. In this regard, it is significant that 37% of the 31 patients classified as idiopathic root dilatation in this report had a history of hypertension. One wonders how many others had undiagnosed hypertension before developing aortic regurgitation. It is generally accepted that chronic hypertension can be associated with increased prominence and dilatation of the aortic root. Finally, as noted by the authors, from the available data it is difficult to separate patients in whom the aortic regurgitation occurred primarily from aortic root dilatation from patients with undiagnosed valvular disease or other causes of aortic regurgitation, in whom the dilatation of the ascending aorta is secondary.—R.C. Schlant, M.D.

Evaluation of Aortic Insufficiency by Doppler Color Flow Mapping

Gilbert J. Perry, Frederick Helmcke, Navin C. Nanda, Christopher Byard, and Benigno Soto (Univ. of Alabama, Birmingham)

J. Am. Coll. Cardiol. 9:952–959, April 1987 3–7

Doppler color flow mapping is a type of echocardiographic technology that permits real-time color-encoded visualization of blood flow. This technique makes it possible to carry out rapid, accurate mapping of the area of a regurgitant jet in multiple planes. Previously, investigators have shown a rough correlation between color Doppler and angiographic estimates of the severity of aortic insufficiency.

The authors have examined the findings in color Doppler echocardiographic studies and aortic angiograms of 29 patients to determine whether any parameters of the regurgitant jet that was visualized by color Doppler study predicted the severity of aortic insufficiency as assessed by angiographic grading.

The maximal length and area of the regurgitant jet were poorly predictive of the angiographic grade of aortic insufficiency. The area of the regurgitant jet in the parasternal short axis view at the level of the high left ventricular outflow tract relative to the area of the left ventricular outflow tract at the same location best predicted the angiographic grade with 23 of 24 patients being correctly classified. However, the jet could be viewed from this approach in only 24 of the 29 patients. The height of the regurgitant jet relative to the height of the left ventricular outflow tract measured from the parasternal long axis view just beneath the aortic valve was shown to correctly classify 23 of the 29 patients.

Mitral stenosis or valve prosthesis (present in 10 patients) did not influence the diagnosis or quantitation of aortic insufficiency by these techniques.

The thickness of the regurgitant stream at its origin relative to the size of the left ventricular outflow tract is a better predictor of the severity of aortic insufficiency as judged by angiographic grading than is the area of the regurgitant jet or the depth to which the jet extends in the left ventricle.

▶ The evaluation of patients with valvular heart disease has been significantly improved by Doppler echocardiography. In this article, the authors evaluate Doppler color flow mapping in the estimation of aortic regurgitation. The authors confirm that the estimation of the severity of aortic regurgitation by either pulsed or color Doppler study of the depth to which the regurgitant jet extends into the left ventricle can be misleading because mild or moderate aortic regurgitation can result in a jet that extends deeply into the left ventricle. They found a much better correlation between the angiographic estimation of the severity of the regurgitant stream and the thickness of the regurgitant stream at its origin in the high left ventricular outflow tract, measured in either one dimension (jet height from the parasternal long-axis view) or two dimensions (short axis area in the high left ventricular outflow tract). The measurements seem to represent a significant advance in our application of color Doppler to the study of patients with valvular heart disease, and it is hoped that the studies will be evaluated further in larger groups of patients by other investigators.

The value of continuous wave Doppler echocardiography was recently reported by Labovitz et al. (*J. Am. Coll. Cardiol.* 8:1341–1347, 1986), Beyer et al. (*Am. J. Cardiol.* 60:852–856, 1987), and Grayburn et al. (*J. Am. Coll. Cardiol.* 10:135–141, 1987). The technical and biologic sources of variability in the mapping of regurgitant color flow jets were critically studied by Wong et al. (*Am. J. Cardiol.* 60:847–851, 1987).—R.C. Schlant, M.D.

Inability to Predict Diagnosis in Febrile Intravenous Drug Abusers

Paul R. Marantz, Mark Linzer, Cheryl J. Feiner, Stuart A. Feinstein, Arthur M. Kozin, and Gerald H. Friedland (Montefiore Med. Ctr., North Central Bronx Hosp., and Albert Einstein College of Med., New York)

Ann. Intern. Med. 106:823–828, June 1987 3–8

Hospitalization is recommended for all febrile intravenous drug abusers. To determine the efficacy of diagnosis in these patients, admission data, laboratory findings, emergency room physician's diagnostic prediction, and final diagnosis were prospectively analyzed for 75 febrile intravenous drug abusers admitted to the emergency room.

The final diagnosis was pneumonia in 37.9%, trivial diagnosis in 26.4%, other conditions in 23.0%, and infective endocarditis in 12.6%. A final diagnosis of endocarditis was associated with pyuria on urinalysis, higher median temperature, and lower median serum levels of sodium and potassium. Prediction of endocarditis by the emergency room physician was not correlated with a final diagnosis of endocarditis. There was a significant association between a prediction of trivial illness and a final diagnosis of a trivial illness. However, no reliable algorithm could be derived.

Although distinguishing between those febrile intravenous drug abusers who require hospitalization and those with trivial illnesses would save time and resources, no reliable method could be derived from these data. Physicians' initial predictions were often wrong. Hospitalization of all febrile intravenous drug abusers should be continued.

▶ Unfortunately, the authors experience is being duplicated in numerous emergency wards (or "rooms") throughout the country, particularly with the increased number of intravenous drug abusers with acquired immunodeficiency syndrome (AIDS). It is very difficult to establish the diagnosis of endocarditis early in these patients, many of whom have no heart murmur when first seen. In a significant number of such patients, echocardiography is very helpful by the identification of vegetations on the tricuspid valve, which is most frequently involved in intravenous drug abusers. Chambers et al. (*Ann. Intern. Med.* 106:833–836, 1987) reported that the use of cocaine was strongly associated with endocarditis in intravenous drug users with fever. This has also been our experience.—R.C. Schlant, M.D.

Myocardial Diseases

Significance of Low Levels of Blood and Hair Selenium in Dilated Cardiomyopathy

Nan Bai-song, Li Chun-sheng, and Chen Li-hua (Tangdu Hosp., Fourth Military Med. College, Xian, China)

Chin. Med. J. 99:948–949, December 1986 3–9

Selenium is a nutritionally important trace element. Selenium deficiency is associated with Keshan disease. The relationship between selenium levels and dilated cardiomyopathy (DCM) was investigated in areas where Keshan disease is not endemic.

The study group consisted of 136 patients with DCM, 87 patients with other heart diseases (OHD), and 132 healthy control subjects. The blood selenium levels of healthy subjects ranged from 0.081 ± 0.027 to 0.147 ± 0.047 μg/ml. The levels in patients with DCM are significantly lower, 0.035 ± 0.010 to 0.045 ± 0.012 μg/ml. The blood selenium levels of patients with OHD were not statistically different from those of the normal subjects. Hair selenium levels in normal subjects ranged from 0.55 ± 0.12 to 0.89 ± 0.27 ppm, while patients with DCM had significantly lower levels, 0.25 ± 0.079 to 0.32 ± 0.11 ppm. The levels of selenium in the hair of patients with OHD were not statistically different from those of normal subjects.

Blood and hair selenium levels, reflecting recent and long-term selenium absorption, respectively, were significantly lower in patients with DCM. This may be characteristic of DCM and should be used in its diagnosis.

▶ In 1935 an epidemic of cardiomyopathy with symptoms of palpitation, dizziness, and vomiting followed by death within a few hours to a few days occurred in a small village of Keshan County in Heilongjiang province in northeast

China. Of the 286 villagers, 57 died of the disease within 2 months. The disease has been noted to occur early in certain rural and mountainous areas of northeast, northern, and southwestern China. In recent years, the incidence of Keshan disease has decreased markedly, perhaps as a result of supplementation with selenium, which is thought by some Chinese investigators to play an important role in its etiology (*Chin. Med. J.* 92:461–482, 1979). The present study suggests that selenium deficiency may also play a role in patients with dilated cardiomyopathy in other areas of China. This would also be a fruitful subject for investigation in other countries. There is also evidence that selenium may prevent Adriamycin-induced cardiotoxicity in the rabbit (Dimitrov et al.: *Am. J. Pathol.* 126:376–383, 1987).—R.C. Schlant, M.D.

Enhancement of Chronic *Trypanosoma Cruzi* Myocarditis in Dogs Treated With Low Doses of Cyclophosphamide

Zilton A. Andrade, Sonia G. Andrade, and Moysés Sadigursky (Centro de Pesquisas Goncalo Moniz, Bahia, Brazil)

Am. J. Pathol. 127:467–473, June 1987 3–10

Most subjects infected with the protozoon, *Trypanosoma cruzi,* which causes Chagas' disease, are asymptomatic. Approximately 30% of these will eventually develop progressive cardiac failure due to chronic diffuse myocarditis. In this study, dogs infected with *T. cruzi* were treated with cyclophosphamide, 50 mg/sq m three times per week for 3 weeks.

Myocarditis developed in all treated animals, typified by fibrinoid, coagulative, and lytic necrosis. Mononuclear cells invaded myocardial fibers; *T. cruzi*-specific immunosuppression did not occur. Infected dogs that were not given cyclophosphamide demonstrated only mild focal myocarditis, with lymphocyte accumulation in interstitial connective tissue.

Administration of cyclophosphamide appears to interfere with maintenance of the latent phase of *T. cruzi* infection in dogs. This may increase the value of the dog model of congestive cardiac failure following *T. cruzi* infection.

▶ The findings that repeated low doses of cyclophosphamide caused an exacerbation in the usually mild myocarditis found in dogs chronically infected with *Trypanosoma cruzi* adds to our knowledge of the very complex role of the immune system in the pathogenesis of Chagas' cardiomyopathy. It will be of interest to note whether or not patients in South America with chronic Chagas' disease develop an acute exacerbation if they acquire AIDS.—R.C. Schlant, M.D.

Response of the Left Ventricle in Idiopathic Dilated Cardiomyopathy to Postextrasystolic Potentiation

Masaru Yamazoe (Niigata Univ., Niigata, Japan)

Am. Heart J. 113:1449–1456, June 1987 3–11

Idiopathic dilated cardiomyopathy (IDC), which is characterized by ventricular dilatation and impaired systolic function, is the final result of many differing disorders. Because postextrasystolic potentiation (PESP), or augmented contractility after a premature contraction, is a good predictor of residual function, the effects of PESP were studied in seven patients with IDC who had cardiac catheterization. All patients had an ejection fraction of 0.40 or less and no coronary artery disease.

The diameter of cardiac muscle fibers was substantially greater than normal. Mean preejection period-left ventricular ejection time (PEP-LVET) ratio was 0.64. Peak systolic aortic pressure was significantly increased with PESP, but peak diastolic aortic pressure declined. The PEP-LVET ratio also decreased with PESP, as LV ejection fraction increased. There was an inverse correlation between the change in PEP-LVET ratio and that in LV ejection fraction. Postextrasystolic changes in regional wall motion differed in each patient.

Considerable residual function may be present in patients with IDC who have a marked rise in LV ejection fraction or a substantial fall in PEP-LVET ratio with PESP. Response to PESP is a safe and accurate means of detecting residual function both in patients with IDC and those with coronary artery disease.

▶ The phenomenon of postextrasystolic potentiation (PESP) has been used clinically for a number of years to detect viable myocardium in patients with coronary artery disease. The present study extends the diagnostic use of PESP to detect residual ventricular function in patients with idiopathic dilated cardiomyopathy. I still think that, someday, someone will develop a technique to use PESP safely as a therapeutic modality in some patients with ventricular failure, even if only for acute use.—R.C. Schlant, M.D.

Coronary Disease, Cardioneuropathy, and Conduction System Abnormalities in the Cardiomyopathy of Friedreich's Ataxia

Thomas N. James, B. Woodfin Cobbs, H. Cecil Coghlan, Walter C. McCoy, and Charles Fisch (Univ. of Alabama, Birmingham, Emory Univ., Atlanta, and Univ. of Indiana, Indianapolis)

Br. Heart J. 57:446–457, May 1987 3–12

Patients with Friedreich's ataxia frequently have heart abnormalities. The author's describe postmortem findings from the hearts of three patients with Friedreich's ataxia who died of congestive heart failure.

In all three patients the heart was enlarged but not dilated. Three or more sites of narrowing without occlusion caused by focal fibromuscular dysplasia were seen in at least two major coronary arteries in each heart. Histologic abnormalities included medial degeneration and fibrosis, intimal proliferation, focal dysplasia, and subintimal or medial deposition of an amorphous material that stained with periodic acid-Schiff. Lesions causing more than 50% narrowing were seen in 5% to 8% of sections from small arteries. There were smaller abnormalities in 35% to 40% of these sections. There was extensive focal degeneration of nerves and ganglia of the conduction system and in the ventricular myocardium. The conduction system was abnormal in all three hearts. The sinus node was most affected, with focal degeneration and fibrosis. Focal fibrosis and bizarrely shaped pleomorphic nuclei were observed in the myocardium.

From this evidence, a multicomponent concept of cardiac pathogenesis in Friedreich's ataxia can be derived. The components are diseases of large and small coronary arteries, cardioneuropathy of nerves and ganglia, and cardiomyopathy. In the conduction system, these components could produce the electrical instability common in this disease. These components also indicate why the heart becomes enlarged, why there is a decline in clinical course, and why the heart eventually fails.

▶ This exquisite study significantly extends our understanding of the multifactorial abnormalities in Friedreich's cardiomyopathy, particularly the interrelations between the coronary artery disease, cardiomyopathy, cardioneuropathy, and molecular faults. The 1987 YEAR BOOK OF CARDIOLOGY contains an abstract of the excellent article by Child et al. (*J. Am. Coll. Cardiol.* 7:1370–1378, 1986), who reviewed the clinical features of a group of 75 patients.—R.C. Schlant, M.D.

Verapamil Prevents the Development of Alcoholic Dysfunction in Hamster Myocardium

Jeffrey S. Garrett, Joan Wikman-Coffelt, Richard Sievers, Walter E. Finkbeiner, and William W. Parmley (Univ. of California, San Francisco)

J. Am. Coll. Cardiol. 9:1326–1331, June 1987 3–13

Ethanol causes acute and chronic depression of cardiac function. Ethanol was added to the drinking water of hamsters in increasing amounts reaching 50% in 5 weeks. A control group received water only. Verapamil, 1.75 mg/ml, was added to the ethanol/water mixture of some of the hamsters to determine if it could protect cardiac function. Hamsters were killed at 5, 7, and 12 weeks, and their hearts were perfused and pressures recorded.

The hearts from the alcohol-treated hamsters had significant reductions of developed pressure, rate of pressure rise, high-energy phosphates, and adenosine compared with the controls. The hamsters given ethanol/verapamil had measurements that were indistinguishable from the control animals.

Oral ingestion of ethanol produced depression of cardiac performance in hamsters. Verapamil prevented development of ethanol-induced cardiac depression and preserved energy metabolism in hamsters drinking 50% alcohol.

▶ The calcium antagonist, verapamil, has also been demonstrated to lessen the development of hereditary cardiomyopathy of the Syrian hamster (Rouleau et al.: *Circ. Res.* 50:405–412, 1982; Jasmin et al.: *Can. J. Physiol. Pharmacol.*

62:891–897, 1984; and Wikman-Coffelt et al.: *Am. J. Physiol., Heart Circ. Physiol.* 250:H22–8, 1986). Hopefully, future investigations will lead to improved forms of therapy to prevent the otherwise relentless progression of many forms of cardiomyopathy in human beings.—R.C. Schlant, M.D.

Hypertrophic Cardiomyopathy: Interrelations of Clinical Manifestations, Pathophysiology, and Therapy (First of Two Parts)

Barry J. Maron, Robert O. Bonow, Richard O. Cannon III, Martin B. Leon, and Stephen E. Epstein (Natl. Insts. of Health, Bethesda, Md.)

N. Engl. J. Med. 316:780–789, March 26, 1987 3–14

Despite advances in our understanding of hypertrophic cardiomyopathy, much uncertainty and debate remain. The pathophysiologic mechanisms that determine the symptoms, the clinical outcome, and the efficacy of drug and surgical therapy were reviewed.

Hypertrophic cardiomyopathy is a primary myocardial abnormality characterized by a hypertrophied and nondilated left ventricle that exists in the absence of a co-existing cardiac or systemic disease capable of producing left ventricular hypertrophy. The distribution of the hypertrophy is usually asymmetric, with all segments of the left ventricular wall not thickened to a similar degree. Patterns and extent of left ventricular hypertrophy vary greatly. In about 55% of patients, hypertrophy is diffuse, involving both septum and large portions of the anterolateral free wall, with the posterior segment of the free wall least affected. Wall thickening may be confined to parts of the ventricle inaccessible to the conventional M-mode echocardiographic beam.

Left ventricular morphology also seems to be a main determinant of the hemodynamic state in hypertrophic cardiomyopathy. Histologic features of the left ventricular myocardium considered to represent possible components of the disease process are cardiac muscle-cell disorganization, myocardial scarring, and abnormalities of the small intramural coronary arteries.

Hypertrophic cardiomyopathy is often familial and transmitted in a pattern consistent with an autosomal dominant trait. Disagreement exists on some of the pathophysiologic mechanisms involved. The left ventricle contracts against a decreased afterload and is thus better described as hyperdynamic rather than hypercontractile. The clinical and pathophysiologic implications of the subaortic gradient have been debated. Decreased distensibility and prolonged relaxation contribute to impaired diastolic filling of the hypertrophied left ventricle. The former results from increases in stiffness of the left ventricular chamber and muscle; the latter is primarily influenced by the inactivation process. Regional myocardial ischemia does occur in hypertrophic cardiomyopathy and may be responsible for chest pain experienced by many patients.

Numerous studies have explored specific facets of hypertrophic cardiomyopathy. Interrelations of clinical manifestations, pathophysiology, and therapy were discussed.

Hypertrophic Cardiomyopathy: Interrelations of Clinical Manifestations, Pathophysiology, and Therapy (Second of Two Parts)

Barry J. Maron, Robert O. Bonow, Richard O. Cannon III, Martin B. Leon, and Stephen E. Epstein (Natl. Insts. of Health, Bethesda, Md.)
N. Engl. J. Med. 316:844–852, April 2, 1987 3–15

Certain aspects of hypertrophic cardiomyopathy continue to be debated. Interrelationships of clinical manifestations, pathophysiology, and therapy were reviewed.

The primary symptoms of hypertrophic cardiomyopathy are exertional angina, dyspnea, fatigue, and impaired consciousness. A direct, one-to-one correlation between a symptom and a single pathophysiologic mechanism does not always exist. Disparities may arise because each pathophysiologic component may produce more than one of its hemodynamic and clinical manifestations, more than one of the disease components usually exist in a given patient, and the relative importance of each component can differ from patient to patient (Fig 3–2). Sudden death occurs most commonly in young patients, 10–30 years of age. Few clinical predictors of sudden death have been identified. Death may result from hemodynamic changes in some patients; the most common precipitating factors appear to be arrhythmias, particularly ventricular tachycardia.

The basic disease process can develop and progress along several pathways, including subaortic obstruction, diastolic dysfunction, and possibly myocardial ischemia. Beta-adrenergic-blocking drugs have been the primary medical therapy for symptomatic patients with obstructive or nonobstructive hypertrophic cardiomyopathy. After an initial improvement, symptoms may recur, mandating higher doses. Other therapeutic agents that have been used are calcium channel blockers, disopyramide, and amiodarone.

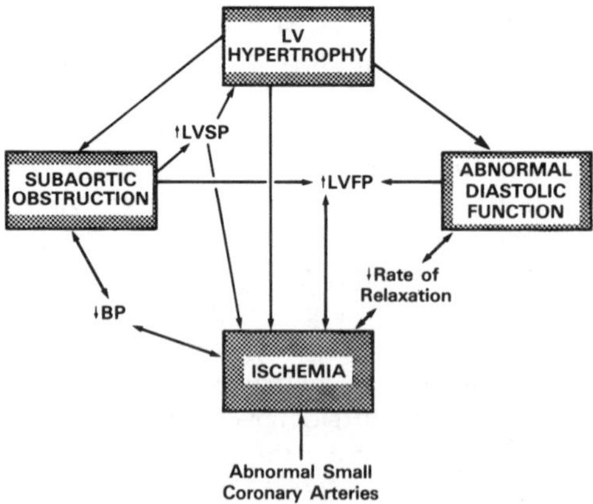

Fig 3–2.—Pathophysiologic and hemodynamic interrelations between left ventricular (LV) hypertrophy, subaortic obstruction, diastolic dysfunction, and myocardial ischemia in hypertrophic cardiomyopathy. The symptoms in any given patient reflect the complex interactions among these pathophysiologic mechanisms. LVSP denotes left ventricular systolic pressure, LVFP, left ventricular filling pressure, and BP, blood pressure. (Courtesy of Maron, B.J., et al.: N. Engl. J. Med. 316:844–852. April 2, 1987.)

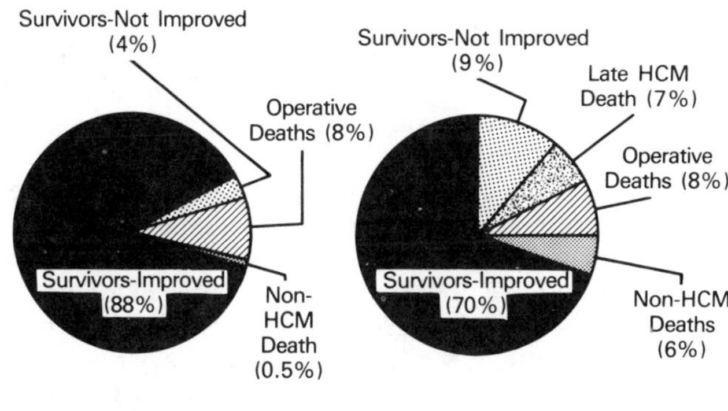

Fig 3–3.—Clinical outcome after ventricular septal myotomy-myectomy in 240 patients with obstructive hypertrophic cardiomyopathy (HCM). (Courtesy of Maron, B.J., et al.: N. Engl. J. Med. 316:844–852, April 2, 1987.)

Surgical intervention relieves the dynamic obstruction to left ventricular outflow, reducing the elevated left ventricular systolic pressures. This has been achieved in about 95% of patients with septal myotomy-myectomy, without compromising global left ventricular function. In the largest series, about 70% of patients reported symptomatic improvement for up to 25 years after surgery (Fig 3–3).

It is not yet possible to construct an accurate profile of the relative contributions of the various pathophysiologic mechanisms to the symptoms of a patient with hypertrophic cardiomyopathy. Such an approach would provide the framework for developing more effective therapies for patients with this disease.

▶ This outstanding two-part review article (Abstracts 3–14 and 3–15) should be carefully studied by anyone caring for a patient with hypertrophic cardiomyopathy to obtain a thorough, up-to-date review of all major facets of this fascinating syndrome. The next abstract (3–16) summarizes an additional, complementary review.—R.C. Schlant, M.D.

Hypertrophic Cardiomyopathy: A 1987 Viewpoint
E. Douglas Wigle (Toronto Gen. Hosp. and Univ. of Toronto)
Circulation 75:311–322, February 1987 3–16

Understanding of the diastolic and rhythm abnormalities in hypertrophic cardiomyopathy (HCM) has increased in the past 30 years; however, the significance of the systolic intraventricular pressure differences remains to be clarified. Most researchers accept that the characteristic pressure gradient, caused by prolonged mitral leaflet-septal contact, represents obstruction to the left ventricular outflow. However, a small group believes there is no hemodynamic evidence of obstruction to outflow and suggest that the intraventricular pressure differences result from very rapid early systolic ejection with resultant cavity obliteration or elimination. The evidence for and against obstruction to left ventricular outflow in obstructive HCM was reviewed, and the important differences between ventricular relaxation and passive chamber stiffness in regulating ventricular diastolic filling were contrasted.

There are four different types of systolic pressure difference that may be seen in this condition. The small early systolic impulse gradient across the aortic valve that results from early systolic flow acceleration may be greater than normal in HCM because of the rapid ejection in early systole but does not extend beyond midsystole. The pressure gradient in midventricular obstruction occurs at the level of the papillary muscles and not in the left ventricular outflow tract at the site of mitral leaflet-septal contact as in obstructive HCM. The obstructive subaortic pressure gradient caused by mitral leaflet-septal contact may be seen (Figs 3–4, left, and 3–5). Cavity obliteration may produce the fourth type of systolic pressure difference (Fig 3–4, right).

Evidence confirms that mitral leaflet-septal contact is the cause of the obstructive subaortic pressure gradient. The time of onset of mitral leaflet-septal contact has been found to not only determine the magnitude of the pressure gradient but also the degree of prolongation of left ventricular ejection time, the percentage of stroke volume obstructed, and the degree of mitral regurgitation. Diastolic filling is compromised by

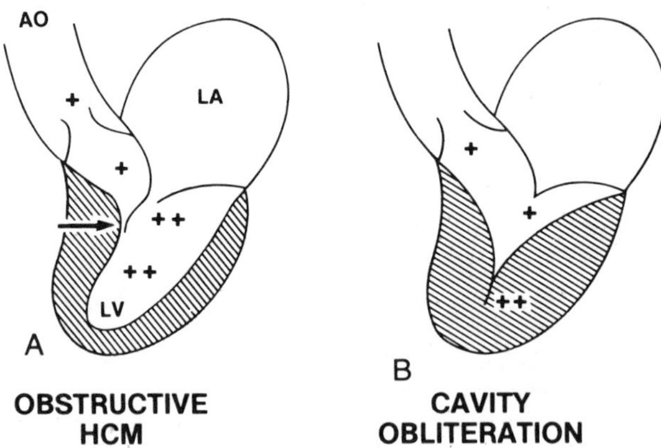

Fig 3–4.—The left ventricular inflow tract pressure concept. **A,** in obstructive HCM, because the obstruction to left ventricular outflow *(arrow)* is caused by anterior mitral leaflet-ventricular septal contact, the intraventricular pressure distal to the stenosis (and proximal to the aortic valve) is low (+), whereas all ventricular pressures proximal to the stenosis, including the one just inside the mitral valve (the inflow tract pressure), are elevated (++). **B,** when an intraventricular pressure difference is recorded because of catheter entrapment by the myocardium in an area of cavity obliteration, the elevated ventricular pressure is recorded only in the area of cavity obliteration (++). The intraventricular systolic pressure in all other areas of the left ventricular cavity, including that in the inflow tract just inside the mitral valve, is low (+) and equal to the aortic systolic pressure. Thus, the inflow tract pressure is elevated in obstructive HCM but not in cavity obliteration. There are now more than 20 characteristic differences between these two types of intraventricular pressure difference. The three areas of the left ventricle represented by the + signs in each of these diagrams are, from above downward, the outflow tract just below the aortic valve (subaortic region), the inflow tract just inside the mitral valve, and the left ventricular apex. AO, aorta; LA, left atrium; LV, left ventricle. (Courtesy of Wigle, E.D.: Circulation 75:311–322, February 1987.)

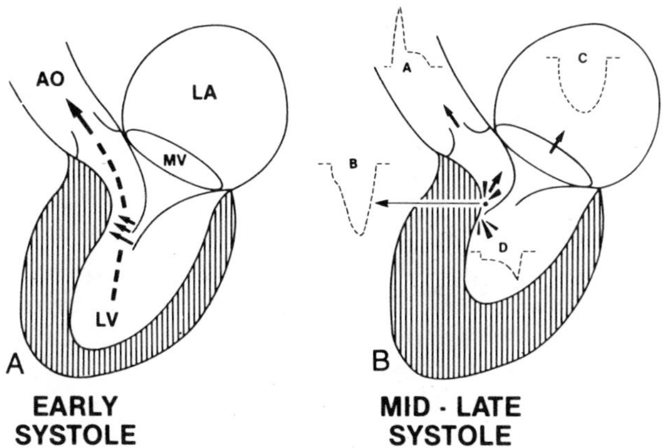

Fig 3–5.—**A,** mechanism of mitral leaflet systolic anterior motion in early systole in obstructive HCM. The ventricular septal hypertrophy causes a narrow outflow tract, as a result of which the ejection velocity is rapid and the path of ejection *(dashed line)* is closer to the mitral leaflets than is normal. These hydrodynamic and anatomical features in obstructive HCM result in Venturi forces *(three short oblique arrows in the outflow tract)* drawing the anterior *(upper two arrows)* and/or posterior *(lower arrow)* mitral leaflet(s) toward the septum (systolic anterior motion). Subsequent mitral leaflet-septal contact results in obstruction to left ventricular outflow and the concomitant mitral regurgitation, as seen on the right. In obstructive HCM with posterior leaflet systolic anterior motion, the posterior leaflet is either longer than the anterior leaflet or the mitral anulus is tilted so that the posterior leaflet extends further into the left ventricular cavity than does the anterior leaflet. AO, aorta; LA, left atrium; MV, mitral valve; LV, left ventricle. **B,** by midsystole, anterior mitral leaflet-septal contact is well established, causing marked narrowing in the left ventricular outflow tract with obstruction to outflow. Proximal to the level of mitral leaflet-septal contact, the converging lines indicate the acceleration of the jet just proximal to the obstruction, as well as the narrowing of the jet width that occurs, presumably caused by mitral leaflet systolic anterior motion. Distal to the obstruction, the arrow and diverging lines indicate the high velocity flow that emanates from the site of mitral leaflet-septal contact, which is directed posterolaterally at a considerable angle from the normal path of aortic outflow. In late systole, although forward flow continues into the outflow tract and aorta, the volume of flow is much less *(smaller aortic arrow)* than early nonobstructed systole (left). The right upper oblique arrow arising from the mitral valve orifice indicates the occurrence of mitral regurgitation. *A,* the integrated Doppler flow signal in the ascending aorta in obstructive HCM (flow toward the transducer). *B, C,* and *D,* the Doppler flow velocity signals that can be recorded from the apex of the left ventricle in obstructive HCM by means of pulsed and/or continuous-wave Doppler (flow away from the transducer); *B,* the higher outflow tract velocities that emanate from the site of mitral leaflet-septal contact and that correspond closely to the simultaneously measured pressure gradients. C, the presence of mitral regurgitation. *D,* the late systolic velocity peak that can be recorded in the apical region of the left ventricle. Although this diagram (right) depicts systolic events after mitral leaflet-septal contact in obstructive HCM, *A, B, C,* and *D* represent flow/velocity signals throughout systole. (Courtesy of Wigle, E.D.: Circulation 75:311–322, February 1987.)

ventricular relaxation impairment and increased passive chamber stiffness.

Hypertrophic cardiomyopathy is a diverse condition in which the presence and severity of the various clinical and pathophysiologic abnormalities appear related to the site and extent of hypertrophic process. Modern cardiologic technology has helped increase understanding of this disorder; much remains to be learned.

▶ This is an excellent review, particularly of the evidence for and against true outflow tract obstruction and of the importance of ventricular relaxation and passive chamber stiffness in the pathophysiology of HCM.—R.C. Schlant, M.D.

Patterns and Timing of Doppler-Detected Intracavity and Aortic Flow in Hypertrophic Cardiomyopathy

Paul G. Yock, Liv Hatle, and Richard L. Popp (Stanford Univ., and Univ. of Trondheim, Norway)

J. Am. Coll. Cardiol. 8:1047–1058, November 1986 3–17

Using combined cardiac Doppler and two-dimensional echocardiography, it is now possible to directly measure and localize abnormal outflow velocities in patients with hypertrophic cardiomyopathy and intracavity pressure gradients. The authors attempted to characterize the patterns of left ventricular outflow and aortic velocities in 25 patients with the echocardiographic diagnosis of hypertrophic cardiomyopathy who also had elevated systolic flow velocities by Doppler study within the left ventricle.

Systematic pulsed and continuous wave Doppler analysis combined with phonocardiography and M-mode echocardiography was used to establish the pattern and timing of outflow in the basal and provoked states. Results indicated that the high velocity left ventricular outflow jet can be reliably discriminated from both aortic flow and the jet of mitral regurgitation using Doppler ultrasound. The Doppler velocity contour responds in a characteristic fashion to provocative influences including extrasystolic and Valsalva maneuver. The onset of mitral regurgitation occurs well before detectable systolic anterior motion of the mitral valve, and left ventricular flow velocities were elevated at the onset of systolic anterior motion of the mitral valve, suggesting a significant contribution of the Venturi effect in displacing the leaflets and chordae. The high velocities of the outflow jets were largely dissipated by the time flow reached the aortic valve. The late systolic flow in the ascending aorta was nonuniform, with formation of distinct eddies that may contribute to "preclosure" of the aortic valve.

Extreme caution must be exercised in extrapolating from Doppler velocity signals to estimations of absolute flow, given the complexity of the flow pattern in this condition.

▶ It is of great interest in patients with HCM that flow in the left ventricular outflow tract and ascending aorta continues throughout systole and that partial closure ("preclosure") of the aortic valve appears to be caused by eddy formation in ascending aorta, together with early deceleration of flow. These studies present compelling evidence against the concept that forward flow into the aorta ceases completely before the end of systole. The fact that the authors found that mitral regurgitation began at the onset of systole argues against the suggestion that the regurgitation is produced by the systolic anterior motion of the anterior mitral valve leaflet.

The finding that the velocity of blood in the left ventricular outflow tract at the level of the mitral leaflet is elevated at the onset of systolic anterior motion is compatible with, but does not prove, a Venturi mechanism being responsible for the anterior motion of the leaflet. While there is now general agreement that the outflow tract is narrowed in patients with hypertrophic cardiomyopathy, additional studies are still necessary to determine in how many (or which) patients there is a true outflow tract "obstruction" and in how many (or which) patients is the pressure gradient across merely the consequence of the increased velocity and the lower pressure mandated by the Bernoulli equation.—R.C. Schlant, M.D.

Differences in Coronary Flow and Myocardial Metabolism at Rest and During Pacing Between Patients With Obstructive and Patients With Nonobstructive Hypertrophic Cardiomyopathy

Richard O. Cannon III, William H. Schenke, Barry J. Maron, Cynthia M. Tracy, Martin B. Leon, John E. Brush, Jr., Douglas R. Rosing, and Stephen E. Epstein (Natl. Insts. of Health, Bethesda, Md.)

J. Am. Coll. Cardiol. 10:53–62, July 1987 3–18

Hypertrophic cardiomyopathy is characterized by hypertrophy of the left ventricle. To determine if elevated intraventricular pressures and subaortic gradients are of pathophysiologic importance in this condition, 50 patients with hypertrophic cardiomyopathy were studied in the basal state and during heart rate pacing. Twenty-three patients had basal obstruction and 27 did not have obstruction.

The patients with basal obstruction had significantly lower basal coronary resistance and higher basal coronary flow in the anterior left ventricle. They also had higher regional myocardial oxygen consumption. Myocardial oxygen consumption and coronary blood flow were also significantly higher at paced heart rates of 100 and 130 beats per minute in patients with obstruction than in patients without obstruction. At rates higher than 130 beats per minute, all patients with obstruction experienced chest pain and an increase in coronary resistance. Patients without obstruction demonstrated signs of ischemia at significantly lower coronary flow, higher coronary resistance, and lower myocardial oxygen consumption than those with obstruction.

Obstruction of left ventricular outflow is associated with high left ventricular systolic pressure and oxygen consumption in patients with obstructive hypertrophic cardiomyopathy, and therefore is of importance in the precipitation of ischemia in these patients. Patients with hypertrophic cardiomyopathy without obstruction may have more impairment of coronary flow during a stress.

▶ The limited coronary reserve in patients with hypertrophic cardiomyopathy may well be responsible not only for angina pectoris but also for cardiac arrhythmias and, potentially, sudden death. Interestingly, patients with little or no obstruction appear to have less impairment of coronary flow from elevation of left ventricular filling pressure than do patients with outflow tract obstruction. Also see the following abstract (3–19).—R.C. Schlant, M.D.

Quantitative Analysis of Narrowings of Intramyocardial Small Arteries in Normal Hearts, Hypertensive Hearts, and Hearts With Hypertrophic Cardiomyopathy

Masaru Tanaka, Hisayoshi Fujiwara, Tomoya Onodera, Der-Jinn Wu, Mitsuo Matsuda, Yoshihiro Hamashima, and Chuichi Kawai (Kyoto Univ., Japan)

Circulation 75:1130–1139, June 1987 3–19

Patients with hypertrophic cardiomyopathy (HCM) and hypertension frequently experience chest pain. Intramyocardial small artery (IMSA) disease is a possible mechanism of myocardial ischemia in these patients. Narrowings of IMSA were measured in 10 hearts from patients with HCM, 4 from patients with HCM that mimics dilated cardiomyopathy (DCM-like HCM), 10 from patients with hypertension, and 15 from normal adults.

The external IMSA calibers were similar in hearts from patients with HCM, hypertension, or controls, but were larger in hearts from patients with DCM-like HCM. The mean percent lumen of IMSAs was reduced in patients with HCM and hypertension and was further reduced in patients with DCM-like HCM compared with normal hearts. The mean IMSA percent lumen was inversely correlated with heart weight, mean size of myocytes, and percent fibrotic area in the septum.

Intramyocardial small artery disease is important in the pathology of patients with HCM and hypertension. It has an even greater impact in patients with DCM-like HCM.

▶ The importance of the small blood vessels in many forms of heart disease, and especially in hypertensive heart disease and many varieties of cardiomyopathy, has been increasingly recognized during the last decade. Both anatomical and functional abnormalities have been recognized that may not only limit coronary vasodilator reserve but may also contribute significantly to myocardial cellular dysfunction and eventually to cell death. It would be important to extend the present studies to other heart specimens that are specially prepared to lessen possible blood vessel postmorten contraction and distortion produced by formalin fixation. Also see the preceding abstract (3–18).—R.C. Schlant, M.D.

Progression of Hypertrophic Cardiomyopathy Into a Hypokinetic Left Ventricle: Higher Incidence in Patients With Midventricular Obstruction

Sayid Fighali, Zvonimir Krajcer, Sidney Edelman, and Robert D. Leachman (St. Luke's Episcopal Hosp. and Texas Heart Inst., Houston)

J. Am. Coll. Cardiol. 9:288–294, February 1987 3–20

It is been shown that hypertrophic cardiomyopathy occasionally progresses into a dilated hypokinetic left ventricle. This process can occur acutely or chronically and can be associated with a marked deterioration in clinical status. The authors studied the pathophysiologic mechanism that is responsible for this process and analyzed the serial clinical and laboratory data for 62 patients.

During a mean follow-up period of 8 years, 5 patients (group A) developed left ventricular hypokinesia, and the remaining 57 (group B) continued to exhibit the clinical and laboratory findings of hypertrophic cardiomyopathy. Three patients developed a dilated left ventricle with generalized hypokinesia, and 2 others had abnormalities of the segmental left ventricular wall motion. None of these 5 patients with left ventricular hypokinesia had fixed coronary artery disease.

Mean age, sex, and duration of follow-up were similar in both groups, as was the presence of coronary myocardial bridges and angina pectoris and an interventricular gradient. In group A 4 of the 5 patients had midventricular obliteration, in group B 4 of the 57 patients had midventricular obliteration.

Segmental or generalized left ventricular hypokinesia can develop in patients with hypertrophic cardiomyopathy in the absence of fixed coronary artery disease. Such hypokinesia can occur after an acute myocardial infarction or can develop gradually without clinical or electrocardiographic evidence of infarction.

The authors note that patients with the midventricular obliteration variant of hypertrophic cardiomyopathy are at higher risk of developing segmental or diffuse left ventricular hypokinesia.

▶ It is of interest that patients with hypertrophic cardiomyopathy who had midventricular obstruction appeared to have a higher risk of progressing to a stage of hypokinesis, which might be either diffuse or more marked in the apical area. Interestingly, the echocardiographic left ventricular end-diastolic diameters of the 5 patients diagnosed as having developed hypokinesis were only 58, 60, 58, 61, and 48 mm with simultaneous fractional changes in echocardiographic left ventricular internal diameter of 34%, 33%, 38%, 31%, and 42% and corresponding angiographic ejection fractions of 35%, 45%, 45%, 30%, and 60%. Thus, several patients did not develop the full picture of dilated cardiomyopathy although they did develop hypokinesis relative to their earlier ventricular function. The progression from hypertrophic to dilated cardiomyopathy has previously been occasionally described by ten Cate and Roelandt, (*Am. Heart J.* 97:762–765, 1979), Beder et al. (*Am. Heart J.* 104:155–156, 1982), Fujiwara et al. (*Jpn. Circ. J.* 48:1210–1214, 1984) and Yutani et al. (*Am. Heart J.* 109:545–553, 1985).

I have known one patient with hypertrophic obstructive cardiomyopathy (HOCM) who also had a bad problem with chronic alcoholism. On several occasions, the patient had documentation of the classic findings of HOCM on physical examination, echocardiography, and cardiac catheterization. On numerous other occasions, however, the patient discontinued propranolol therapy and began to drink heavily. This produced transient dilatation and hypokinesis of the left ventricle together with loss of all evidence of outflow tract obstruction. Interestingly, this challenging patient very much enjoyed participating in the oral examinations formerly conducted by the Board of Cardiovascular Diseases at Grady Memorial Hospital. I suspect that chronic alcoholism may be a major contributing cause of left ventricular dysfunction in many patients with other forms of cardiac disease.—R.C. Schlant, M.D.

Regional Left Ventricular Asynchrony and Impaired Global Left Ventricular Filling in Hypertrophic Cardiomyopathy: Effect of Verapamil

Robert O. Bonow, Dino F. Vitale, Barry J. Maron, Stephen L. Bacharach, Terri M. Frederick, and Michael V. Green (Natl. Insts. of Health, Bethesda, Md.)

J. Am. Coll. Cardiol. 9:1108–1116, May 1987 3–21

Many patients with hypertrophic cardiomyopathy have impaired left ventricular relaxation and filling. The relation between spatial and temporal nonuniformity and impaired global ventricular diastolic filling has not been extensively studied in hypertrophic cardiomyopathy, and the potential for regional heterogeneity reversal during medical therapy has not been explored. The authors investigated the influence of regional heterogeneity on left ventricular relaxation and filling in 48 patients with hypertrophic cardiomyopathy and sinus rhythm.

The patients were studied with radionuclide angiography before and after undergoing 1–2 weeks of verapamil therapy, 320–640 mg per day. Left ventricular regional function was evaluated by subdividing the ventricular region of interest into 20 sectors and quadrants from which regional time-activity curves were derived. Diastolic asynchrony was measured as the regional variation in timing between minimal volume and peak filling rate. Heterogeneity in the magnitude of rapid diastolic filling was measured as the regional variation in percent contribution of the atrial systole to end-diastolic volume. Patients were then compared with 28 healthy subjects.

Patients with hypertrophic cardiomyopathy had greater regional variation in timing and magnitude of rapid filling than control subjects (35 ± 24 vs. 12 ± 6 ms and 10 ± 6 vs. 7 ± 4%, respectively). Verapamil reduced the regional variation in timing and magnitude of rapid filling (to 21 ± 16 ms and to 7 ± 3%, respectively). These regional changes indicated more uniform regional diastolic performance after verapamil and were associated with improved global diastolic filling. Global rapid filling increased both in rate and magnitude, and time to peak filling rate decreased.

The beneficial effect of verapamil on left ventricular diastolic function in hypertrophic cardiomyopathy may be mediated by reduced regional asynchrony.

► This is an important contribution to our understanding of the mechanism of the benefits produced by verapamil therapy in patients with hypertrophic cardiomyopathy. At present, such therapy is usually reserved for those patients who do not respond satisfactorily to therapy with the β-blocker, propranolol. Also see Abstracts 3–15 and 3–16.—R.C. Schlant, M.D.

Sensitivity and Specificity of the Echocardiographic Features of Cardiac Amyloidosis

Rodney H. Falk, Jonathan F. Plehn, Thomas Deering, Edgar C. Schick, Jr., Paul

Boinay, Alan Rubinow, Martha Skinner, and Alan S. Cohen (Boston City Hosp. and Univ. Hosp., Boston Univ.)
Am. J. Cardiol. 59:418–422, February 1987 3–22

Although increased myocardial echogenicity has been described as being highly suggestive of cardiac amyloid in adults, no study has systematically addressed its prevalence in amyloidosis nor the interobserver variability in its interpretation. To determine whether echogenicity is a specific feature of cardiac amyloid or whether any other feature was of diagnostic value, 31 patients with documented cardiac amyloidosis were compared with 39 control subjects with left ventricular hypertrophy from nonamyloid heart disease.

The two-part investigation sought first to determine whether increased myocardial echogenicity distinguished blindly interpreted echocardiograms of the two patient groups, and then to examine echocardiograms in a blinded but more detailed manner. Increased myocardial echogenicity was present in 16 patients when a single short-axis view was examined. It had a sensitivity of 63% and a specificity of 74% for the diagnosis of amyloidosis.

When the complete echocardiograms were reviewed in 15 patients, an improved sensitivity of 87% and specificity of 81% based on echogenicity were observed (table). Increased atrial septal thickness was found in 60% of amyloid patients and no controls. The combination of increased myocardial echogenicity and increased atrial thickness was 60% sensitive and 100% specific for amyloidosis diagnoses. A ratio of ECG voltage to left ventricular cross-sectional area less than 1.5 was 82% sensitive and 83% specific for amyloid, excluding 2 patients with left bundle-branch block.

This study confirms the value of increased echogenicity for diagnosing cardiac amyloid. The voltage/mass ratio in symptomatic amyloid patients clearly distinguished them from those with true LV hypertrophy.

PRESENCE OF INDIVIDUAL FEATURES SUGGESTIVE OF CARDIAC AMYLOIDOSIS*

	Amyloid (n = 15)		Control (n = 16)	
	≥2/3 Observers	All Observers	≥2/3 Observers	All Observers
IME	13 (87)	9 (60)	3 (19)	0
IAST	9 (60)	4 (27)	0	0
IME + IAST	9 (60)	3 (20)	0	0
IRVT	4 (27)	2 (13)	1 (16)	0

*Numbers in parentheses are percentages. IAST = increased atrial septal thickness; IME = increased myocardial echogenicity; IRVT = increased right ventricular thickness.

(Courtesy of Falk, R.H., et al.: Am. J. Cardiol. 59:418–422, February 1987.)

Differentiation of Cardiac Amyloidosis and Hypertrophic Cardiomyopathy: A Comparison of Familial Amyloidosis With Polyneuropathy and Hypertrophic Cardiomyopathy by Electrocardiography and Echocardiography

Peter Eriksson, Christer Backman, Anders Eriksson, Sture Eriksson, Kjell Karp, and Bert-Ove Olofsson (Univ. of Umeå, Umeå, Sweden)

Acta Med. Scand. 221:39–46, 1987 3–23

Because it may be clinically important to differentiate cardiac amyloidosis from hypertrophic cardiomyopathy, 29 patients with familial amyloidosis and polyneuropathy were compared with 22 patients with hypertrophic cardiomyopathy. Amyloidosis was diagnosed clinically and from finding amyloid in a skin or rectal mucosal biopsy specimen. The diagnosis of cardiomyopathy was based on a nondilated, hypertrophied left ventricle without other cardiac or systemic disorder.

Low QRS voltage was seen only in patients with amyloidosis. Voltage criteria of hypertrophy were fulfilled by 59% of patients with cardiomyopathy but in none of those with amyloidosis. Asymmetric (ventricular) septal thickening occurred in both groups, but thickened heart valves were seen only in patients with amyloidosis. Strongly reflective myocardial echoes also occurred only in patients with amyloidosis. Systolic anterior motion of the mitral valve was seen only in hypertrophic cardiomyopathy.

The use of left ventricular mass, systolic anterior motion, thickened heart valves, and a granular sparkling myocardial appearance on echography led to a correct classification of more than 90% of both groups of patients.

Cardiac amyloidosis can be diagnosed accurately by noninvasive findings and histopathologic documentation of amyloid at a site other than the heart.

▶ The echocardiographic study of 31 patients with cardiac amyloidosis by Falk et al. (Abstract 3–22) evaluates criteria for the identification of this specific type of heart muscle disease, which can present with a syndrome of restrictive cardiomyopathy but can also mimic hypertrophic cardiomyopathy. They found that the combination of increased myocardial echogenicity (earlier referred to as "granular sparkling") and thickening of the atrial septum was present in 60% of patients with amyloid but in only 1 of 39 control patients with left ventricular hypertrophy. They did not report on the finding of thickening of the heart valves.

On the other hand, Eriksson et al. (Abstract 3–23), who studied 29 patients with familial amyloidosis and polyneuropathy, found that the combination of granular sparkling appearance of the myocardium and thickened heart valves to be the best predictor of amyloidosis rather than hypertrophic cardiomyopathy. They found asymmetrical hypertrophy of the ventricular septum in 38% of their patients with amyloidosis but did not comment on thickening of the atrial septum. Both studies confirmed the observation that patients with amyloidosis often have normal or low QRS voltage, particularly considering the increase in left ventricular mass.

We should keep the findings of these two studies in mind in order to suspect and diagnose amyloid heart disease earlier in its course. Although there is no specific therapy for amyloidosis, there is some preliminary evidence that colchicine might slow the development of primary amyloidosis (Cohen et al.: *Am. J. Med.* 82:1182–1189, 1987).—R.C. Schlant, M.D.

Echocardiographic Features of Idiopathic Hemochromatosis

Lyle J. Olson, William P. Baldus, and A. Jamil Tajik (Mayo Clinic and Found.)

Am. J. Cardiol. 60:885–889, Oct. 1, 1987 3–24

Cardiac involvement is considered the chief cause of death from idiopathic hemochromatosis. Seventeen men and 7 women with this diagnosis underwent echocardiographic assessment in 1978–1985. Mean age of the 24 was 48 years. All but 2 of 21 liver biopsy specimens showed fibrosis or cirrhosis.

Echocardiographic findings were abnormal in 7 of 19 patients without valvular, ischemic, or hypertensive heart disease, and 12 had normal echographic findings. These groups were not distinguished by age, gender, or laboratory markers of iron overload. Chamber dilatation and global systolic dysfunction were observed, but increased wall thickness was not. The patients with echocardiographic abnormalities also had abnormal ECG findings and radiographic findings of cardiomegaly. Four of these 7 patients died of congestive heart failure within 30 months of echocardiographic study.

A spectrum of cardiac dysfunction is present in patients with idiopathic hemochromatosis. Patients with severe left ventricular dysfunction have substantially poorer survival than others. The findings show the importance of early detection when left ventricular dysfunction may be preventable or reversible.

▶ The diagnosis of idiopathic hemochromatosis is especially important since it is one of the very few types of myocardial disease in which therapy (phlebotomy) has been demonstrated to improve left ventricular function (Skinner et al.: *Br. Heart J.* 35:466–468, 1983; Candell-Riera et al.: *Am. J. Cardiol.* 52:824–829, 1983; Dabestani et al.: *Am. J. Cardiol.* 54:153–159, 1984). While most patients present as dilated cardiomyopathy, occasional patients have had the syndrome of restrictive cardiomyopathy (Cutler et al.: *Am. J. Med.* 69:923–928, 1980).

Although hemochromatosis is usually less severe in women, it is of interest that 7 of 24 patients in the present series were women, including 3 of 7 patients with cardiac dysfunction. The 3 women in this group were 58, 67, and 80 years of age. Since the incidence of idiopathic hemochromatosis has been estimated to be 2 to 3 per 1,000 and heterozygotes may constitute 10% of the population (Edwards et al.: *Ann. Intern. Med.* 93:519–525, 1980), it behooves all of us to keep a sharp eye out for this potentially treatable form of heart muscle disease.—R.C. Schlant, M.D.

Restrictive Cardiomyopathy Versus Constrictive Pericarditis: Role of Endomyocardial Biopsy in Avoiding Unnecessary Thoracotomy

Mark H. Schoenfeld, Edward W. Supple, G. William Dec, Jr., John T. Fallon, and Igor F. Palacios (Massachusetts Gen. Hosp. and Harvard Univ.)
Circulation 75:1012–1017, May 1987 3–25

It is extremely difficult to differentiate between restrictive cardiomyopathy and constrictive pericarditis. Nevertheless, the distinction between the two diagnoses is of critical importance, for the two disease entities require different management and have different prognoses. Efforts to separate the two diagnoses by means of noninvasive methods have not been successful, and a definitive differential diagnosis between the two disorders still requires exploratory thoracotomy for pericardial evaluation.

Transvenous endomyocardial biopsy has been proved useful in the diagnosis of myocardial disease in patients with symptoms of heart failure of undetermined origin. A study was done to assess the utility of right ventricular endomyocardial biopsy in defining the need for exploratory thoracotomy in patients with symptomatic heart failure resulting from constrictive or restrictive physiology.

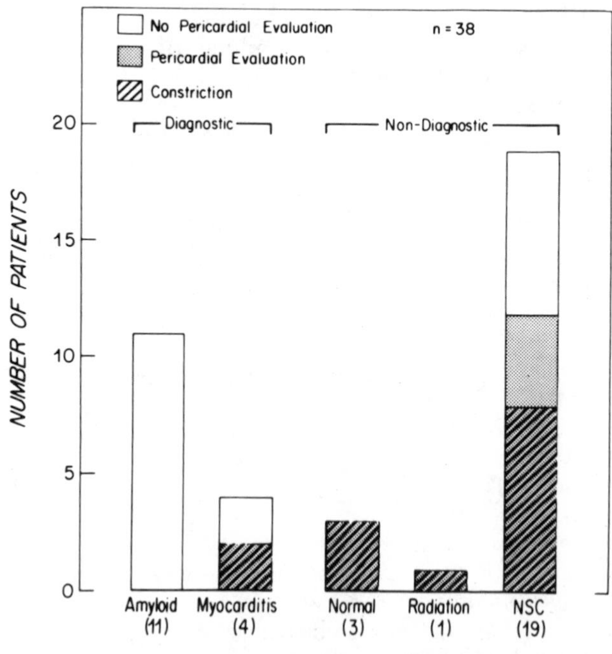

Fig 3–6.—Pathologic diagnosis by right ventricular endomyocardial biospy in 38 patients with severe constrictive/restrictive syndrome (group D). The presence of constriction at the time of pericardial evaluation in 18 of these patients is also shown. NSC, nonspecific changes. (Courtesy of Schoenfeld, M.H., et al.: Circulation 75:1012–1017, May 1987.)

The study comprised 54 patients, 32 men and 22 women aged 22–89 years, who had evidence of constrictive/restrictive physiology. All patients underwent right heart catheterization with right ventricular endomyocardial biopsy and measurement of cardiac output. The patients were subdivided into two groups: group I included 38 patients with profound symptoms of heart failure who were scheduled for exploratory/therapeutic thoracotomy, and group II included 16 patients with milder symptoms.

In group I, endomyocardial biopsy identified a specific source of restrictive cardiomyopathy in 15 patients (39%), namely cardiac amyloidosis (n = 11) and myocarditis (n = 4). Of the remaining 23 patients with normal or nonspecific biopsy findings, 15 underwent thoracotomy and 3 were autopsied, which showed that 14 of 18 patients (77%) had constrictive pericarditis (Fig 3–6). In group II, biopsy findings showed that 4 (25%) of 16 patients had a specific form of restrictive cardiomyopathy, 6 had nonspecific changes, and 6 had normal biopsies.

Endomyocardial biopsy identifies a large subset of patients in whom exploratory thoracotomy should be avoided because of specific forms of restrictive cardiomyopathy (which can be well identified by endomyocardial biopsy).

► The hemodynamic findings of cardiac catheterization often do not distinguish between patients with constrictive pericarditis and those with restrictive cardiomyopathy. Echocardiography was performed in 39 of the 54 patients but was not distinctly helpful. Pericardial thickening was observed in 9 patients, of whom 2 were found not to have constriction intraoperatively. On the other hand, 5 patients thought to have normal pericardial thickness by echocardiography were found to have pericardial constriction at the time of pericardial evaluation.

In patients with the syndrome of constrictive pericarditis-restrictive cardiomyopathy, right ventricular endocardial biopsy is reasonably safe and often clinically useful when performed by experienced operators, although many patients with negative or nondiagnostic changes on endomyocardial biopsy still require exploratory thoracotomy to rule out pericardial constriction. It should be noted that 2 patients in this series who had myocarditis on biopsy were subsequently found to have pericardial constriction as well, indicative of their having had a pancarditis.—R.C. Schlant, M.D.

Pericardial Diseases

Management of Tuberculous Pericarditis

John M. Quale, Gregg Y. Lipschik, and Albert E. Heurich (State Univ. of New York, Brooklyn)

Ann. Thorac. Surg. 43:653–655, June 1987 3–26

Tuberculous pericarditis is found in about 1% of patients with tuberculosis, and mortality in recent series is about 5%. Data on 17 patients who were seen between January 1980 and July 1986 with this diagnosis were reviewed. Mean age of the 17 was 54 years. All had positive pericardial biopsy specimen, or evidence of active extrapericardial disease along with major pericardial effusion or thickening. All had constitutional symptoms, but pericardial signs were infrequent and findings on ECGs usually were nonspecific. Only 7 of 13 patients had a positive tuberculin skin test result. Echocardiography was useful in both diagnosis and management.

Three of 13 patients with effusive pericarditis had medical treatment only and improved, but 1 had later evidence of pericardial thickening. The other 10 patients had surgery as well, usually creation of a pericardial window. One patient required complete pericardiectomy subsequently. Two of 4 patients with constrictive pericarditis died before diagnosis of overwhelming tuberculosis. The other 2 patients did well after treatment.

Tuberculous pericarditis is far from being extinct. Echocardiography is helpful in diagnosing effusive pericarditis and in expediting treatment. The role of steroids remains uncertain. If a major effusion is present in a patient with suspected tuberculous pericarditis, creation of a pericardial window precludes the need for steroid therapy. The authors believe it is not likely that steroids will lower the incidence of late constrictive pericarditis.

▶ The general management of patients with tuberculous pericarditis described is very similar to that now widely employed in the United States. Instead of the creation of a subxiphoid pericardial window, patients with recurrent large effusions may also be treated by pericardiocentesis, which is much more safely performed when guided by two-dimensional echocardiography (Kopecky et al.: *Am. J. Cardiol.* 58:633–635, 1986), followed by percutaneous pericardial catheter drainage. While corticosteroids may often enhance the reabsorption of pericardial fluid, such therapy has not been proven to be of clear benefit either in the short-term management of many patients with pericardial effusion/tamponade or in the prevention of constrictive pericarditis. On the other hand, corticosteroids do appear to temporarily benefit some acutely ill patients with large pericardial effusions who do not respond well to triple-drug therapy for tuberculosis and to pericardiocentesis and drainage. Many of these patients will require pericardiectomy after 4–8 weeks of therapy.—R.C. Schlant, M.D.

Management of Malignant Pericardial Effusion and Tamponade

Oliver W. Press and Robert Livingston (Univ. of Washington and Fred Hutchinson Cancer Research Ctr., Seattle)

JAMA 257:1088–1092, Feb. 27, 1987 3–27

Neoplastic cardiac tamponade is commonly considered a rare condition. An incidence of 11.6% among cancer autopsies has been reported. There is, however, no agreement on its optimal management. While some investigators favor pericardiocentesis with or without sclerotherapy, others advocate surgical decompression and radiation therapy as the treat-

RELATIVE FREQUENCY OF VARIOUS NEOPLASMS IN 789 PATIENTS WITH PERICARDIAL METASTASES

Primary Malignancy	No. (%) of Cases*
Lung	288 (36.5)
Breast	176 (22.3)
Leukemia and lymphoma†	136 (17.2)
Sarcomas	28 (3.5)
Melanoma	21 (2.7)
Stomach	16 (2.0)
Carcinoma of unknown origin	16 (2.0)
Renal	15 (1.9)
Gynecologic	13 (1.6)
Head and neck cancer	11 (1.4)
Colorectal	9 (1.1)
Other	60 (7.6)
Total	**789 (99.8)‡**

*Series describing cardiac metastases specifying pericardial involvement have been omitted. Some cases were described in more than one reference; these have been listed only once in the above tabulation.

†Of the 136 cases of hematologic malignancy, 32 cases were leukemia, 88 were lymphoma, and 16 were not specified.

‡Percentages do not add up to 100% because of rounding.

(Courtesy of Press, O.W., and Livingston, R.: JAMA 257:1088–1092, Feb. 27, 1987.)

ment of choice. Most of the documented cases of pericardial metastasis have occurred secondary to primary lung cancer (36.5%), followed by primary breast cancer (22.3%) and leukemia and lymphoma (17.2%) (table).

Most patients with cardiac and pericardial metastases are clinically asymptomatic. Clinical findings in patients with pericardial metastases who are symptomatic include dyspnea, cough, chest pain, orthopnea, weakness, dysphagia, syncope, and palpitations. These patients usually have nonspecific signs often erroneously attributed to advanced malignancy or congestive heart failure. Echocardiography is the most useful laboratory test for confirming pericardial effusion.

A review of all published data on the treatment of acute neoplastic cardiac tamponade has shown that pericardiocentesis effectively relieves symptoms in 90% of cases, with acceptable risk if performed in a controlled environment. Subxiphoid pericardiotomy is a safe alternative that can be performed under local anesthesia.

It is hoped that neoplastic cardiac tamponade will be recognized earlier in the future, since several effective, durable treatments for this condition are now available.

▶ The long-term management of malignant pericardial effusions varies with the type of tumor involved and other factors. Some hematologic malignancies can be treated by systemic chemotherapy or external radiation, or both. Most malignancies producing symptomatic pericardial effusions can be controlled by the intrapericardial installation of 500–1,000 mg of tetracycline hydrochloride in 20 ml of saline, which is readily instilled through a percutaneous pericardial catheter following the intrapericardial administration of 100 mg of lidocaine. The tetracycline is retained for 1–2 hours and then drained through the catheter. Such therapy may be repeated for 2–3 days (Shepherd et al.: *Am. J. Cardiol.* 60:1161–1166, 1987).

Subxiphoid pericardiectomy is often still very effective and in some patients may be safer than pericardiocentesis. On the other hand, the creation of a pleuropericardial window through an anterior thoracotomy or sternotomy should usually be reserved for patients requiring exploration of other intrathoracic disease, and radical pericardiectomy should be employed only for constrictive pericarditis. External beam radiation is effective in cases of extremely radiosensitive tumors.—R.C. Schlant, M.D.

Disturbances of Cardiac Rhythm and Conduction

Unexplained Sinus Bradycardia: Clinical Significance and Long-Term Prognosis in Apparently Healthy Persons Older Than 40 Years

Donald D. Tresch and Jerome L. Fleg (Natl. Inst. of Aging, Baltimore)
Am. J. Cardiol. 58:1009–1013, November 1986 3–28

Sinus bradycardia (SB) in healthy young adults at rest is common and is considered a manifestation of enhanced vagal tone, often associated with endurance training. However, the significance of SB in clinically healthy, non–endurance-trained, middle-aged and older people is unknown. Sinus bradycardia in this age group was explored in a study of 1,172 healthy volunteers enrolled in the Baltimore Longitudinal Study of Aging.

Of these 1,172 volunteers, 47 persons, aged 58 ± 13 years, with SB of less than 50 beats per minute were identified by resting ECG. They were then compared with a control group matched for age and sex. The prevalence of unexplained SB was about 4% and nearly identical in men and women. At a mean follow-up of 5.4 years, 43% of the group with SB had associated conduction abnormalities, compared with 19% of the control group. Conduction abnormalities seen were first-degree atrioventricular block, left-axis deviation, and complete or incomplete right bundle-branch block (Table 1).

On maximal treadmill exercise testing, performed in 44 patients within 1 year of their most recent examination showing SB, mean maximal heart rate was 157 ± 18 beats per minute; that of control subjects was 163 ± 19 beats per minute. Exercise duration was 11 ± 2.8 minutes in the control subjects and 9.7 ± 3.1 minutes in subjects with SB. No subjects with SB had syncope, high-degree atrioventricular block, or other manifestation of sick sinus syndrome during the follow-up period. Eight percent of subjects with SB and 11% of control subjects had angina pectoris, myocardial infarction, congestive heart failure, or cardiac death during the observation period (Table 2). This difference was not significant.

TABLE 1.—ASSOCIATED ELECTROCARDIOGRAPHIC CONDUCTION ABNORMALITIES *

ECG Findings	Sinus Bradycardia (n = 47)	Control (n = 47)
PR interval >0.20 sec	7 (15%)	2 (4%)
Complete right BBB	5 (11%)	1 (2%)
Incomplete right BBB	6 (13%)	5 (11%)
Left-axis deviation	9 (19%)	5 (11%)
Any of the above	22 (47%)	12 (26%)*

*$P < .05$. BBB = bundle branch block.

(Courtesy of Tresch, D.D., and Fleg, J.L.: Am. J. Cardiol. 58:1009–1013, November 1986.)

TABLE 2.—NEW CARDIAC EVENTS OF ABNORMALITIES IN SUBJECTS WITH FOLLOW-UP*

Event or Abnormality	Sinus Bradycardia (n = 37)	Control (n = 37)
Positive treadmill test	7	5
Positive thallium scan	3 (n = 22)	2 (n = 31)
Angina pectoris	1	3
Myocardial infarction	2	1
Congestive heart failure	0	1
Cardiac death	1	1
Any of the above	11	9

*None of these differences is statistically significant.

(Courtesy of Tresch, D.D., and Fleg, J.L.: Am. J. Cardiol. 58:1009–1013, November 1986.)

This study demonstrated that SB in apparently healthy, nonathletic people older than 40 years is associated with certain abnormalities of atrioventricular or intraventricular conduction. However, it is not associated with chronotropic incompetence with exercise, nor does it appear to adversely affect long-term cardiovascular morbidity or mortality.

▶ The data from this study are reassuring to physicians who find sinus bradycardia in patients between 40 and 90 years of age. It will be important to continue to follow these (and many other) patients since the mean follow-up in this study was only 5.4 ± 3.8 years (median, 4.6).—R.C. Schlant, M.D.

Usefulness of Anticoagulant Therapy in the Prevention of Embolic Complications of Atrial Fibrillation

Denis Roy, Etienne Marchand, Pierre Gagné, Michel Chabot, and Richard Cartier (Univ. of Montreal)

Am. Heart J. 112:1039–1043, November 1986 3–29

Prevention of cardiac embolism is an important concern. This article reviews the usefulness of anticoagulant therapy in the prevention of em-

Incidence of Embolic Events per 100 Patient-Years From Chronic or Paroxysmal Atrial Fibrillation With or Without Anticoagulation Therapy*

	Patient-year follow-up	*Number of embolic events*	*Incidence/100 patient-years*
Without anticoagulation	549	30	5.46
Paroxysmal AF	431	23	5.33
Chronic AF	118	7	5.93
With anticoagulation	284	2	0.70
Paroxysmal AF	188	2	1.06
Chronic AF	97	0	0.0
Total	833	32	3.84

*AF, atrial fibrillation.
(Courtesy of Roy, D., et al.: Am. Heart J. 112:1039–1043, November 1986.)

bolism. The occurrence of embolism was studied retrospectively in 254 patients with atrial fibrillation who either received or did not receive anticoagulation therapy.

During a follow-up period of 833 patient-years, there were 32 embolism events. Thirty of the embolisms occurred in the patients who did not receive embolism therapy during follow-up (table). The incidence of embolism was eight times more frequent in this group, which is statistically significant. This incidence was not affected by the presence of mitral valve disease. The rate of anticoagulation therapy complications was acceptable.

In the population used in this study, anticoagulation therapy reduced the risk of embolism. It appears, then, that anticoagulants should not be limited to patients with mitral valve disease.

▶ The results of this study should be contrasted with those of Kopecky et al. (*N. Engl. J. Med.* 317:669–674, 1987), which suggested that the routine use of coumadin anticoagulation is not justified for all patients younger than 60 years with lone atrial fibrillation. On the other hand, Wolf et al. (*Arch. Intern. Med.* 147:1561–1564, 1987) found in Framingham that chronic nonrheumatic atrial fibrillation was a significant contributor to stroke, and especially in the elderly.

I tend to favor long-term coumadin therapy for many, but not all, patients with chronic atrial fibrillation especially when associated with mitral valve disease or dilated cardiomyopathy, unless there are contraindications or reasons to question the compliance of the patient. In most instances, it is probably satisfactory to use low doses of coumadin to maintain the prothrombin time at only 1.3–1.5 times control unless the patient has a prosthetic mitral valve or other indications for a higher degree of anticoagulation. In patients with mechanical heart valves the addition of dipyridamole (75 mg three times a day) to coumadin therapy appears to be useful in preventing thromboembolic phenomena. In patients with atrial fibrillation who are not given coumadin, enteric-coated aspirin (325 mg daily) is frequently given, although there are no good data currently available to support this practice.—R.C. Schlant, M.D.

Prevention of Atrial Fibrillation or Flutter by Acebutolol After Coronary Bypass Grafting

Patrick Daudon, Thierry Corcos, Iradj Gandjbakhch, Jean-Pierre Levasseur, Annik Cabrol, and Christian Cabrol (Hôpital de la Pitie and the Univ. Pierre et Marie Curie, Paris)

Am. J. Cardiol. 58:933–936, November 1986 3–30

Supraventricular tachyarrhythmias occur postoperatively in 11% to 100% of patients undergoing coronary artery bypass grafting (CABG). These tachyarrhythmias may have deleterious hemodynamic effects and may require urgent drug therapy or even electric cardioversion. The authors evaluated whether acebutolol, a cardioselective β-blocking drug, prevents supraventricular tachyarrhythmias after CABG.

The study population included 100 consecutive patients, aged 30–77 years, who had undergone CABG. Exclusion criteria included contraindications to β-blocking drugs, left ventricular aneurysm, major renal failure, history of cardiac arrhythmia, and cardiac arrhythmia during the immediate postoperative period. From 36 hours after surgery until discharge, 50 patients received acebutolol 200 mg administered orally twice daily. The 50 patients in the control group did not receive β-blocking drugs after surgery. The two groups were comparable in angina functional class, ejection fraction, number of diseased vessels, antianginal therapy before CABG, number of bypassed vessels, and duration of cardiopulmonary bypass. Each of the patients was clinically evaluated twice daily and had continuous ECG monitoring and daily ECGs. A 24-hour continuous ECG was recorded in the last 20 patients. Atrial tachyarrhythmias developed in 20 patients (40%) in the control group (17 patients had atrial fibrillation and 3 had atrial flutter), but in none of the patients in the acebutolol group.

It is concluded that acebutolol is efficacious in the prevention of supraventricular tachyarrhythmias after CABG.

► It is interesting that of the 39 patients in the control group who were receiving β-blocking drugs preoperatively, 18 (46%) had atrial arrhythmia postoperatively when they did not receive a β-blocker. On the other hand, only 2 of the 11 patients in the control group who were not receiving a β-blocker drug preoperatively had such arrhythmias when they did not receive β-blocker therapy postoperatively. In general, it is usually best to continue β-blocker therapy in patients undergoing coronary artery bypass graft surgery or, if they have not been on such therapy, to initiate it preoperatively when possible.

It is uncertain whether or not there is any advantage among the available β-blockers for this purpose. Lamb et al. (*Eur. Heart J.* 9:32–36, 1988) have recently reported that atenolol started 72 hours before operation was effective in reducing supraventricular arrhythmias following elective coronary artery bypass surgery in patients with good left ventricular function. Three of the four studies in which digoxin was used prophylactically to prevent perioperative atrial fibrillation or flutter have also shown a benefit; in general, however, β-adrenoreceptor blocking drugs are usually preferable and satisfactory.—R.C. Schlant, M.D.

Potassium/Magnesium Depletion in Patients With Cardiovascular Disease

Thomas Dyckner and Per Ola Wester (Nacka Hosp., Nacka, and Univ. Hosp., Umeå, Sweden)

Am. J. Med. 82 (Suppl. 3A):11–17, March 20, 1987 3–31

Hypokalemia occurs in up to half of the patients with cardiovascular disease who receive thiazide therapy. Hypokalemia also is seen in acutely ill patients, presumably in association with increased sympathoadrenal activity, and it is related to an increased risk of serious arrhythmias and higher mortality in patients with acute myocardial infarction. It often is assumed that supplemental potassium normalizes potassium status, but this may not be the case. Supplies of intracellular potassium are not readily repleted if magnesium deficiency is present.

Hypomagnesemia is reported in about 40% of hypokalemic patients and in nearly the same proportion of patients with heart failure who receive diuretic therapy. The infusion of magnesium alone increases muscle levels of magnesium and potassium and lowers the frequency of ventricular beats. Both potassium and magnesium are conserved by potassium-sparing agents.

Because the tissue and serum levels of magnesium are not correlated, and correlations for levels of potassium are weak, it is suggested that abnormalities of these electrolytes be prevented and that deficiencies be promptly corrected. In patients for whom the consequences of deficiency would be serious, depletion of both substances can be prevented by administering a potassium–magnesium-sparing diuretic.

▶ Since an increased incidence of ventricular ectopic beats and an increased risk of sudden death may occur in patients receiving chronic diuretic therapy, the findings of this article, which was part of a supplement on "Potassium/Magnesium: Is Your Patient at Risk of Sudden Death?" (*Am. J. Med.* 82 (Suppl. 3A):1–53, March 20, 1987), should be considered in the management of all patients requiring diuretic treatment and other high risk groups such as chronic alcoholism.

There are a number of other, smaller, preliminary reports of the beneficial effect of intravenously administered magnesium in patients with acute myocardial infarction in respect to arrhythmias, size of infarction, and mortality. (Morton et al.: *Magnesium* 3:346–352, 1984; Smith et al.: *Int. J. Cardiol.* 12:175–180, 1986; Rasmussen et al.: *Lancet* 1:551–552, 1986; and Rasmussen et al.: *Clin. Cardiol.* 10:351–353, 1987). The results of all of these studies need to be confirmed by larger, well-controlled clinical trials. I think the importance of magnesium depletion will be increasingly recognized in the coming years. See also the next article (Abstract 3–32).—R.C. Schlant, M.D.

Magnesium in the Prevention of Lethal Arrhythmias in Acute Myocardial Infarction

Abraham S. Abraham, David Rosenmann, Mordechai Kramer, Jonathan Balkin,

Monty M. Zion, Hannan Farbstein, and Uri Eylath (Shaare Zedek Med. Ctr. and Hebrew Univ., Jerusalem, Israel)
Arch. Intern. Med. 147:753–755, April 1987 3–32

The authors had previously found that acute myocardial infarction patients have altered lymphocyte potassium (K) and magnesium (Mg) concentrations. Higher K levels are associated with acute arrhythmias, while high Mg levels are associated with a lower level of arrythmias. The effects of intravenous (IV) magnesium sulfate in 94 patients with acute myocardial infarction were studied in a prospective, randomized, double-blind, placebo-controlled trial.

Of the 48 patients who were given one 2.4-gm dose of magnesium sulphate, 14.6% had potentially lethal arrhythmias during the first 24 hours. Of 46 patients receiving placebo, 34.8% had potentially lethal arrhythmias. The majority of the arrhythmias in the placebo group occurred within 2 hours, while in the Mg group, none occurred for more than 4 hours. After Mg treatment, the serum Mg level rose 16.5%, and lymphocyte Mg concentrations increased 72%.

Magnesium appears to be effective and safe in reducing the incidence of potentially lethal arrythmias in patients with acute myocardial infarction. The correct dosage and regimen, as well as the long-term effects, remain to be determined.

▶ The importance of both potassium and magnesium in the pathogenesis of cardiac arrhythmias has become more and more evident in the last two decades. The results of this study suggest that magnesium sulfate may be of prophylactic value in the prevention of cardiac arrhythmias in patients with acute myocardial infarction. At present, it would seem prudent to correct either hypokalemia or hypomagnesemia in patients with acute myocardial infarction (or in other high-risk groups of patients) to prevent potentially fatal cardiac arrhythmias. Although the present results are very encouraging, additional studies are necessary, however, before one can recommend the routine administration of magnesium for arrhythmia prophylaxis in patients following acute myocardial infarction.

It would be interesting to compare the prophylactic value of lidocaine, magnesium, the combination of lidocaine and magnesium, and placebo in a large group of patients after acute myocardial infarction. Rasmussen et al. (*Arch. Intern. Med.* 148:329–332, 1988), who employed an intravenous loading test of magnesium chloride, found that some patients with ischemic heart disease had severe magnesium deficiency and that the deficiency was more marked in patients receiving long-term diuretic treatment. They also found that the serum magnesium concentration correlated poorly with magnesium retention. See also the preceding article (Abstract 3–31).

Hollenberg and Hollifield have recently edited a symposium entitled "Potassium/Magnesium Depletion: Is Your Patient at Risk of Sudden Death?" (*Am. J. Med.* 82 (Suppl. 3A):1–53, March 20, 1987). The authors of the present article have previously published data suggesting that lymphocyte cation concentrations reflect myocardial interstitial concentrations better than serum levels (Abraham et al.: *Am. J. Med.* 8:983–988, 1986). Perhaps we will soon need to monitor both serum and lymphocyte cation concentrations, although the techniques for the latter are still relatively difficult for most hospital laboratories. Also see Abstract 3–42.—R.C. Schlant, M.D.

Prognosis of Ventricular Arrhythmias in Relation to Sudden Cardiac Death: Therapeutic Implications

Borys Surawicz and Richard L. Roudebush (Indiana Univ. VA Med. Ctr., Indianapolis)

J. Am. Coll. Cardiol. 10:435–447, August 1987 3–33

Ambulatory ECG monitoring has generated data regarding ventricular arrhythmias. The author reviewed data to determine whether ventricular arrhythmias can be used to predict sudden cardiac death.

The frequency and complexity of ventricular arrhythmias increase with age and heart disease severity. Neither simple nor complex arrhythmias increase the risk of sudden cardiac death in subjects without heart disease or in those with heart disease but with normal myocardial function. Ventricular arrhythmia is not an independent predictor of sudden cardiac death after myocardial infarction.

In patients with preserved ventricular function, the use of antiarrhythmic drugs is not indicated. Treatment of asymptomatic or mildly symptomatic ventricular arrhythmias is not likely to reduce the incidence of sudden cardiac death. Ventricular arrhythmias are predictors of sudden cardiac death in patients with obstructive cardiomyopathy, nonsustained ventricular tachycardia, and non-Q wave myocardial infarction survivors; prophylactic therapy is justified for these patients.

▶ The identification of patients with ventricular arrhythmias who should be treated and who should not be treated is a major challenge to cardiology. While this study provides some general guidelines, there is a need for more detailed guidelines, data for which are not available. The problem is compounded by the potential proarrhythmic and other side effects of all available agents (see Abstract 3–34) and by the fact that arrhythmias vary spontaneously without treatment. For example, Pratt et al. (*Am. J. Cardiol.* 56:67–72, 1985) found that in patients with symptomatic but not life-threatening arrhythmias, the number of premature ventricular complexes (PVCs) decreased by 50%, of pairs by 65%, and of ventricular tachycardia by 85% during periods of placebo treatment. Hopefully, the ongoing Cardiac Arrhythmia Suppression Trial (CAST) will provide additional guidelines for the management of patients who survive a myocardial infarction but have PVCs.—R.C. Schlant, M.D.

Proarrhythmic Effects of Antiarrhythmic Drugs During Programmed Ventricular Stimulation in Patients Without Ventricular Tachycardia

Phillip K. Au, Anil K. Bhandari, Randall Bream, Douglas Schreck, Rukhsana Siddiqi, and Shahbudin H. Rahimtoola (Univ. of Southern California, Los Angeles)

J. Am. Coll. Cardiol. 9:389–397, February 1987 3–34

Antiarrhythmic drugs have the capacity to produce ventricular arrhythmias or to aggravate existing arrhythmias. The authors evaluated the proarrhythmic effects of class IA antiarrhythmic drugs during programmed ventricular stimulation in 24 consecutive patients with frequent ventricular premature beats whose baseline study revealed no inducible sustained ventricular arrhythmias.

Sequential stimulation studies using up to three extrastimuli were carried out after administration of procainamide, quinidine, and disopyramide on different days. They defined proarrhythmic response as induction of one or more of the following: sustained monomorphic ventricular tachycardia; sustained polymorphic ventricular tachycardia; ventricular fibrillation; or reproducibly inducible nonsustained monomorphic ventricular tachycardia. During 55 antiarrhythmic drug trials in the 24 patients, 6 patients had a proarrhythmic response. Thus, 11% of drug trials led to a proarrhythmic response, and 25% of the patients responded to one of the drugs tested. A proarrhythmic response to one drug did not predict a similar response to another drug of the same class.

Although the 6 patients with a proarrhythmic response did not differ significantly from the other 18 patients with regard to underlying heart disease, ECG, or baseline 24-hour ambulatory ECG characteristics, they did have a higher incidence of digoxin usage, a shorter baseline right ventricular effective refractory period, and a smaller increment in effective refractory period during antiarrhythmic drug testing. Two of these 6 patients were observed to have clinical occurrence of sustained ventricular arrhythmias while taking an antiarrhythmic agent; all others have continued to do well during a mean follow-up of 9 months.

These results indicate that antiarrhythmic agents may induce ventricular tachyarrhythmias in patients with ventricular premature beats but no prior ventricular tachycardia. This should be taken into consideration when treating patients with ventricular arrhythmias of uncertain prognostic significance.

▶ This is a good study that again documents a proarrhythmic response in a substantial proportion (25%) of patients with premature ventricular contractions treated with class IA antiarrhythmic drugs. All physicians who treat patients with cardiac arrhythmias should consider the potential hazards of such therapy before initiating it. It should be noted that the definition of a proarrhythmic effect varies considerably. Accordingly, the incidence of such an effect can vary depending on the criteria one chooses to use.—R.C. Schlant, M.D.

Influence of Left Ventricular Dysfunction on Flecainide Therapy

Angelo A.V. de Paola, Leonard N. Horowitz, Joel Morganroth, Sheila Senior, Scott R. Spielman, Allan M. Greenspan, and Harold R. Kay (Hahnemann Univ., Philadelphia)

J. Am. Coll. Cardiol. 9:163–168, January 1987 3–35

Flecainide acetate, a benzamide compound with antiarrhythmic action, has been shown to have electrophysiologic properties and to be effective

CONGESTIVE HEART FAILURE DURING FLECAINIDE THERAPY

Previous Functional Class*	No. of Patients	CHF On Flecainide	Death
	Patients With an EF of 30% or Less		
I	18	1	0
II	8	1	0
III/IV	7	5	3
	Patients With an EF Over 30%		
I	35	0	0
II	3	0	0
III/IV	5	0	0

*New York Heart Association functional classification for congestive heart failure (CHF).

(Courtesy of de Paola, A.A.V., et al.: J. Am. Coll. Cardiol. 9:163–168, January 1987.)

in suppressing ventricular arrhythmias. In animals and humans, flecainide has been reported to exert myocardial depressant action, but the clinical importance of this finding has not been clearly defined. A study was done to investigate the influence of left ventricular dysfunction on the results of flecainide therapy in patients with refractory ventricular arrhythmias.

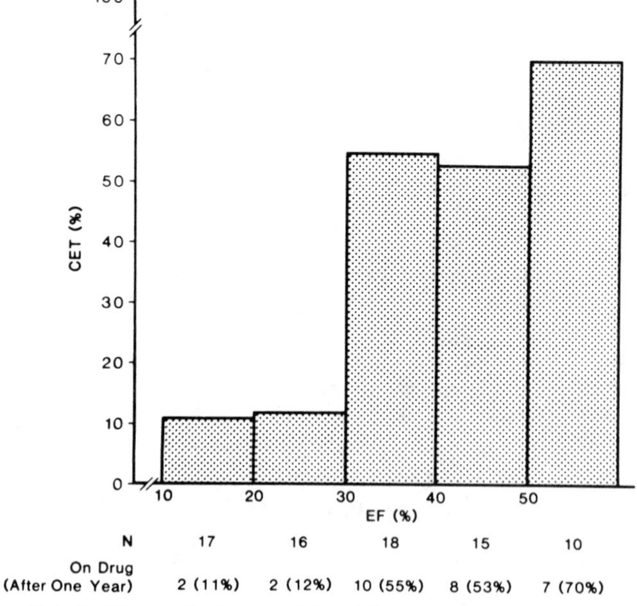

Fig 3–7.—Clinical efficacy and tolerance (CET) of flecainide as a function of EF. Patients were grouped by EF on the abscissa. After 1 year, CET was significantly greater in patients with EF greater than 30% compared with patients with an EF of 30% or less. (Courtesy of de Paola, A.A.V., et al.: J. Am. Coll. Cardiol. 9:163–168, January 1987.)

The 40 patients with sustained ventricular tachycardia and 36 patients with nonsustained ventricular tachycardia were treated with a mean oral dose of 150 mg of flecainide twice a day. The mean plasma concentration was 720 ng/ml. The baseline radionuclide left ventricular EF was 30% or less in 33 patients and more than 30% in 43 patients. Compensated heart failure was present in 23 patients before therapy; the EF was 30% or less in 15 and more than 30% in 8. New or worsened congestive heart failure was seen in 7 patients receiving flecainide therapy, all of whom had an EF of 30% or less (table). Six of these patients had a history of heart failure; of these, 3 died. The only independent variable that significantly affected the clinical efficacy and tolerance (CET) of flecainide was EF (Fig 3–7). After 1 year of therapy, the CET was 58% in patients with an EF greater than 30% and 12% in those with an EF of 30% or less.

Congestive heart failure can occur in patients receiving flecainide therapy, especially those with a history of congestive heart failure and an EF of 30% or less. The CET of flecainide was also found to be significantly lower in patients with an EF of 30% or less.

▶ The message here is not to use flecainide in patients with an ejection fraction less than 30% unless the patient is hospitalized and does not respond to other agents. Disopyramide may also produce significant depression of left ventricular function.—R.C. Schlant, M.D.

Nitrous Oxide and Dysrhythmias

Michael F. Roizen, Glenn O. Plummer, and J. Lance Lichtor (Univ. of California, San Francisco, Anesthesia Service Med. Group, San Diego, Calif., and Univ. of Chicago)

Anesthesiology 66:427–431, March 1987 3–36

Nitrous oxide is often used as an adjunct anesthesia agent. The authors describe a patient in whom nitrous oxide induced atrioventricular junctional rhythm (AVJR). This phenomenon was investigated in an additional nine patients.

Man, 24, scheduled for bone grafting, was given 10 mg of diazepam and 10 mg of morphine sulfate. After 1.5 hours, he was brought to the operating room and given 100% oxygen. He was then given 700 μg of fentanyl, 3 mg of d-tubocurarine, 300 mg of thiopental, and 120 mg of succinylcholine. After endotracheal intubation, he was given 1800 μg of fentanyl. Ventilation with 90% oxygen and 10% nitrous oxide was instituted. After 90 minutes, his heart rate increased, systolic blood pressure rose, and the patient began to move. In response, nitrous oxide was increased to 70%. Within 3 minutes, AVJR had replaced normal sinus rhythm. Nitrous oxide was stopped, and within 3 minutes normal sinus rhythm was reestablished. This pattern was repeated six times.

The relationship between nitrous oxide and AVJR was examined in nine patients, with nitrogen substituted for nitrous oxide during periods of AVJR. Five patients developed AVJR whenever nitrous oxide was administered, and returned to normal sinus rhythm after nitrogen was substituted. In one patient, sinus rhythm did not return for 30 minutes. In another patient, after the initial AVJR and return to normal sinus rhythm, AVJR did not return. In two patients, AVJR returned to sinus rhythm initially after nitrogen was substituted, but did not return subsequently.

These ten patients demonstrate that nitrous oxide can cause AVJR in the presence of a narcotic or volatile anesthetic. Further studies of this phenomenon are necessary to determine the frequency with which this occurs.

▶ Since nitrous oxide is so widely used in anesthesia and has even been recommended to treat the pain of myocardial ischemia (Kerr, F., et al.: *Lancet* 1:63–66, 1972), it is important that the findings in this report be confirmed or disproven. Initially, one is tempted to think that the phenomenon could not be very frequent or it would have been noted previously.—R.C. Schlant, M.D.

Amiodarone

Jay W. Mason (Univ. of Utah)
N. Engl. J. Med. 316:455–466, Feb. 19, 1987 3–37

Amiodarone is an antiarrhythmic agent that remains in the body following long-term treatment. It has been noted to interact with many other drugs (Table 1). Amiodarone prolongs repolarization in myocardial tissue and has a depressant effect on the sinus and atrioventricular nodes. Intravenously administered amiodarone reduces cardiac contractility, but it may improve cardiac performance by increasing coronary flow and lowering systemic vascular resistance.

Amiodarone is relatively effective and safe in the treatment of supraventricular arrhythmias and ventricular arrhythmias. More than half

TABLE 1.—Interactions of Amiodarone With Other Drugs

Drug	Result of Interaction	Reference Nos.
Pharmacokinetic interactions		
Aprindine	Increased aprindine concentration	34
Digoxin	Increased digoxin concentration	35–38
Flecainide	Increased flecainide concentration	39
Phenytoin	Increased phenytoin concentration	40,41
Procainamide	Increased procainamide concentration	42
Quinidine	Increased quinidine concentration	3,42
Warfarin	Increased warfarin concentration and effect	43–46
Pharmacodynamic interactions		
Catecholamines	α- and β-Adrenergic antagonism	47–51
Diltiazem	Sinus arrest and hypotension	52
Propranolol	Bradycardia, sinus arrest	53
Quinidine	Torsades de pointes ventricular tachycardia	3,54

(Courtesy of Mason, J.W.: N. Engl. J. Med 316:455–466, Feb. 19, 1987.)

TABLE 2.—REPORTED SIDE EFFECTS OF AMIODARONE*

Cardiac	Neurologic
Sinus bradycardia	Central nervous system
Heart block	Peripheral neuropathy
Congestive failure	**Ocular**
Proarrhythmia	Corneal deposits
PM capture failure	Impaired vision
Increased DFT	**Dermatologic**
Pulmonary	Photosensitivity
Dysfunction	Blue discoloration
Pneumonitis	**Thyroid**
Asthma exacerbation	Hypothyroidism
Gastrointestinal	Hyperthyroidism
Increased transaminases	**Other**
Hepatitis	Epididymitis
Intolerance	Increased blood glucose
Renal	Increased triglycerides
Renal dysfunction	

*PM denotes artificial pacemaker; DFT, cardiac defibrillation threshold.

(Courtesy of Mason, J.W.: N. Engl. J. Med. 316:455–466, Feb. 19, 1987.)

of patients with previously refractory ventricular tachyarrhythmia can be expected to respond at 1 year. Many adverse effects have been documented, including exacerbations of arrhythmia, hepatitis, pneumonitis, and worsening of congestive heart failure (Table 2). Prompt withdrawal of treatment leaves drugs in the body, and it has been suggested that amiodarone not be used if alternatives are available.

The precise role of amiodarone in the management of sustained, life-threatening ventricular tachycardia or fibrillation remains to be established. Further work is needed in comparing amiodarone with other drugs and placebo for efficacy and in elucidating the causes of toxicity from amiodarone.

▶ It is important that all physicians who may treat patients with amiodarone be thoroughly familiar with its many side effects, its many interactions with other drugs, and the incidence of major adverse effects. For the present, I agree with Jay Mason that "the decision to initiate therapy with amiodarone and the responsibility for monitoring its use should be left to cardiologists who specialize in arrhythmia management in centers where all therapies are available." Also see the following abstract (3–38).—R.C. Schlant, M.D.

Thyroid Dysfunction During Chronic Amiodarone Therapy

Stewart G. Albert, Larry E. Alves, and Edward P. Rose (St. Louis Univ., St. Louis, and Memorial Hosp., Belleville, Il.)

J. Am. Coll. Cardiol. 9:175–183, January 1987 3–38

Amiodarone is an iodinated organic compound with substantial antiarrhythmic properties; it may also interfere with normal thyroid hormone dynamics. The authors analyzed clinical and laboratory features of 99 patients receiving long-term amiodarone therapy to determine which individuals may be at a high risk for developing amiodarone-induced thyroid dysfunction.

The study group included 68 men and 31 women who were followed up for an average of 27 months. There were no differences in age, sex, dose of amiodarone, type of severity of underlying heart disease, or baseline serum throxine levels in patients who developed hypothyroidism (32 patients) or hyperthyroidism (5 patients) or who remained euthyroid (62 patients). Although the baseline serum thyrotropin levels were statistically higher in patients who became hypothyroid, there was considerable overlap with the other patient groups. Serum reverse triiodothyronine correlated directly with serum thyroxine levels and was not an independent variable. There was no pattern to the time course for development of thyroid dysfunction, which occurred in 49% of those followed up and developed as early as 1 month or as late as after 3 years of amiodarone therapy.

There are few guidelines for replacement therapy in patients with amiodarone-induced hypothyroidism. The L-thyroxine dosage was adjusted cautiously in these high-risk individuals to achieve serum thyroxine levels within the reference range of euthyroid individuals taking amiodarone. Normalization of serum thryotropin would have required excessively high doses of L-thyroxine. Serum cholesterol levels increased in the entire group during the course of amiodarone administration and remained elevated. This degree of hypercholesterolemia is clinically significant, especially in persons with underlying heart disease. The cause and type of hypercholesteremia were not determined.

Amiodarone may cause abnormalities of thyroid function testing in all individuals. There were no clinical features useful for predicting who would develop thyroid dysfunction.

▶ This is yet another warning of potentially serious side effects of amiodarone. One hopes that the search chemists are very busy modifying its molecule and searching for an analog that maintains most of its benefits but with fewer of its many disadvantages and hazards. Also see the preceding abstract (3–38). —R.C. Schlant, M.D.

The Signal-Averaged Electrocardiogram as a Screening Test for Inducibility of Sustained Ventricular Tachycardia in High Risk Patients: A Prospective Study

Peter C. Nalos, Eli S. Gang, William J. Mandel, Marc L. Ladenheim, Yoram Lass, and Thomas Peter (Cedars-Sinai Med. Ctr., Los Angeles)

J. Am. Coll. Cardiol. 9:539–548, March 1987 3–39

Recently, signal averaging of the surface ECG has been shown to be a useful technique in identifying patients at risk for ventricular tachycardia and sudden death. The authors prospectively assessed the clinical value of the signal-averaged ECG in a large group of consecutive high-risk patients referred for programmed ventricular stimulation, using a standardized stimulation protocol.

The study group included 100 patients with presenting diagnoses of syncope (38 patients), nonsustained ventricular tachycardia (24 patients), sustained ventricular tachycardia (25 patients), and sudden cardiac arrest (13 patients). When programmed ventricular stimulation was used, 71 patients (group 1) did not have and 29 patients (group II) did have inducible sustained monomorphic ventricular tachycardia. The two groups were compared using the signal-averaged ECG with filtering at high pass corner frequencies of 67 and 100 Hz. The signal-averaged ECG was considered normal if all of the following criteria were satisfied: the total filtered QRS complex duration was greater than 120 ms; the duration of the terminal QRS complex of less than or equal to 20 μV was greater than or equal to 30 ms; and at least one deflection (late potential) was present in this region.

Differences between groups I and II in these three measures were highly significant. The sensitivity and specificity of signal averaging for predicting the induction of sustained ventricular tachycardia were 93% and 94%, respectively. Using stepwise logistic regression analysis, the signal-averaged ECG was identified as the best predictor of induction of sustained monomorphic ventricular tachycardia, independent of left ventricular ejection fraction, presence of ventricular aneurysm, myocardial infarction, and other clinical variables.

The signal-averaged ECG is a sensitive and specific test for the induction of sustained monomorphic ventricular tachycardia, having independent predictive value.

▶ This study contributes to the literature indicating the potential clinical value of the signal-averaging ECG in a specific group of highly selected patients. Buckingham et al. (*Am. J. Cardiol.* 59:568–592, 1987) found that the presence of late potentials by signal averaged electrocardiography was useful in identifying patients with prior sustained ventricular tachycardia (VT) independent of ventricular function. Buxton et al. (*Am. J. Cardiol.* 60:80–85, 1987) found that the signal-averaged ECG measurements in patients with anterior myocardial infarction and inducible sustained VT or with nonsustained VT did not differ from those in patients without such findings, whereas the measurements in patients with inferior infarction and spontaneous nonsustained VT were intermediate between the control group without arrhythmias and the control group with sustained VT. Kuchar et al. (*Am. J. Cardiol.* 58:949–953, 1986) and Gang et al. (*Am. J. Cardiol.* 58:1014–1020, 1986) have reported the value of the technique in the study of patients with syncope due to ventricular tachycardia.

There is a great need for larger studies to further document the value of this technique in other groups of patients and also to determine better both the optimal technique for recording signal-averaging ECG (high and low pass filter levels, etc.) and the criteria for defining an abnormal signal-averaged ECG. There is considerable variation between the characteristics of the commercially available instruments and a need for well-established criteria. One hopes that as this promising technique develops further, there will be sufficient data on which such standards can be based and incorporated into the instruments. In addition, the cost-benefit ratio of this new, investigative procedure needs to be better defined before the procedure is applied widely.—R.C. Schlant, M.D.

Automatic Implantable Cardioverter-Defibrillator: Patient Survival, Battery Longevity and Shock Delivery Analysis

Mark D. Gabry, Richard Brodman, Debra Johnston, Rosemary Frame, Soo G. Kim, Lawrence E. Waspe, John D. Fisher, and Seymour Furman (Montefiore Med. Ctr., Bronx, N.Y.)

J. Am. Coll. Cardiol. 9 :1349–1356, June 1987 3–40

Automatic implantable cardioverter-defibrillators (AICD) are used to reduce mortality in patients with malignant ventricular tachycardias. The authors describe the use of 36 AICDs in 22 patients over a 44-month period.

Five patients died during this period. Two patients died suddenly, 1 died of congestive heart failure, 1 died of respiratory failure, and 1 died of catheter sepsis. Eleven patients received one or more countershocks during the follow-up period. Nine patients also received unnecessary shocks. In the absence of the AICD, the hypothetical cumulative survival would have been 34 ± 14.1%, instead of the actual rate of 59 ± 16.8%. No AICD lasted longer than 22 months. There were 12 battery depletions during this time. The number of shocks did not affect the life of the unit. Six units remained active 7–17 months after the AICD elective replacement indicator showed inactivity.

The AICD prolongs the life of patients with intractable arrhythmias. However, there are problems with the current AICDs. The device gives unnecessary shocks, its battery has a very limited life, it is not programmable, its replacement indicator is not reliable, and it has an inadequate follow-up system.

▶ This exciting field is developing rapidly, with new and improved devices frequently becoming available. Further data are needed to help physicians select patients to have this very expensive device implanted.—R.C. Schlant, M.D.

The Management of Preexcitation Syndromes

Hein J.J. Wellens, Pedro Brugada, and Olaf C. Penn (Academic Hosp. of Maastricht, Univ. of Limberg, Maastricht, The Netherlands)

JAMA 257:2325–2333, May 1, 1987 3–41

New techniques, such as epicardial mapping and programmed stimulation of the heart, have made a better understanding of ventricular preexcitation possible. These methods are reviewed and their use in the treatment of patients with preexcitation syndromes is discussed.

There are several pathways by which a part or the whole ventricle can

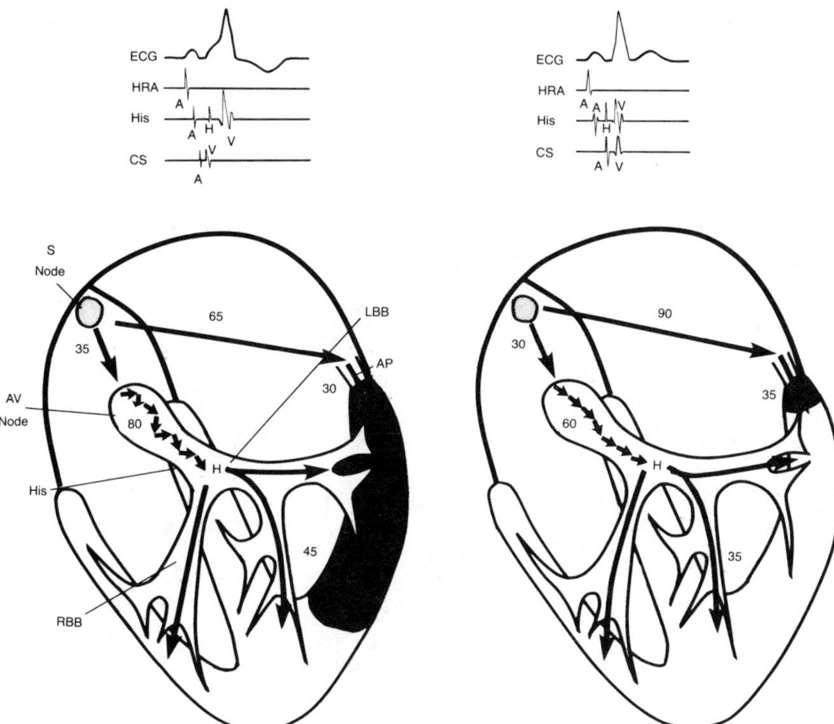

Fig 3–8.—Factors determining degree of preexcitation in left-sided accessory atrioventricular (AV) pathway during sinus rhythm. On *left*, because of shorter conduction time from sinus node (S node) to ventricle over accessory pathway (65 + 30 = 95 ms vs 35 + 80 + 45 = 160 ms over normal AV conduction system), important part of ventricle is preexcited, resulting in ECG with short PR interval, clear delta wave, and widened QRS complex *(top of figure)*. This is in contrast with situation on *right* where activation of ventricle starts simultaneously over normal AV conduction system (30 + 60 + 35 = 125 ms) and accessory pathway (90 + 35 = 125 ms). This leads to ECG with longer PR interval, hardly any delta wave, and a more narrow QRS complex *(top of figure)*. RBB, right bundle branch; LBB, left bundle branch; HRA, high right atrium; CS, coronary sinus; H, His bundle; and AP, accessory pathway. (Courtesy of Wellens, H.J.J., et al.: JAMA 257:2325–2333, May 1, 1987.)

TABLE 1.—OLD AND NEW NOMENCLATURE OF ACCESSORY CONNECTIONS

Nomenclature			
Old	**Symbol in Fig 1**	**New**	**Connections**
Kent's bundle	K	Accessory atrioventricular pathway	Atrium to ventricle
Mahaim fiber	M_1	Nodoventricular pathway*	Atrioventricular node to ventricle
Mahaim fiber	M_2	Fasciculoventricular pathway	His bundle or bundle branch to ventricle
Atrio-Hissian fiber	A	Atriofascicular bypass tract	Atrium to His bundle
James fiber	J	Intranodal bypass tract	Atrium to atrioventricular node

*The fiber may insert into the bundle branch and is then called a nodofascicular fiber.
(Courtesy of Wellens, H.J.J., et al.: JAMA 257:2325–2333, May 1, 1987.)

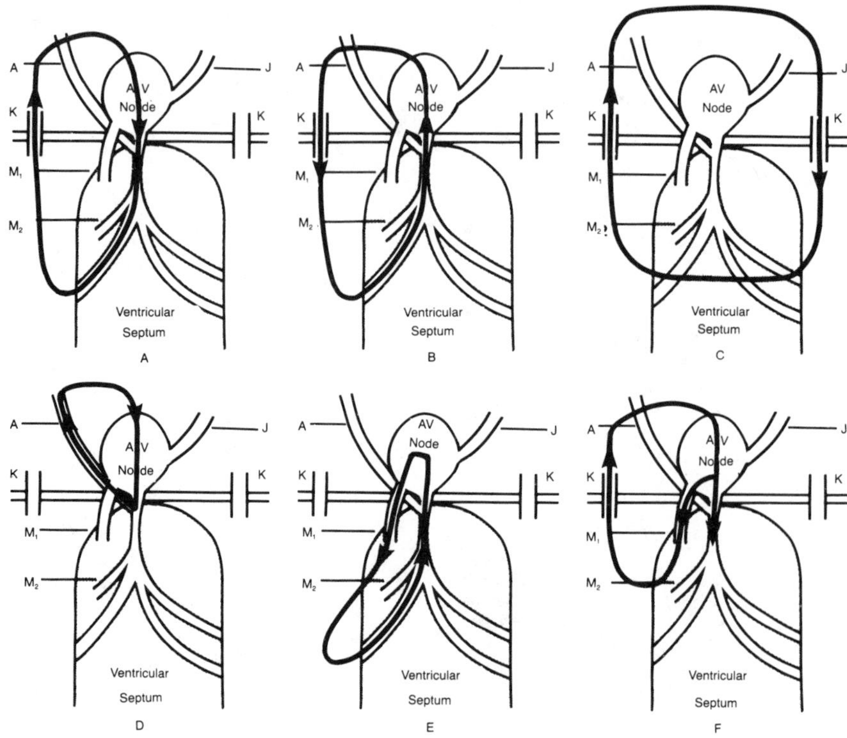

Fig 3–9.—Some examples of possible reentry circuits in patients with accessory connections. **A,** classic orthodromic circus movement tachycardia using atrioventricular (AV) node–His pathway in anterograde and accessory pathway in retrograde direction. **B,** antidromic circus movement tachycardia showing reversed direction of tachycardia shown in **A. C,** tachycardia circuit using one accessory AV pathway for anterograde and another accessory AV pathway for retrograde conduction. **D,** circuit using AV node and atriofascicular bypass tract. **E,** tachycardia circuit with anterograde conduction over nodoventricular fiber and retrograde conduction over bundle branch–His system. **F,** circus movement tachycardia with anterograde conduction over nodoventricular fiber and retrograde conduction over accessory AV pathway. (Courtesy of Wellens, H.J.J., et al.: JAMA 257:2325–2333, May 1, 1987.)

be activated earlier than expected (Table 1). The most common type is an accessory atrioventricular (AV) pathway or Kent's bundle. In case of ventricle activation over two pathways, a fusion QRS complex results on ECG whose configuration depends on the contribution of each of the two activation fronts (Fig 3–8). An ECG showing a classic Wolff-Parkinson-White syndrome is not always present.

The ECG form depends on the amount of ventricular muscle activated over the accessory AV pathway. Important factors to consider include the location of the accessory pathway, site of atrial impulse formation in relation to the location of the accessory pathway, atria size, and transmission characteristics of the AV node and accessory AV pathway. Pathways leading to ventricular preexcitation may be incorporated in several different types of reentry circuits (Fig 3–9). The circus movement tachycardia and atrial fibrillation are the most common types of arrhythmias in patients with preexcitation. In circus movement tachycardia, a critically

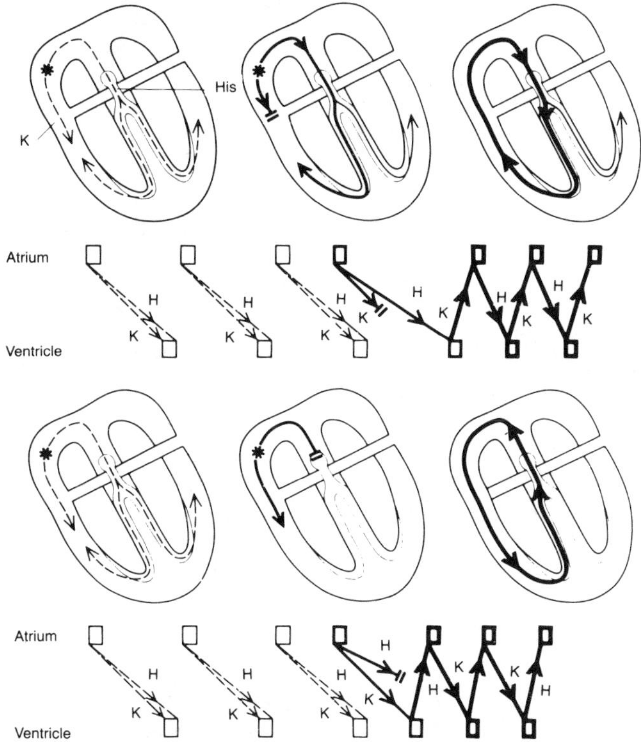

Fig 3–10.—Mode of initiation of circus movement tachycardia by atrial premature beat. Critically timed atrial premature beat during atrial pacing leads in *upper panel* to unidirectional block in accessory pathway. Atrioventricular (AV) conduction over AV node–His pathway is followed by othrodromic circus movement tachycardia. Initiation of reversed (antidromic) type of circus movement tachycardia is shown in *lower panel*. Electrocardiogram during orthodromic circus movement tachycardia will show disappearance of delta wave, while delta wave will become more prominent during antidromic circus movement tachycardia. K, accessory pathway; H, His bundle. (Courtesy of Wellens, H.J.J., et al.: JAMA 257:2325–2333, May 1, 1987.)

timed atrial premature beat that finds the accessory pathway to be refractory is conducted from atrium to ventricle over the AV node-His pathway only and returns from ventricle to atrium over the accessory pathway (Fig 3–10).

It is now known how different drugs affect the properties of the AV node-His pathway and the accessory AV pathway (Fig 3–11). The necessity and mode of treatment depend on the incidence and severity of the tachycardia attacks. Certain patient maneuvers should be attempted if the problem is a rare circus movement tachycardia without serious hemodynamic consequences (Table 2). If these fail, patients should take a medication such as quinidine or disopyramide phosphate by mouth and wait for the arrhythmia to subside. Certain steps should be taken in treating persistent arrhythmia or preventing a recurrent one (Table 3).

Depending on the electrophysiologic properties of the accessory connection and of the accessory pathway and other cardiac structures, atrial

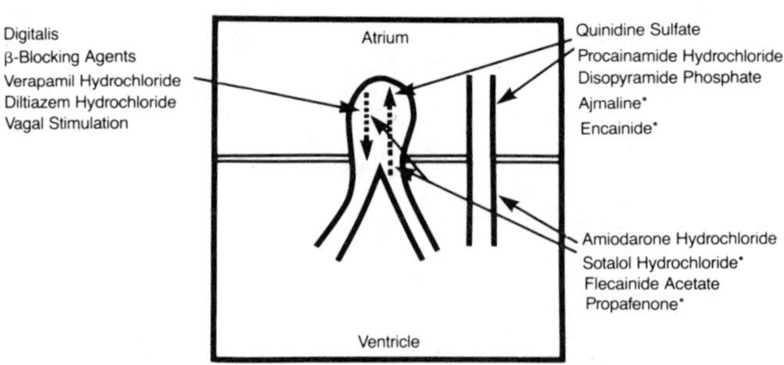

Fig 3–11.—Site of prolongation of refractory period in atrioventricular nodal–His pathway and accessory atrioventricular pathway by different drugs. Note that several drugs have effect on both pathways. Note also that some drugs, for example quinidine sulfate, lengthen refractory period of accessory pathway and refractory period in retrograde direction in His–AV node pathway. Drugs indicated by an asterisk are investigational in the United States. (Courtesy of Wellens, H.J.J., et al.: JAMA 257:2325–2333, May 1, 1987.)

fibrillation and circus movement tachycardia may result in a relatively benign arrhythmia or a life-threatening situation. To effectively diagnose ventricular preexcitation, physicians need an understanding of the different possible accessory connections of the cardiac conduction system and their effect on the ECG.

TABLE 2.—Maneuvers Used to Interrupt a Supraventricular Tachycardia

Valsalva	"Upside-down position" (legs against the wall)
Squatting (Valsalva maneuver)	"Dive reflex" (immersion of the face in cold water)
"Gag" reflex (finger in the throat)	

(Courtesy of Wellens, H.J.J., et al.: JAMA 257:2325–2333, May 1, 1987.)

TABLE 3.—Treatment of Tachycardia in Patients With Preexcitation

Circus Movement Tachycardia	Atrial Fibrillation
Treatment during an attack	Treatment
Vagal maneuvers	Hemodynamically intolerable: direct current shock
Verapamil hydrochloride, 10 mg intravenously	Hemodynamically tolerated: procainamide, ajmaline, disopyramide phosphate
Diltiazem hydrochloride,* 0.25 mg/kg intravenously	Prophylaxis
Adenosine phosphate, 37.5 μg/kg intravenously, same dosage may be repeated at 1-min intervals	Amiodarone
Ajmaline,* 1 mg/kg intravenously	Sotalol*
Procainamide hydrochloride, 10 mg/kg intravenously	Quinidinelike drugs plus β-blocking agent
Pacing	
Direct current shock	
Prophylaxis	
Amiodarone hydrochloride	
Class Ic drugs: Propafenone*, Flecainide acetate, Encainide*	
Sotalol hydrochloride*	
Quinidinelike drugs	

*Drugs marked by an asterisk are investigational in the United States.
(Courtesy of Wellens, H.J.J., et al.: JAMA 257:2325–2333, May 1, 1987.)

▶ This is a very important article that elegantly and practically summarizes the modern diagnosis and management of preexcitation syndromes. Many advances have been made in this field in recent years, and I would urge physicians to reread this article whenever they see a patient with a preexcitation syndrome. Also see the following two abstracts (3–42 and 3–43).—R.C. Schlant, M.D.

The Localization Bypass Tracts in the Wolff-Parkinson-White Syndrome From the Surface Electrocardiogram

G. Veerender Reddy and Leo Schamroth (VA Med. Ctr., Wilmington, Del., and Univ. of the Witwatersrand, Johannesburg, Republic of South Africa)

Am. Heart J. 113:984–993, April 1987 3–42

The bypass tracts of the Wolff-Parkinson-White syndrome can be located anywhere along the atrioventricular (AV) ring. Although ten potential sites have been described, more than 90% of such tracts occur at four sites: right lateral pathway (18%), left lateral pathway (46%), right and left posteroseptal pathways (26%), and right and left anteroseptal pathways (10%). Left lateral pathways are most common, and anteroseptal pathways are least common. These sites can be localized fairly accurately from the surface ECG.

Localization is based on analysis of the delta-wave and QRS deflections. It is best derived from a 12-lead ECG showing maximal preexcitation. A normal PR interval does not necessarily suggest preexcitation through a Mahaim fiber. The main QRS deflection is the dominant and terminal part of the QRS complex and excludes the delta wave. Right lateral pathways tend to have mean manifest QRS axes in the region of −60 degrees (a marked left axis deviation). Posteroseptal pathways tend to have mean manifest QRS axes in the region of 0 degrees counterclockwise to −30 degrees (a moderate left axis deviation). The polarity of the main QRS deflection in leads V_1–V_3, taken in conjunction, are important distinguishing features for locating the bypass sites. The polarity of the delta waves in the horizontal plane is not as definitive as the polarity in the frontal plane. Negative delta waves in leads V_5 and V_6 may indicate a left lateral bypass tract. Generally, the delta wave is isoelectric in lead V_1 and often in V_2 in right-sided pathways. The delta wave is positive in lead V_1 in left-sided accessory pathways. Evaluation of the delta-wave polarity alone in lead V_1, however, is usually not helpful; it should be considered in conjunction with the QRS complex in lead V_1 and the delta wave and QRS complex in lead V_2 (table).

Accurate localization of the bypass tracts of the Wolff-Parkinson-White syndrome has largely been done by electrophysiologic studies in the past. However, criteria for localizing the bypass tracts from the conventional 12-lead ECG have become increasingly clear in recent years.

▶ This is an excellent review and summation of criteria to localize accurately the most frequent types of ventricular preexcitation through accessory bypass

POLARITY OF DELTA WAVES AND QRS COMPLEXES

Pathway	*Delta wave* *Lead V_1*	*QRS complex* *Lead V_1*	*Lead V_2*
Right posteroseptal	Isoelectric or negative	Dominantly negative	Positive
Left posteroseptal	Positive (always)	Dominantly positive or equiphasic	Positive

(Courtesy of Reddy, G.V., and Schamroth, L.: Am. Heart J. 113:984–993, April 1987.)

tracts from the conventional 12-lead ECG. Many cardiologists will recognize that the left lateral accessory pathway is equivalent to type C of Pick and Lagendorf; the right lateral accessory pathway is equivalent to type B of Rosenbaum; and the left posteroseptal pathway is equivalent to type A of Rosenbaum. With the increasing use of techniques to interrupt such pathways, the noninvasive localization of pathways assumes greater importance, although the conclusions must still be confirmed by electrophysiologic study prior to any invasive, therapeutic procedure. Also see the preceding and succeeding abstracts (3–41 and 3–43).—R.C. Schlant, M.D.

Sotalol in Patients With Wolff-Parkinson-White Syndrome

Klaus-Peter Kunze, Michael Schlüter and Karl-Heinz Kuck (Univ. Hosp. Eppendorf, Hamburg, West Germany)

Circulation 75:1050–1057, May 1987 3–43

Sotalol is a β-blocking agent with class III antiarrhythmic action. The effects of intravenously (1.5 mg/kg of body weight) and orally (240–320 mg per day) administered sotalol were investigated in 17 patients with an accessory atrioventricular (AV) pathway.

Both forms of sotalol caused significant increases in sinus cycle length, AV nodal conduction time, and myocardial and accessory pathway refraction length. Before sotalol treatment, AV reciprocating tachycardia was inducible and sustained in 15 patients. After sotalol therapy, AV tachycardia was still inducible in 14 patients; however, it was no longer sustained in 10 of these patients. Follow-up of 16 patients receiving orally administered sotalol was 1–43 months; 15 of these patients were clinically free of symptoms or experienced major improvement. In the other patient, sotalol was discontinued because of recurrent supraventricular tachycardia.

Orthostatic hypotension occurred in 5 patients, and sotalol withdrawal was necessary in 1 of these patients. Programmed electrical stimulation predicted clinical outcome with intravenously administered sotalol correctly 63% of the time and with orally administered sotalol 86% of the time. Exercise testing and Holter monitoring did not have predictive value.

Long-term treatment with sotalol is effective in patients with Wolff-Parkinson-White syndrome and supraventricular tachycardia.

► The management of patients with the Wolff-Parkinson-White syndrome and regular supraventricular tachycardia has been a difficult clinical problem. On the basis of this study, as well as those of Simon (*J. Clin. Pharmacol.* 19:547–556, 1979) and of Touboul et al. (*Am. Heart J.* 114:545–550, 1987) sotalol should also be considered in the treatment of patients with the Wolff-Parkinson-White syndrome who have episodes of regular supraventricular tachycardia certainly before amiodarone. Also see abstracts 3–41 and 3–42.—R.C. Schlant, M.D.

Electrophysiologic Testing and Follow-up of Patients With Aborted Sudden Death

Michael Eldar, Mary Jane Sauve and Melvin M. Scheinman (Univ. of California, San Francisco)

J. Am. Coll. Cardiol. 10:291–298, August 1987 3–44

Patients whose sudden cardiac death has been prevented have a 45% rate of recurrent cardiac death within 2 years. Clinical, electrophysiologic, and follow-up data were analyzed for 108 patients with aborted sudden death to determine the efficacy of standard therapy. Seventy-five patients, had inducible ventricular arrhythmias (group I) and 33 patients had no inducible arrhythmias (group II).

In 17 patients, treatment guided by electrophysiologic testing was used. Standard treatment included quinidine, procainamide, disopyramide, lidocaine, phenytoin, and verapamil. In 13 patients in group I, their arrhythmias became noninducible and 4 patients had sustained arrhythmias that became nonsustained after therapy. There was a significantly higher rate of sudden death and recurrent ventricular tachycardia in the patients with inducible arrhythmias. In the entire patient group, the incidence of sudden death during a mean 2-year follow-up period was 11%, and 15% had recurrence of ventricular tachycardia. Amiodarone was used to treat 64 patients; 6 (6%) of these patients died suddenly and 9 (14%) had recurrent tachycardia.

There was a significant recurrence of life-threatening ventricular arrhythmias in patients with aborted sudden death who were given standard therapy. This indicates the limitations of standard therapy for these patients.

▶ All of the 108 patients in this study underwent drug-free invasive electrophysiologic studies. In 69% of the patients with aborted sudden death, ventricular arrhythmia could be induced but inducibility could be suppressed in only 20%, making it difficult to assess the role of therapy guided by electrophysiologic testing. Nevertheless, I believe one should consider such invasive testing and guided therapy in most patients with aborted sudden death. In patients whose condition is not controlled by other drugs, amiodarone may be useful, as well as the use of an automatic implantable cardioverter-defibrillator (AICD) device as described in Abstract 3–40.—R.C. Schlant, M.D.

Spontaneous Arrhythmia Detected on Ambulatory Electrocardiographic Recording Lacks Precision in Predicting Inducibility of Ventricular Tachycardia During Electrophysiologic Study

Craig M. Pratt, Beth C. Thornton, Sharon A. Magro, and Christopher R.C. Wyndham (Baylor College of Med. and The Methodist Hosp., Houston)

J. Am. Coll. Cardiol. 10:97–104, July 1987 3–45

The relationship of spontaneous ventricular arrhythmia to ventricular tachycardia induced during programmed electrical stimulation was investigated in 80 patients. These patients had sustained ventricular tachycardia, sudden death followed by resuscitation, ventricular fibrillation, or syncope. All patients were monitored by ambulatory electrocardiography and received programmed electrical stimulation.

Programmed electrical stimulation induced ventricular tachycardia, which required intervention in 53 patients. Ambulatory ECG results could not be used to predict which patients would develop ventricular tachycardia during stimulation. Of the 53 patients in whom tachycardia developed during stimulation, 25% did not have any spontaneous arrhythmia, 28% had no couplets, and 55% did not have nonsustained ventricular tachycardia that was detected by ECG.

Ambulatory ECG recording of spontaneous ventricular arrhythmia could not be used to predict which patients were likely to suffer ventricular tachycardia during programmed electrical stimulation.

▶ This study emphasizes the limitations of ambulatory ECG recordings in predicting which patients will have ventricular tachycardia induced during programmed electrical stimulation. The authors found that the combination of a clinical presentation of sustained ventricular tachycardia, confirmed coronary artery disease and a left ventricular ejection fraction of less than 30%, had a better positive predictive value than did any ambulatory ECG criterion in predicting the inducibility of sustained ventricular tachycardia.—R.C. Schlant, M.D.

Miscellaneous Topics

Sudden Death Risk in Overt Coronary Heart Disease: The Framingham Study

William B. Kannel, L. Adrienne Cupples, Ralph B. D'Agostino (Boston Univ.)
Am. Heart J. 113:799–811, March 1987 3–46

Because sudden death is a common feature of coronary disease, further insights are needed into the way it evolves in the high-risk segment of the population with clinically overt coronary heart disease (CHD). Occurrence of sudden death was examined in participants in the Framingham Study who developed CHD under observation.

A cohort of 5,209 subjects, aged 30–62 years on entry into the study, were surveyed for 30 years. Death within minutes in subjects without potentially lethal illness was considered sudden coronary death. At the time of initial examination, 5,127 people were free of overt CHD. Over the 30 years of follow-up, 760 men and 574 women developed overt CHD. Of

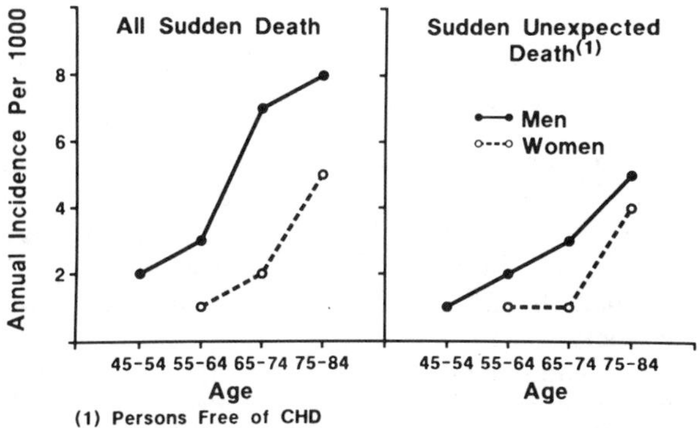

Fig 3–12.—Incidence of sudden death by age and sex: 30-year follow-up, Framingham Study. (Courtesy of Kannel, W.B., et al.: Am. Heart J. 113:799–811, March 1987.)

TABLE 1.—RISK OF SUDDEN DEATH IN RECOGNIZED VS. UNRECOGNIZED MYOCARDIAL INFARCTION: 30-YEAR FOLLOW-UP, FRAMINGHAM STUDY, SUBJECTS 33 to 87 YEARS OF AGE

	10-year age-adjusted mortality rate/1000 at risk			
	All CHD deaths		*Sudden deaths*	
Myocardial infarction	*Men*	*Women*	*Men*	*Women*
Unrecognized	26	20	10	5
Recognized	27	22	12	5

(Courtesy of Kannel, W.B., et al.: Am. Heart J. 113:799–811, March 1987.)

TABLE 2.—RISK FACTORS FOR SUDDEN DEATH IN SUBJECTS WITH CHD: 30-YEAR FOLLOW-UP, FRAMINGHAM STUDY, SUBJECTS 35 to 94 YEARS OF AGE*

	Standardized logistic coefficients	
Risk factors	*Men*	*Women*
Age	0.007	0.592 †
Systolic blood pressure	−0.014	0.104
Cholesterol	0.084	−0.165
Cigarettes	−0.002	0.215
Glucose intolerance	−0.024	0.325 ‡
ECG-LVH	0.376 §	0.108
VPC	0.201 ‡	−0.027
Cardiac failure	0.224 †	0.225 ‖

**LVH* indicates left ventricular hypertrophy; *VPC*, ventricular premature contractions.
†$P < .01$.
‡ $P < .05$.
§$P < .001$.
‖$P < .08$.
(Courtesy of Kannel, W.B., et al.: Am. Heart J. 113:799–811, March 1987.)

the 1,019 deaths among men and 857 deaths among women, 515 men and 379 women died of cardiovascular disease, and 350 men and 196 women died of CHD. There were 160 sudden deaths among the men and 73 among women. The sudden death risk was increased 6.7 times in those with sustained clinically manifest CHD compared with those without an interim event.

The incident of sudden death in those without prior CHD doubled with each decade past age 45 (Fig 3–12). The relative risk was comparable in both sexes, but CHD did not eliminate the female advantage over men. For subjects with unrecognized myocardial infarction, sudden death

TABLE 3.—ELECTROCARDIOGRAPHIC CONTRIBUTORS TO SUDDEN DEATH IN SUBJECTS WITH OVERT CHD: 30-YEAR FOLLOW-UP, FRAMINGHAM STUDY*

	Standardized logistic regression coefficients	
ECG abnormality	*Men*	*Women*
ECG-MI	0.391†	0.355‡
ECG-LVH	0.336†	0.153
IV block	0.180§	0.294‡
NSA-ECG	0.265‡	0.261

*Concurrent covariates: age, systolic blood pressure, cholesterol, cigarettes, glucose, atrioventricular block, heart rate, cardiac failure. MI indicates myocardial infarction; LVH, left ventricular hypertrophy; IV, intraventricular; and NSA, nonspecific abnormality.

†$P < .001$

‡$P < .05$

§$.05 < P < .10$.

(Courtesy of Kannel, W.B., et al.: Am. Heart J. 113:799–811, March 1987.)

risk was just as great as for those sustaining a symptomatic recognized myocardial infarction (Table 1). Myocardial infarction imposed a greater sudden death risk than angina pectoris, and CHD onset put younger subjects at equal risk of sudden death as older subjects. Forty percent of sudden deaths occurred in the 4% of the cohort with overt CHD. The proportion of coronary attacks presenting as sudden death was 13% for subjects aged 35–64 years and 20% for those aged 65–94 years. The fraction of CHD deaths termed sudden death was lower in those with than without interim CHD.

After onset of CHD, none of the major modifiable CHD risk factors were predictive of sudden death in men (Fig 3–13, Table 2); in women, diabetes was a predisposing factor. In those with established CHD, factors that reflect ischemic myocardial damage were main predictors of sudden death. Electrocardiographic abnormalities indicating myocardial

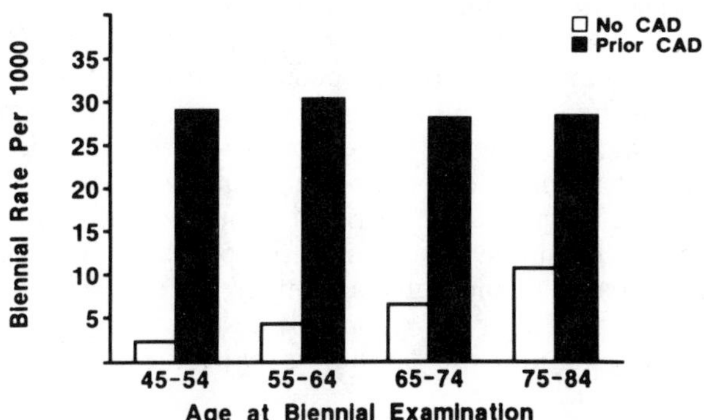

Fig 3–13.—Risk of sudden death by coronary disease status: 30-year follow-up, men in the Framingham Study. (Courtesy of Kannel, W.B., et al.: Am. Heart J. 113:799–811, March 1987.)

infarction, left ventricular hypertrophy, conduction disturbance, or repolarization abnormality were significant predictors (Table 3).

The proportion of CHD deaths presenting as sudden deaths has not declined in subjects with prior CHD in 30 years, despite a national decline in overall CHD mortality.

▶ In our attempts to identify persons most likely to experience sudden death, it is significant to note that in 28% of men and 35% of women in Framingham who developed a myocardial infarction (and thereby markedly increase their risk of sudden death), the infarction went unrecognized and was diagnosed by "routine" electrocardiography. The risk of sudden death in these patients with "silent" myocardial infarction was as high as that of patients who survived symptomatic myocardial infarction.

In addition to the major problem of identifying individuals most likely to experience sudden death, a second problem is proving that treatment of a high-risk group of individuals actually does decrease the incidence of sudden death. On the basis of the data in this report, one could argue in favor of periodic, "routine" ECGs in selected subsets of patients to identify those who have had silent myocardial infarction, although the cost-benefit ratio would likely be very high.—R.C. Schlant, M.D.

Induction of Lateralized Sympathetic Input to the Heart by the CNS During Emotional Arousal: A Possible Neurophysiologic Trigger of Sudden Death

Richard D. Lane and Gary E. Schwartz (Yale Univ.)

Psychosom. Med. 49:274–284, May–June 1987 3–47

Activation of strong emotion is associated with sudden cardiac death. Ventricular fibrillation usually precedes death. The authors describe a mechanism for the induction of fatal arrythmias by intense emotion.

Sympathetic input to the heart is lateralized. The right cardiac nerve innervates the anterior surface of sinoatrial and atrioventricular nodes and the anterior surfaces of the ventricles, while the left cardiac nerve innervates the posterior surface of the heart. The right cerebral hemisphere is superior to the left in recognizing emotion, while the left side of the brain is relatively more active during positive emotional states. Thus, it is hypothesized that persons who have more lateralized CNS activity during emotional arousal may generate more lateralized sympathetic input to the heart. Activation on one side of the brain would generate an imbalance in sympathetic input to the heart favoring the other side. Using this model, sudden death is more likely to occur in the presence of intense negative emotion, which activates the right hemisphere relatively more strongly.

This model has not yet been rigorously tested. However, if correct, it could be used to determine the psychological profile of persons at risk for sudden cardiac death.

▶ The hypothesis presented by the authors is both fascinating and of great potential importance, both at a basic level and eventually at a clinical level. Would it be possible, for example, to identify individuals by psychophysiologic testing who manifest greater laterality of CNS function and greater cardiovascular reactivity during emotional arousal and to test whether or not such individuals have a higher risk of sudden cardiac death? The future will undoubtedly bring exciting explorations of the many complex interactions between brain, heart, and body, including the hypothesis put forth in this study.—R.C. Schlant, M.D.

Esophageal Electrocardiography in Acute Cardiac Care: Efficacy and Diagnostic Value of a New Technique

Miles Shaw, James T. Niemann, Richard J. Haskell, Robert J. Rothstein, and Michael M. Laks (Univ. of California, Los Angeles, and Harbor-UCLA Med. Ctr., Torrance)

Am. J. Med. 82:689–696, April 1987 3–48

Previous methods of esophageal ECG recording have proved impractical for routine use in the acute care setting. Esophageal "pill" electrocardiography, in which signals from the esophageal electrodes are electrically filtered and amplified, avoids many of these problems. Little discomfort is involved, and the surface ECG can be recorded simultaneously.

The pill technique was evaluated in 48 acutely ill patients who swallowed a system that consisted of a bipolar electrode pair (3 × 20 mm) attached to Teflon wires (0.5 mm in diameter) in a gelatin capsule. After the patient swallowed the system, recording electrodes were placed posterior to the left atrium. A preamplifier system with a low-frequency filter and a standard 3-channel ECG recorder were used.

Only 2 of 50 eligible patients were unable to swallow the capsule. Several patients who were thought to have sinus tachycardia actually had atrial flutter or other arrhythmias. Atrial flutter was ruled out in other patients in whom esophageal ECG recording showed sinus, ventricular, or supraventricular tachycardia. The diagnosis also was changed in several patients who were thought to have an atrioventricular nodal reentrant rhythm from the surface ECG findings. No complications resulted from esophageal electrocardiography. Technicians were able to perform the procedure with minimal training.

The esophageal pill ECG technique markedly improves diagnostic accuracy in acute cardiac care. Consequently, the management of tachyarrhythmias is improved. The procedure carries no complications.

▶ This simple technique is clearly occasionally of great value in establishing the proper diagnosis of many tachyarrhythmias. It is worth emphasizing that all of the 50 patients with tachyarrhythmias who were studied had absent or equivocal atrial activity on surface ECG. In 25 (52%) of the 48 patients who were able to swallow the pill electrode, the original diagnosis based on the 12-lead ECG was found to be incorrect. Perhaps more importantly, the findings from esophageal recording altered management in 19 (40%) of the 48 patients.

I believe this technique will be widely used in the diagnosis of patients with selected tachyarrhythmias of uncertain type. The use of the pill electrode and transesophageal rapid atrial pacing is also frequently effective in the termination of atrial flutter (Falk and Morgan: *Chest* 92:110–114, 1987).—R.C. Schlant, M.D.

Effects of Enalapril on Mortality in Severe Congestive Heart Failure: Results of the Cooperative North Scandinavian Enalapril Survival Study (CONSENSUS)

CONSENSUS Trial Study Group

N. Engl. J. Med. 316:1429–1435, June 4, 1987 3–49

The efficacy of the angiotensin-converting enzyme inhibitor enalapril in severe congestive heart failure was studied by a double-blind technique in 253 patients in New York Heart Association functional class IV. Half the patients received enalapril in a starting dose of 5 mg twice daily with increases up to 20 mg twice daily.

Mortality after 1 year was 52% in the placebo group and 36% in enalapril-treated patients (Fig 3–14). Sudden cardiac deaths were similarly frequent in the two groups, but mortality from progressive heart failure was reduced 50% in the enalapril-treated group. Functional class improved about twice as often in the enalapril-treated group. Systolic blood pressure fell more in the enalapril-treated patients than in the placebo group. Increased serum levels of potassium were more frequent in the enalapril-treated patients.

Enalapril considerably reduces mortality in patients in severe conges-

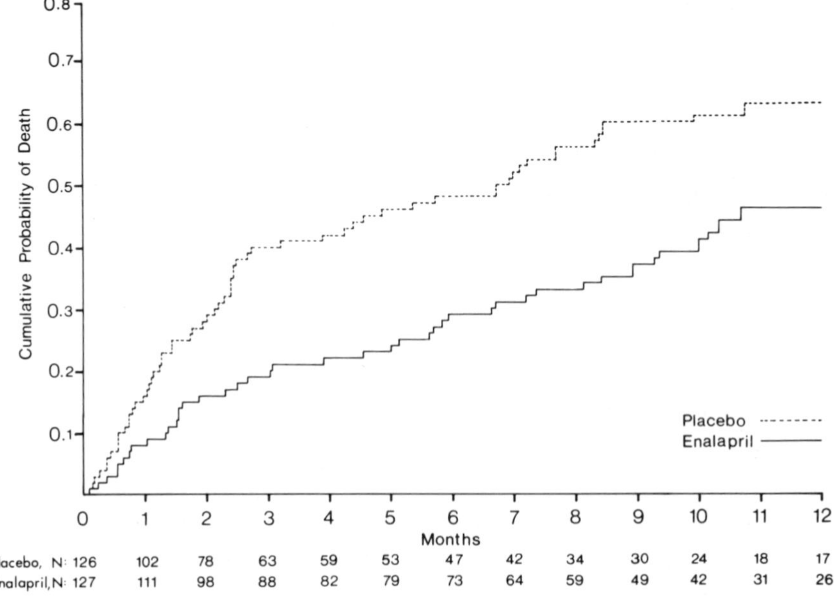

Fig 3–14.—Cumulative probability of death in placebo and enalapril groups. (Courtesy of CONSENSUS Trial Study Group: N. Engl. J. Med. 316:1429–1435, June 4, 1987.)

tive heart failure. The drug is well tolerated, but treatment should begin with low doses, particularly in high-risk patients. The decreased mortality in enalapril-treated patients is explained by a reduction in deaths from progressive heart failure, not a reduction in sudden deaths.

▶ This is an important study that complements studies (Furberg and Yusuf: *Am. J. Cardiol.* 55:1110–1113, 1985) showing that the addition of the other currently available ACE-inhibitor, captopril, improves the quality of life and may prolong life in patients with chronic congestive heart failure. It is important to note that enalapril was *added* to conventional therapy and not used in place of such therapy. This was also true in most of the patients in the studies reviewed by Furberg and Yusuf and in the Veterans Administration Cooperative Study, which used isosorbide dinitrate and hydralazine (Cohn et al.: *N. Engl. J. Med.* 314:1547–1552, 1986).

In this study, 92% of the patients treated with enalapril received digitalis, 98% furosemide (mean daily dose, 210 mg), 50% spironolactone (mean daily dose, 80 mg), 47% isosorbide dinitrate, and 33% an anticoagulant agent. In the group of patients also receiving other vasodilators, the reductions in crude mortality was only from 48% to 42% ($P = .11$). Although one might have expected a decrease in sudden death in the patients receiving enalapril, perhaps because of its tendency to cause patients to retain potassium, there was no difference in the incidence of sudden cardiac death between the two treatment groups.

The addition of an angiotensin-converting enzyme inhibitor, either captopril or enalapril, to standard therapy with digoxin and diuretics represents a major advance in our therapy of patients with heart failure due to systolic left ventricular heart failure. I would emphasize that the ACE-inhibitors are used in addition to, and not in place of, digitalis and diuretics.

We do not yet have strong data of benefit from the early therapy of patients with aortic or mitral regurgitation before there are symptoms or any detectable evidence of ventricular dysfunction, although such benefit would appear highly likely. There is now an ongoing study that is looking at the possible benefit of ACE-inhibitor therapy in patients with minimal or no symptoms but with significant left ventricular dysfunction.—R.C. Schlant, M.D.

Physiologic Hypertrophy: Effects on Left Ventricular Systolic Mechanics in Athletes

Steven D. Colan, Stephen P. Sanders, and Kenneth M. Borow (Children's Hosp., Boston, and Univ. of Chicago)

J. Am. Coll. Cardiol. 9:776–783, April 1987 3–50

Physiologic hypertrophy due to intense athletic participation results in normal, reduced, and augmented overall left ventricular performance. Rather than representing true differences in left ventricular contractility, these data may reflect the variable degree of ventricular dilatation and increased wall thickness that occur with different types of exercise. Thus, the resultant altered loading conditions may diminish the ability of the usual indices of left ventricular function to accurately assess the left ventricular contractile state. The authors used load-independent contractility indices to test three groups of elite athletes with distinct patterns of myocardial hypertrophy.

The study group included 11 swimmers, 11 long-distance runners, 11 power lifters, and 33 age-matched control subjects. Compared with control subjects, all athletes had increased left ventricular mass, even when values were normalized for body surface area. The runners had a dilated left ventricle and normal wall thickness, the swimmers had a mildly dilated ventricle with increased wall thickness, and the power lifters had normal cavity size with substantially increased wall thickness. Peak systolic wall stress was normal in runners and swimmers, but was reduced in power lifters, whereas end-systolic stress was low in swimmers and power lifters, but normal in runners. The minute stress-time integral, a measure of myocardial oxygen consumption, was normal in runners and swimmers, but was markedly reduced in lifters.

In runners, fractional shortening was significantly reduced with normal velocity of shortening, whereas swimmers and power lifters had marked augmentation of fractional shortening and velocity of shortening. When the rate-corrected velocity of shortening–end-systolic stress relation was examined, both swimmers and power lifters had normal contractility with augmented systolic performance due to reduced afterload. A comparison of runners and control subjects demonstrated normal afterload but reduced preload in runners, which was manifested as reduced fractional shortening with normal afterload and contractile state.

These data indicate that physiologic hypertrophy results in marked alterations in left ventricular loading conditions with secondary changes in systolic performance. When load-independent indices are used, the left ventricular contractile state is found to be normal in young athletes, despite increased left ventricular mass. Different types of exercise are associated with distinct patterns of left ventricular hypertrophy and dilation, necessitating individual assessment of preload and afterload in the interpretation of indices of left ventricular function.

▶ This study confirms the findings of previous studies indicating that young athletes generally maintain systolic function measured by load-independent indices. But it also confirms previous findings (Morganroth et al.: *Ann. Intern. Med.* 82:521–524, 1975; Roeske et al.: *Circulation* 53:286–291, 1976; Gilbert et al.: *Am. J. Cardiol.* 40:528–533, 1977; Longhurst et al.: *J. Appl. Physiol.* 48:154–162, 1980; Kanakis et al. *Chest* 78:618–621, 1981; and Kuel et al.: *Circ. Res.* 48(suppl. 1):162–170, 1981) that different types of exercise (endurance vs. high-resistance training) produce significant differences in left ventricular hypertrophy and function. These findings potentially may occasionally have clinical relevance in advice given to athletes and may also have basic importance in the study of the factors that initiate and maintain different types of cardiac hypertrophy—a very important and fundamental aspect of cardiology. —R.C. Schlant, M.D.

4 Coronary Artery and Other Heart Diseases, Heart Failure

Introduction

Exciting advances are occurring in the management of patients with coronary artery disease, and some of these are highlighted in the following selections. The role of thrombolysis, with or without PTCA, in the setting of an acute myocardial infarction has been the focus for several important trials which are included in this year's selection. The recently reported results of the ISIS-II trial demonstrating a marked reduction in mortality after myocardial infarction with a combination of aspirin and streptokinase have not been published as a paper yet, so this important study will not appear in these pages until the next volume. The literature on PTCA unrelated to myocardial infarction also continues to expand with as yet no direct comparison between CABG and PTCA in terms of efficacy, safety, and cost. Fortunately, several randomized trials are under way in North America and abroad which will be awaited with great interest.

The changing environment of health care policy and economics is clear to all engaged in clinical practice. Included in this year's selection are two papers on the appropriateness of use of several cardiovascular procedures which should be reviewed carefully. The objective study of quality of care and utilization of procedures, obviously interrelated topics, should be encouraged with full participation by the medical profession in planning and reporting such results. The application of scientific principles to such studies is crucial.

Robert L. Frye, M.D.

Myocardial Infarction

Effect of Intravenous Streptokinase on Left Ventricular Function and Early Survival After Acute Myocardial Infarction

Harvey D. White, Robin M. Norris, Michael A. Brown, Morimasa Takayama, Andrew Maslowski, Nigel M. Bass, John A. Ormiston, and Toby Whitlock (Green Lane, Middlemore, and Auckland Hosps., Auckland, New Zealand)

N. Engl. J. Med. 317:850–855, Oct. 1, 1987 4–1

The effects of early treatment with streptokinase were assessed in a double-blind study of 219 consecutive patients seen within 4 hours of the onset of chest pain that was caused by a first myocardial infarction. The

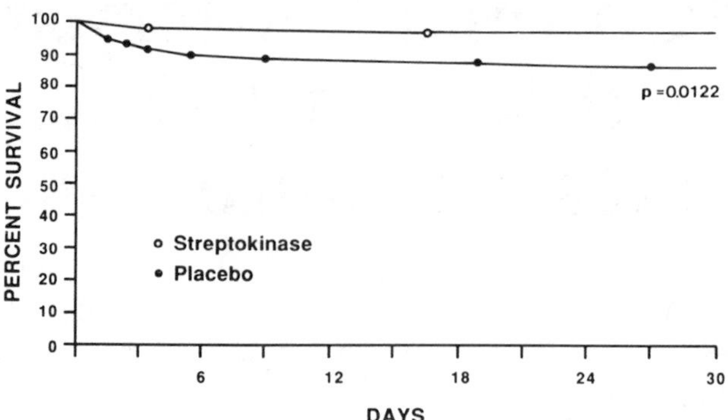

Fig 4–1.—Thirty-day actuarial survival curves for patients with first infarctions who were treated with streptokinase or placebo. (Courtesy of White, H.D., et al.: N. Engl. J. Med. 317:850–855, Oct. 1, 1987.)

patients, all younger than 70 years, were assigned to receive 1.5 million units of streptokinase or a placebo intravenously over 30 minutes. The infusion was followed by aspirin-dipyridamole and heparin for 48 hours.

Left ventricular ejection fraction was significantly higher in the streptokinase-treated patients and end-systolic volume was smaller. Segmental wall motion was better in the study group. Only 1 streptokinase-treated patient who also received propranolol died, compared with 4 placebo-treated patients who received propranolol.

Overall mortality was 13% in the placebo group and 2.5% in the streptokinase group (Fig 4–1). No significant adverse effects were noted. Reinfarction was infrequent. Seven streptokinase-treated patients and 6 in the placebo group had surgery in the first 30 days.

It is concluded that early infusion of streptokinase is an effective treatment for evolving initial myocardial infarction. Early mortality is lowered, and left ventricular function is improved in treated patients, compared with those who are given placebo. Benefit is seen in patients with either anterior or inferior infarction and independently of whether or not propranolol is given. Reinfarction has been infrequent and adverse effects are uncommon, even when streptokinase is combined with propranolol.

Effects of Early High-Dose Streptokinase Intravenously on Left Ventricular Function in Acute Myocardial Infarction

Jean-Pierre Bassand, René Faivre, Olivier Becque, Chantal Habert, Marc Schuffenecker, Pierre-Yves Petiteau, Jean-Claude Cardot, Josette Verdenet, Michel LaRoze, and Jean-Pierre Maurat (Univ. Hosp. and Faculty of Medicine, Besancon, France)

Am. J. Cardiol. 60:435–439, Sept. 1, 1987 4–2

A series of 107 patients aged 70 years and younger with a first acute transmural myocardial infarction were randomized within 5 hours of the onset of symptoms to receive standard heparin therapy or intravenous doses of streptokinase. After 2 weeks the patency of the infarct vessel and left ventricular (LV) function were assessed. Fifty-five patients received heparin, 500 IU/kg daily, intravenously and 52 received streptokinase, 1.5 million units, followed by infusion of heparin.

There were 7 hospital deaths in the heparin group and 4 in the streptokinase group. About two thirds of the infarct vessels were patent in both groups, and LV ejection fractions did not differ significantly. Function was better in streptokinase-treated patients with anterior wall infarction than in those who were given heparin only. Mortality after a mean of nearly 2 years was 18% in the heparin group and 10% in the streptokinase group. Four patients in the streptokinase group and 2 in the heparin group successfully underwent coronary angioplasty.

Early infusion of streptokinase may significantly preserve LV function in patients with anterior wall infarction, but it may be less appropriate for use in inferior wall infarction. Preservation of ventricular function presumably results from early reperfusion of the infarct vessel.

▶ These two small but well-documented randomized trials of intravenously administered streptokinase document preservation of left ventricular function with such therapy (Abstracts 4–1 and 4–2). Different conclusions are reached regarding the benefits in the setting of inferior wall infarction. Both, however, are well done studies and should be reviewed carefully.—R.L. Frye, M.D.

A Multicenter, Randomized, Placebo-Controlled Trial of a New Form of Intravenous Recombinant Tissue-Type Plasminogen Activator (Activase) in Acute Myocardial Infarction

Eric J. Topol, Douglas C. Morris, Richard W. Smalling, Richard R. Schumacher, Charles R. Taylor, Akira Nishikawa, Henry A. Liberman, Désiré Collen, Margaret E. Tufte, Elliott B. Grossbard, and William W. O'Neill (Univ. of Michigan Med. Ctr., Ann Arbor, Emory Univ., Atlanta, Univ. of Texas Health Science Ctr., Houston, Methodist Hosp., Indianapolis, Univ. of Vermont, Burlington, and Genetech, Inc., South San Francisco)

J. Am. Coll. Cardiol. 9:1205–1213, June 1987 4–3

The first recombinant tissue plasminogen activator (t-PA) made available in small quantities for clinical testing was a two-chain form. It has demonstrated efficacy in acute myocardial infarction, but clot selectivity at moderate doses was relative versus absolute. A new, predominantly single chain t-PA is now being manufactured in large amounts for clinical use. This multicenter, randomized, double-blind, placebo-controlled study evaluated the thrombolytic efficacy of this product in 100 patients with acute myocardial infarction. Minor objectives of the study were the effect of t-PA on the coagulation and fibrinolytic proteins, bleeding complications, and the role of coronary angioplasty.

Patients were randomized on a 3:1 basis to receive either t-PA or placebo, respectively. Tissue plasminogen activator was administered intravenously at a dose of 0.75 mg/kg body weight over the first hour and 0.25 mg/kg per hour over the next 2 hours up to a maximum of 105 mg.

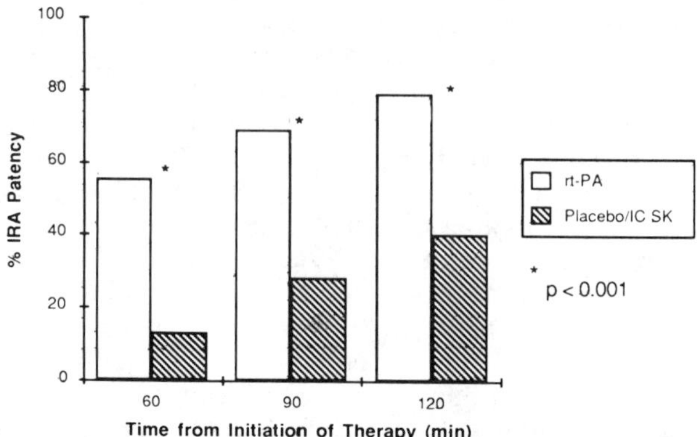

Fig 4–2.—Comparison of infarct-related vessel (IRA) patency for the two treatments as a function of time. At the three times of angiographic evaluation, there was a significant increase in patency of tissue plasminogen activator *(open columns)* compared with placebo/intracoronary streptokinase (IC SK)-treated *(hatched columns)* patients. *$P < .001$. (Courtesy of Topol, E.J., et al.: J. Am. Coll. Cardiol. 9:1205–1213, June 1987.)

The infarct-related vessel was assessed by coronary arteriography at 60, 90, and 120 minutes after the start of study drug. After determining the infarct-related vessel patency at the first angiogram, the blind was broken. Patients in the placebo group who had persistent occlusion could receive intracoronary streptokinase (SK). Any patient showing hemodynamic deterioration was eligible for emergent coronary angioplasty. Blood samples were collected before infusion and 45 minutes, 2 and 6 hours, and 1 and 7 days after the start of treatment.

The mean time from symptom onset to start of treatment was 3.6 hours. At the first angiogram, 40 (57%) of 70 patients in the t-PA group had infarct-related vessel patency compared with 3 (13%) of 23 placebo-treated patients. Streptokinase was administered to 17 patients in the placebo group. At 90 minutes, 49 (69%) of 71 t-PA-treated patients had patency of the infarct-related artery compared with 5 (24%) of 21 controls, respectively ($P < .001$; Fig 4–2). The final angiogram showed vessel patency in 59 (79%) of 75 t-PA patients and in 10 (40%) of 25 placebo/SK patients. All differences between groups were statistically significant. There was no significant difference in the incidence of moderate or severe bleeding episodes occurring in the t-PA (39%) versus placebo/SK (32%) groups. A nadir value of less than 100 mg/dl fibrinogen occurred in significantly fewer t-PA patients (11%) compared to the SK-treated group (40%).

This study demonstrated the efficacy of a new t-PA for producing infarct vessel recanalization with significantly less fibrinogen depletion than intracoronary streptokinase. Additional studies are needed to determine the optimal regimen for sustaining vessel patency and reducing time to recanalization without producing hematologic complications.

▶ An example of further improvements in thrombolytic drugs. This will be an ongoing area of investigation in cardiovascular medicine with an overall goal of a highly clot-specific lytic agent. As noted by the investigators, further studies will be necessary to define the appropriate dose of this particular agent.—R.L. Frye, M.D.

A Randomized Trial of Immediate Versus Delayed Elective Angioplasty After Intravenous Tissue Plasminogen Activator in Acute Myocardial Infarction

Eric J. Topol, Robert M. Califf, Barry S. George, Dean J. Kereiakes, Charles W. Abbottsmith, Richard J. Candela, Kerry L. Lee, Bertram Pitt, Richard S. Stack, William W. O'Neill, and the Thrombolysis and Angioplasty Myocardial Infarction Study Group (Univ. of Michigan, Duke Univ., Riverside Methodist Hosp., Columbus, Ohio, and Christ Hosp., Cincinnati)

N. Engl. J. Med. 317:581–588, Sept. 3, 1987 4–4

Although early administration of streptokinase decreases mortality in patients with acute myocardial infarction, it has also been associated with a higher incidence of reinfarction and early postinfarction angina. Recombinant tissue-type plasminogen activator, more effective than streptokinase in establishing reperfusion of viable, jeopardized myocardium, carries the potential for an even higher frequency of recurrent ischemic events. Percutaneous transluminal coronary angioplasty has been shown useful for primary or adjunctive recanalization of the infarct-related artery; however, proper timing of angioplasty after thrombolysis is not yet known. The efficacy of immediate coronary angioplasty after acute myocardial infarction was compared with elective angioplasty at 7–10 days in patients initially treated with intravenous tissue plasminogen activator.

The plasminogen activator, 150 mg, was given 2.95 ± 1.1 hours after the onset of symptoms in 386 patients with acute myocardial infarction. Patency of the coronary artery serving the infarct area was demonstrated by coronary angiography in 288 patients, or 75%, 90 minutes later. Bleeding problems were common. An average drop in hematocrit level of 11.7 ± 6.5 points from baseline to nadir was noted, and 70 patients needed transfusion not related to bypass surgery. After successful thrombolysis, 197 patients with a patent but severely stenotic vessel suitable for angioplasty were randomly assigned to receive immediate angioplasty or deferred angioplasty if indicated 7–10 days later.

Reocclusion occurred in 11% of the 99 patients in group 1 and 13% of the 98 in group 2. Neither group had a significant improvement in global left ventricular function. Regional wall motion in the infarct zone improved similarly in both groups (Fig 4–3). Of those in the deferred angioplasty group, 16% required emergency angioplasty for recurrent ischemia. Of those in the immediate angioplasty group, 5% required emergency repeated angioplasty. In 14% of those receiving deferred angioplasty, the stenosis was substantially reduced by the 7-day follow-up angiography, obviating the need for angiography.

In patients with initially successful thrombolysis and suitable

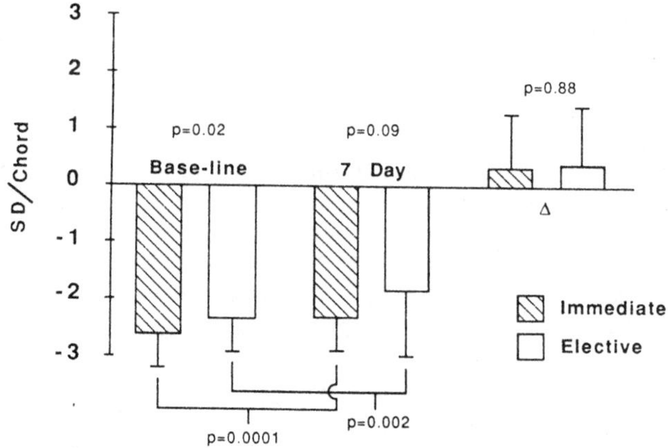

Fig 4–3.—Regional wall motion in the infarct zone in the immediate-angioplasty group and the elective-angioplasty group. A baseline difference between the two groups was demonstrated. Both the immediate- and elective-angioplasy strategies led to significant improvement in regional wall motion from baseline to the 7-day repeat study, and there was no difference in the magnitude of the improvement. (Courtesy of Topol, E.J., et al.: N. Engl. J. Med. 317:581–588, Sept, 3, 1987.)

coronary-artery anatomy, immediate angioplasty has no clear advantage over deferred elective angioplasty.

▶ This is an extremely important report dealing with the appropriate use of angioplasty after a thrombolytic therapy in the setting of acute myocardial infarction. From these studies and also the results of TIMI II, immediate angioplasty did not have any clear advantage over deferred elective angioplasty of the infarct-related artery.—R.L. Frye, M.D.

Thrombolysis in Myocardial Infarction (TIMI) Trial, Phase I: A Comparison Between Intravenous Tissue Plasminogen Activator and Intravenous Streptokinase: Clinical Findings Through Hospital Discharge

J.H. Chesebro, G. Knatterud, R. Roberts, J. Borer, L.S. Cohen, J. Dalen, H.T. Dodge, C.K. Francis, D. Hillis, P. Ludbrook, J.E. Markis, H. Mueller, E.R. Passamani, E.R. Powers, A.K. Rao, T. Robertson, A. Ross, T.J. Ryan, B.E. Sobel, J. Willerson, D.O. Williams, B.L. Zaret, and E. Braunwald (TIMI Coordinating Ctr., Baltimore)

Circulation 76:142–154, 1987 4–5

The authors report the angiographic and clinical results of the Thrombolysis in Myocardial Infarction (TIMI) Trial, phase I. The efficacy and side effects of intravenously administered recombinant tissue-type plasminogen activator (rt-PA) were compared with those of intravenously given streptokinase (SK) in a randomized, double-blind trial in 290 patients with myocardial infarction and occlusion documented by coronary arteriography.

Within 90 minutes of therapy, occluded arteries had opened in 62% of

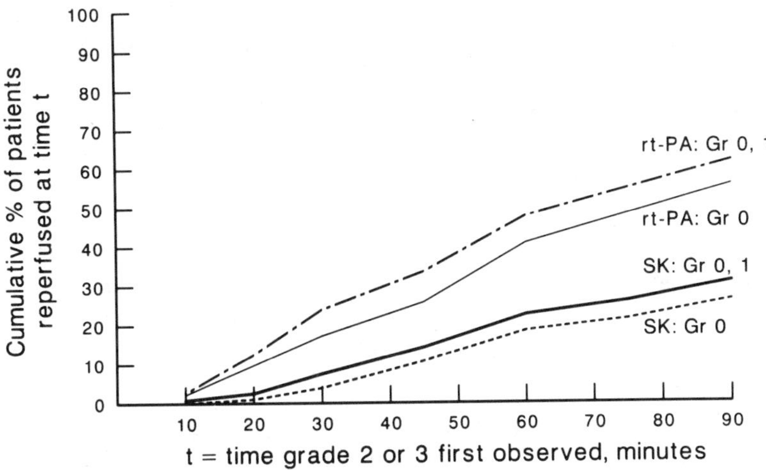

Fig 4–4.—The proportion of successfully reperfused (grade 2,3) infarct-related arteries reperfused at time t (ordinate) vs. time t in minutes at which grade 2, 3 reperfusion was first observed (abscissa) for rt-PA and SK groups at seven time intervals of angiographic observation up to 90 minutes after the start of thrombolytic therapy. Patients with baseline grade 0 (93 rt-PA– and 103 SK-treated patients) and baseline grade 0,1 (113 rt-PA– and 119 SK-treated patients) perfusion. The reocclusion of four arteries in the rt-PA group and two in the SK group within 90 minutes is not tabulated in this comparison. At each time interval rt-PA reperfused at least twice as many arteries as SK. (Courtesy of Chesebro, J.H., et al.: Circ. 76:142–154, 1987.)

the 113 patients in the rt-PA group and in 31% of the 119 patients in the SK group. Seven angiograms were obtained during this 90-minute period, and at each one twice as many occluded arteries had opened in the rt-PA group (Fig 4–4). Patients treated with SK had greater reductions in circulating fibrinogen and plasminogen and a significantly greater increase in circulating fibrin split products at 3 and 24 hours than did those treated with rt-PA. The incidence of bleeding, blood transfusions, and reocclusions were similar in the two groups.

In patients with acute myocardial infarction, rt-PA reopened twice as many occluded infarct-related arteries as did SK during the first 90 minutes of therapy. Therefore, rt-PA is effective as a first step in myocardial salvage.

▶ These data are from the early phase of the TIMI Trial documenting an advantage of intravenously given t-PA in comparison with intraveously given streptokinase in terms of lysis of clot in the infarct-related artery. This was with 80 mg of t-PA, and subsequent studies in TIMI have utilized a higher dose of t-PA. Thus, the in clot lysis differences may be greater with higher doses of t-PA. It is clear there is some effect on circulating clotting factors with the t-PA used in the TIMI Trial, and the further development of thrombolytic agents that are more clot-specific will undoubtedly evolve. The advances in thrombolysis are most exciting and are reflected not only by the above studies, but by the other important observations from a number of groups throughout this section.—R.L. Frye, M.D.

A Prospective Placebo-Controlled Double-Blind Multicenter Trial of Intravenous Streptokinase in Acute Myocardial Infarction (ISAM): Long-Term Mortality and Morbidity

Rolf Schröder, Karl-Ludwig Neuhaus, Alain Leizorovicz, Thomas Linderer, Ulrich Tebbe, for the ISAM Study Group (Freie Universität Berlin, Georg-August-Universität, Göttingen, West Germany, and Hôpital Neuro-Cardiologique, Lyon, France)

J. Am. Coll. Cardiol. 9:197–203, January 1987 4–6

Intravenous (IV) streptokinase infusion was first used to treat acute myocardial infarction in 1959. Since that time many studies have been carried out, and recently, data on in-hospital mortality and morbidity in two randomized, large-scale multicenter trials of high-dose, brief-duration intravenous administration of streptokinase were published. However, long-term results have not been reported. The ISAM study was a prospective German Swiss-Canadian controlled double-blind multicenter trial, evaluating the effect of 1.5 million IU of streptokinase or placebo administered intravenously over 60 minutes within 6 hours after the onset of symptoms of myocardial infarction.

The authors assessed long-term mortality and morbidity of 1,741 patients with acute myocardial infarction who were treated with IV streptokinase or placebo as part of the ISAM study. At the 7-month follow-up, it was found that 94 (10.9%) of the 859 patients in the streptokinase group and 98 (11.1%) of the patients in the placebo group had died; at an average follow-up of 21 months, 14.4% of the streptokinase group and 16.1% of the placebo group had died. These differences were not found to be statistically significant. However, it was observed that the long-term mortality was slightly higher in patients with anterior myocardial infarction and streptokinase treatment (20.1% vs. 18.4%) and

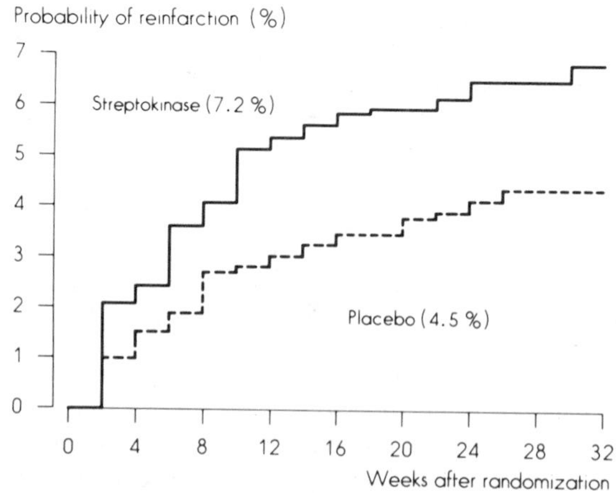

Fig 4–5.—Seven-month probability of reinfarction in patients allocated to streptokinase or placebo treatment. Log-rank test: chi-square = 4.52, P = .02. (Courtesy of Schröder, R., et al.: J. Am. Coll. Cardiol. 9:197–203, January 1987.)

lower in patients with inferior myocardial infarction (10.2% vs. 14.2%). Those patients who had had a previous myocardial infarction had a higher long-term mortality rate with streptokinase (34.9% vs. 21.5% with placebo). At 7 months, there were significantly more cases of reinfarction in the streptokinase group (7.2% vs. 4.5%) (Fig 4–5).

Despite a significant limitation of infarct size by intravenous streptokinase, long-term mortality is only slightly reduced and reinfarction is significantly more frequent. These findings suggest the need for complementary therapy, such as revascularization procedures after thrombolysis.

▶ This is an extremely important study documenting the importance of dealing with the infarct-related artery following successful thrombolytic therapy in the prevention of reinfarction. Dr. Schröder and colleagues have contributed importantly to our knowledge in this area. Other studies quoted in this section deal with the appropriate timing of revascularization procedures after thrombolysis.—R.L. Frye, M.D.

Mortality and Morbidity Rates of Patients Older and Younger Than 75 Years With Acute Myocardial Infarction Treated With Intravenous Streptokinase

Allan S. Lew, Hanoch Hod, Bojan Cercek, Prediman K. Shah, and William Ganz (Cedars-Sinai Med. Ctr., Los Angeles, and the Univ. of California at Los Angeles)

Am. J. Cardiol. 59:1–5, Jan. 1, 1987 4–7

Elderly patients generally do not receive early thrombolytic therapy for acute infarction because of fear of serious hemorrhagic complications. Experience with such treatment in 120 consecutive patients with acute infarction was reviewed, where no upper age limit was set for patient inclusion. An intravenous infusion of 750,000 units of streptokinase was followed by a continuous heparin infusion aimed at producing a partial thromboplastin time of 100 seconds. Twenty-seven patients with delayed signs of reperfusion received a second streptokinase infusion.

Fourteen (12%) patients died, 11 of cardiac causes. Mortality rose sharply in patients aged 75 years and older. Older patients had more extensive myocardial necrosis. Reocclusion of the infarct vessel was more frequent, as was three-vessel coronary artery disease. Past infarction also was more frequent in patients aged 75 and older. Significant independent predictors of mortality were patient age, healed past infarction, and peak creatinine-kinase-MB. Serious hemorrhagic complications were more than twice as frequent in older patients, 2 of whom had intracranial bleeding. Five of 17 patients with serious hemorrhagic complications died.

Patients aged 75 years and older with acute myocardial infarction have increased mortality and a higher risk of serious hemorrhagic complications following intravenous thrombolytic therapy than do younger patients. Mortality is not reduced in elderly patients, and they should not routinely receive streptokinase intravenously. Women and patients with diabetes or hypertension in particular should not be treated in this way.

▶ This is an important study and should be read carefully by all who use thrombolytic therapy. Since the major clinical trials have excluded patients aged 75 years and older, these observations are of particular importance in that they document an increased mortality rate with the use of intravenous thrombolytic therapy in patients older than 75 years related to a major increment in hemorrhagic complications, particularly in women. As noted in several other studies quoted in this section, there are unique features to the treatment and complication rates of women with coronary disease as compared with men, and this needs attention in planning further studies.—R.L. Frye, M.D.

A Community-Wide Assessment of the Use of Pulmonary Artery Catheters in Patients With Acute Myocardial Infarction

Joel M. Gore, Robert J. Goldberg, David H. Spodick, Joseph S. Alpert, and James E. Dalen (Univ. of Massachusetts, Worcester)

Chest 92:721–727, October 1987 4–8

Trends in the use of flow-directed pulmonary artery catheters were studied in 3,263 patients who were seen at 16 hospitals with confirmed acute myocardial infarction in 1975, 1978, 1981, and 1984. Hemodynamic monitoring with a pulmonary artery catheter increased progressively and significantly over time. Seven percent of patients were catheterized in 1975 and 20% were catheterized in 1984. All but 4% of patients who were catheterized had heart failure, hypotension, or cardiogenic shock.

The in-hospital case fatality rate for patients in congestive failure was 45% when a pulmonary artery catheter was used and 25% when no catheter was used. The respective figures for hypotensive patients were 48% and 32%, and for those in cardiogenic shock the respective figures were 74% and 79%. Catheterization was associated with a longer hospital stay, regardless of whether acute clinical complications developed. The long-term outlook for survivors of complicated infarction was not influenced by whether a pulmonary artery catheter had been used during hospitalization.

No benefit from the use of a pulmonary artery catheter was apparent in this community-wide study of patients who were hospitalized with acute myocardial infarction. A randomized trial of efficacy is needed, especially in view of current interest in containing costs. The benefit of other diagnostic measures in patients with myocardial infarction also should be evaluated.

▶ Gore and colleagues have stimulated discussion regarding the use of hemodynamic monitoring in patients with myocardial infarction. The observational nature of the study is emphasized. However, the data presented have been utilized by others (Robin, E.: *Chest* 92:727, 1987) to suggest that "thousands of patients have died and are currently dying because of complications associated with use of the PA catheter in acute myocardial infarction." This is an extraordinary conclusion (not by the authors of the original study), since Gore and coauthors in fact provide no specific data to *prove* the higher death rates were specifically caused by the use of the catheter. An association, as demonstrated in the Gore's study, obviously does not prove the catheters were the cause of death. Acceptance of statistical adjustment for risks need to be interpreted with caution since unrecognized variables or imprecise classification of patients may occur in such a retrospective observational study.

Before mounting a huge clinical trial, it would seem more important to document in Gore's sample of patients the precise complications associated with the catheter and an analysis of the deaths that occurred before concluding they are all catheter related.—R.L. Frye, M.D.

Spatial Distribution and Prognostic Significance of ST Segment Potential Determined by Body Surface Mapping in Patients With Acute Inferior Myocardial Infarction

Stephen J. Walker, Anthony J. Bell, Michael G. Loughhead, Peter S. Lavercombe, and David Kilpatrick (Royal Hobart Hosp., Hobart, Tasmania, and Univ. of Tasmania)

Circulation 76:289–297, August 1987 4–9

A more aggressive approach to acute myocardial infarction requires the early identification of patients at high risk after infarction. Standard ECG examination may not be a sensitive means of quantifying anterior ST depression, because of limited chest wall sampling. Body surface maps were recorded at admission in 100 patients who had acute inferior infarction. The degree of maximal ST segment elevation and maximal depression, as well as levels of ST depression on the standard 12-lead ECG, were analyzed against morbidity and mortality after a median follow-up of 14 months.

The values obtained by subtracting maximum ST elevation from maximum depression correlated with the outcome. In addition, maximum ST depression correlated with complications and mortality, and increasing levels of ST depression on the 12-lead ECG correlated with mortality. Patients with marked anterior negativity had a mortality of 37%, compared with 5% for all other patients. Limited angiographic and autopsy data suggested that coronary artery disease correlated with the results of mapping.

Body surface mapping can identify patients at high risk after acute inferior myocardial infarction. The standard ECG is less useful, because the standard leads cover a region of steep voltage gradient, and small changes in lead position can result in large changes in the displayed potentials.

▶ This interesting article provides new information regarding the prognostic value of the initial ECG at the time of acute inferior wall infarction. This is an important effort since identifying the patient with inferior infarct who may be at higher risk for mortality and other complications is a difficult one. As pointed out by these investigators, prior correlations between the ST segment elevations in the inferior leads versus ST segment depressions in the early precordial leads by standard electrocardiography have resulted in conflicting data. By body surface mapping, it would appear that patients with a higher expected mortality can be identified, but as noted by the authors, such a conclusion needs further defense by additional detailed studies with combined body surface maps and coronary arteriography.

The fact that such studies are under way is reassuring, and the results will be awaited with great interest. It is important to reemphasize that this is not an idle question, since even in the GISSI trial there was no apparent benefit of thrombolytic therapy in patients with inferior wall myocardial infarction. Identification of the truly high-risk patients with inferior wall infarction and selecting those for thrombolytic therapy would be of real help clinically in refining the indications for thrombolytic therapy in the setting of inferior wall infarction.—R.L. Frye, M.D.

Left Ventricular End-Systolic Volume as the Major Determinant of Survival After Recovery From Myocardial Infarction

Harvey D. White, Robin M. Norris, Michael A. Brown, Peter W.T. Brandt, Ralph M.L. Whitlock, and Christopher J. Wild (Green Lane Hosp., Auckland, New Zealand)

Circulation 76:44–51, July 1987 4–10

The functional state of the left ventricle is the most important predictor of long-term survival after recovery from acute infarction. The end-systolic volume (ESV) and end-diastolic volume (EDV) might be better measures of prognosis than ejection fraction, an arithmetic term based on these two values. This was studied in 605 men younger than 60 years 1–2 months after myocardial infarction. A first infarction occurred in 443 patients, and recurrent infarction occurred in 162 others. There were 101 cardiac deaths, 71 of which were sudden.

Multivariate analysis showed that ESV had greater predictive value for survival than EDV or ejection fraction (Fig 4–6). Stepwise analysis indicated that, after the relation of survival with ESV had been fitted, neither EDV nor ejection fraction provided significant added predictive information. The severity of coronary occlusions and stenoses was of only borderline significance. Continued smoking was an independent risk factor for survival.

End-systolic volume appears to be the primary predictor of survival after myocardial infarction. It is better than ejection fraction when this is less than 50% or when the ESV is less than 100 ml. Treatment is aimed at both limiting infarct size and preventing ventricular dilation. Studies monitoring blood pressure, heart rate, and contractility in the days and weeks following infarction will help determine the effects of interventions in the healing phase.

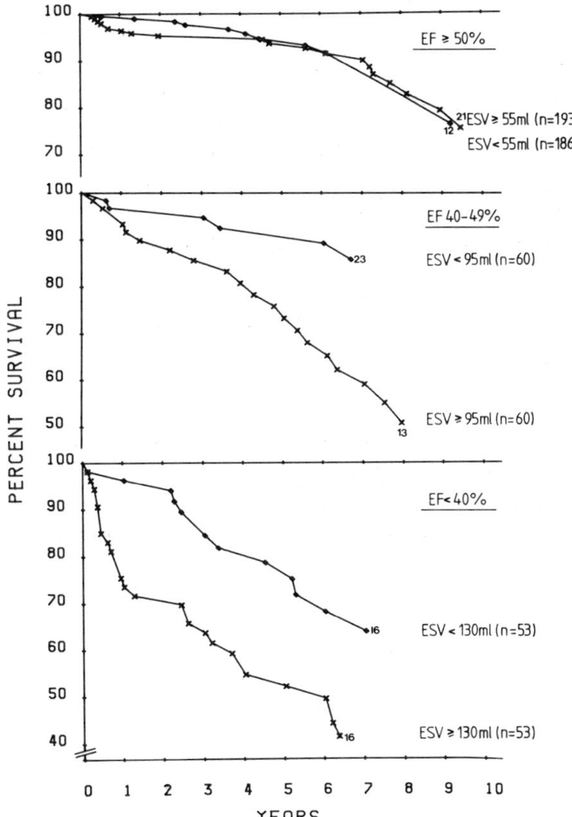

Fig 4–6.—Actuarial curves constructed for three groups of EF (≥50%, 40% to 49%, and <40%), each group being subdivided according to whether ESV was above or below the median for that group. Predictive value for ESV is apparent only when EF is less than 50%, mortality for patients with EFs of 40% to 49% but ESV below the median being no worse than that for patients with EFs of 50% and above. (Courtesy of White, H.D., et al.: Circulation 75:44–51, July 1987.)

▶ An interesting study that further documents the importance of ventricular dilatation as a risk factor emphasizing left ventricular end-systolic volume in patients after myocardial infarction.—R.L. Frye, M.D.

Right Ventricular Myocardial Infarction With Anterior Wall Left Ventricular Infarction: An Autopsy Study

Henry S. Cabin, K. Soni Clubb, Frans J. Th. Wackers, and Barry L. Zaret (Yale Univ.)

Am. Heart J. 113:16–23, January 1987 4–11

Right ventricular myocardial infarction has been associated exclusively with inferior wall left ventricular myocardial infarction. With anterior infarction, right ventricular dysfunction, when present, has been attributed to increased right ventricular afterload due to severe left ventricular dysfunction. However, early necropsy studies of myocardial infarction demonstrated right ventricular infarction with anterior as well as inferior left ventricular myocardial infarction. The authors attempted to resolve this contradiction by determining the frequency and pathologic characteristics of anterior biventricular necrosis.

All hearts at the Yale Cardiovascular Pathology Study Unit with anterior myocardial infarction studied over a 3-year period were examined for evidence of right ventricular necrosis or scar. Of 97 hearts with anterior myocardial infarction, 13 (13%) had anterior right ventricular myocardial infarction. The right ventricular infarcts involved 10% to 50% of the circumference of the right ventricular free wall from base to apex. The associated left ventricular infarcts were all anteroseptal and large and involved 36% to 67% of the total area of the left ventricular free wall and septum. Nine of these 13 patients underwent equilibrium radionuclide angiography and 6 had demonstrable right ventricular regional and global dysfunction.

Right ventricular myocardial infarction does occur with anterior wall left ventricular infarction, and right ventricular dysfunction may be demonstrable by radionuclide angiography. Further investigation is necessary to define the hemodynamic characteristics, clinical importance, and therapeutic implications of anterior right ventricular myocardial infarction.

▶ A clear demonstration of the potential importance of right ventricular infarction in the setting of anterior wall infarctions. As noted by the authors, further study will be necessary to document differences in hemodynamics associated with the anatomical location of the infarction.—R.L. Frye, M.D.

Association Between Transient Pulmonary Congestion During Acute Myocardial Infarction and High Incidence of Death in Six Months

Edward M. Dwyer, Jr., Henry Greenberg, Robert B. Case, and the Multicenter Postinfarction Research Group (St. Lukes-Roosevelt Hosp. Ctr. and Columbia Univ., New York)

Am. J. Cardiol. 58:900–905, November 1986 4–12

The clinical characteristics, postinfarction course, and clinical details of 57 patients who died within 6 months following acute myocardial infarction (AMI) were compared with those of 44 patients who died in the subsequent 18 months. Total patient selection came from 866 patients younger than 70 years who had no other life-threatening conditions.

Analysis of the death rate showed an average annualized 15% rate for the first 3 months and 12% for the following 3 months. For the remaining 3-month periods to 24 months, the death rate declined to an annualized value of 3% to 5%. The group of patients who died in the first 6 months had a similar history and characteristics as those who died after 6 months. Thirty of the 57 who died early had pulmonary congestion compared with 9 of 44 who died later. Closely associated with pulmonary congestion was sinus tachycardia. Many patients with pulmonary edema during AMI were subsequently observed to have a normal radionuclide ejection fraction, regardless of survival outcome. More patients who died early were experiencing their first infarction, with anterior infarction significantly greater than inferior ones.

No correlation of early death was seen with more severe left ventricular dysfunction, more malignant arrhythmias, or more severe ischemia. The incidence of rehospitalization and reinfarction among patients who died early was not significantly different from those who died late, nor was there a statistical difference in instantaneous death rate. The causes of death were similar except in the category of arrhythmia, which was seen more often in those who died late.

At the time of infarction, pulmonary congestion may represent a combination of irreversible infarction, in some patients, and reversible ischemic asynergy. It is the ischemic region that has the potential of recurrent ischemia and early death. A high incidence of signs or symptoms of ischemia was seen at the time of death (55%), although no difference existed between those who died early and those who died late. While pulmonary congestion is associated with the high and early mortality in the patients studied, the exact reason is not clear, and such congestion should be considered a warning signal of poor prognosis, regardless of the ventricular function.

▶ Another intriguing study documenting the importance of pulmonary congestion in the presence of essentially normal global left ventricular systolic function as a predictor of subsequent mortality in patients with myocardial infarction. Rapapport initially described a similar pattern in a smaller group of patients. Unfortunately, no measures of diastolic function are available, and it does seem likely these patients have an ischemic "stiff" ventricle regardless of the measure of systolic function of the ventricle.—R.L. Frye, M.D.

Mechanism of Atropine-Resistant Atrioventricular Block During Inferior Myocardial Infarction: Possible Role of Adenosine

Robert C. Wesley, Jr., Bruce B. Lerman, John P. DiMarco, Robert M. Berne, and Luiz Belardinelli (Univ. of Virginia, Charlottesville)

J. Am. Coll. Cardiol. 8:1232–1234, November 1986 4–13

Ischemia-induced atrioventricular (AV) block may be caused by the production of adenosine, a metabolite that accumulates during hypoxia and ischemia. Adenosine antagonism has been shown to reverse experimental AV node block in dogs. This case report describes the use of aminophylline, an adenosine antagonist, to reverse atropine-resistant AV node block in a patient.

Woman, 62, with diabetes mellitus and controlled hypertension had a 3-day history of faintness, weakness, and fatigue, without chest pain, coinciding with the discontinuation of metoprolol ingestion. An ECG showed a new Q wave in lead III, ST elevation in leads III and aVF, and complete heart block (narrow QRS complex) with a junctional escape rate of 50 beats per minute. Atropine had no effect on AV node conduction. On day 3, the third-degree and 2:1 second-degree AV block were reversed by the administration of aminophylline. As the level of aminophylline decreased, high AV node block recurred, until spontaneous resolution on the seventh day.

This case report demonstrates that aminophylline, a competitive antagonist of adenosine, is able to reverse AV node block that is unresponsive to atropine. These findings suggest that this block accompanying acute inferior infarction was not of parasympathetic origin. Such adenosine antagonists are potential candidates for the treatment of symptomatic ischemia-induced bradyarrhythmias.

▶ A provocative bedside observation that appears to have not only practical clinical importance but to provide a thought-provoking role for adenosine independent of parasympathetic tone in AV nodal block associated with myocardial ischemia and infarction.—R.L. Frye, M.D.

Electrocardiographic Evolution of Posterior Acute Myocardial Infarction: Importance of Early Precordial ST Segment Depression

William E. Boden, Robert E. Kleiger, Robert S. Gibson, David J. Schwartz, Kenneth B. Schechtman, Robert J. Capone, Robert Roberts, and the Diltiazem Reinfarction Study Group (Wayne State Univ.)

Am. J. Cardiol. 59:782–787, April 1, 1987 4–14

Precordial ST segment depression is characteristic of anterior non-Q-wave acute infarction. Fifty of 544 patients with infarction, which was confirmed by creatine kinase (CK)-MB testing, and without Q waves had isolated ST depression of 1 mm or more in two or more contiguous precordial leads.

Electrocardiographic evidence of posterior infarction developed in 23 of the 50 study patients. Posterior infarction evolved by study day 3 in 18 cases. No patient had an abnormal reelevation of CK-MB within 2 weeks of hospital admission. The patients in whom signs of posterior infarction developed had higher mean peak CK values and greater mean precordial ST segment depression than those who did not. The former patients all had horizontal ST segment depression and upright precordial T waves, whereas those with anterior infarction had downsloping ST depression and precordial T wave inversion.

Early ST segment depression in leads V_1-V_4 during evolving acute infarction may signal ischemia of the posterior wall. Patients with reciprocal precordial ST segment elevation should be considered eligible for early thrombolytic therapy. Exclusion of such patients, especially those with circumflex coronary artery obstruction and an appreciable area at risk of infarction, makes it difficult to extrapolate findings of potential benefit from acute thrombolysis to all anatomical subtypes of infarction.

▶ Another interesting electrocardiographic observation on the importance of recognizing evolving posterior wall myocardial infarction.—R.L. Frye, M.D.

Serial Acquisition of Data to Predict One-Year Mortality Rate After Acute Myocardial Infarction

Paul A. Tibbits, Judy E. Evaul, Robert E. Goldstein, Stephen J. Boccuzzi, Terry M. Therneau, Roger Parker, Dean Wong, and the Multicenter Postinfarction Research Group

Am. J. Cardiol. 60:451–455, Sept. 1, 1987 4–15

Predictors of long-term outcome were sought in a series of 866 patients who were younger than 70 years and had acute myocardial infarction with no serious complicating illness. The chief end point was 1-year cardiac death. There were 65 cardiac deaths and 21 nonfatal repeat infarctions during a mean 12-month follow-up.

Twenty-one variables had high predictive value on univariate analysis. Multivariate analysis and analysis of receiver-operator characteristic curves yielded an initial group of independent predictors comprising rales, left bundle-branch block, and symptomatic status a month before admission. Predictions were not improved by adding data on ambulatory monitoring or serum chemistry. Radionuclide ejection fraction contributed independently to predictions of mortality. However, the addition of data on the radionuclide scans and exercise tests was not clinically significant.

Although risk prediction can be improved by predischarge testing in patients who have specific symptoms or signs of cardiac dysfunction, costly tests should not be universally applied for prognostic purposes after acute myocardial infarction. No algorithm for selective testing has yet been validated, and at present individual patient characteristics must be considered to select tests efficiently.

▶ This is an extremely important study that should be reviewed carefully by all physicians managing patients with acute myocardial infarction. The approach is one that needs to be followed in other studies that attempt to predict prognosis after acute myocardial infarction. This relates to an attempt to define clearly the *incremental* value, if any, of additional testing beyond certain clinical variables present at the time of admission to the coronary care unit. While there was additional statistical value that could be demonstrated of a measure of left ventricular function, this was not large, and the most important variable in regard to exercise testing was whether or not the test was performed.

The fact that the overwhelming dominance of the entry clinical criteria in predicting subsequent prognosis must raise questions about the need for "across the board" uncritical application of a multitude of tests in patients following myocardial infarction. The distinction between individual variables that may have prognostic value and the incremental value of such variables given an overall baseline clinical status of a patient cannot be overemphasized.—R.L. Frye, M.D.

Prevalence, Characteristics and Significance of Ventricular Tachycardia Detected by 24-Hour Continuous Electrocardiographic Recordings in the Late Hospital Phase of Acute Myocardial Infarction

J. Thomas Bigger, Joseph L. Fleiss, Linda M. Rolnitzky, and the Multicenter Post-Infarction Research Group (The Columbia-Presbyterian Med. Ctr., New York, and other participating institutions)

Am. J. Cardiol. 58:1151–1160, Dec. 1, 1986 4–16

The prevalence and significance of ventricular tachycardia (VT) in the late hospital phase of acute myocardial infarction (AMI) is uncertain. The authors used data from the Multicenter Post-Infarction Program (a large, representative sample of the post-AMI population), and investigated VT after AMI to determine the prevalence of VT; to determine the relation between VT and other postinfarction predictors; to compare the mortality rates for patients with VT to those for patients without VT; to determine the characteristics of VT and their association with mortality; and to determine the strength of association between VT and mortality after adjusting for other risk predictors.

A 24-hour continuous ECG recording 11 ± 3 days after AMI in 820 of 867 participants in the Multicenter Post-Infarction Program. Ninety patients (11%) had unsustained VT, and 2 (0.2%) had sustained VT. In 53 (58%) of 92 patients with VT, there was only 1 episode of VT in the recording. There were 26 (28%) patients in whom the longest episode of VT was 3 consecutive complexes; 56 patients (61%) in whom it was 4 to 10 complexes; and 10 patients (11%) in whom it was more than 10 consecutive complexes. Most of the episodes of VT began long after the T wave. The occurrence of VT was strongly related to the frequency of ventricular premature complexes in the 24-hour recording; 46% of patients having at least 100 ventricular premature complexes per hour had VT.

The 92 patients who had VT were compared with 728 patients who did not have VT, and several variables were markedly more common in the VT group, including age older than 60 years, previous AMI, history of angina pectoris, occurrence of VT or ventricular fibrillation in the coronary care unit, left ventricular ejection fraction less than 30%, rales greater than bibasilar in the coronary care unit, and use of antiarrhythmic drugs, digitalis, or diuretics at the time of discharge from the hospital. The cumulative probability of surviving 3 years was 0.67 for patients with VT and 0.85 for patients without VT. Although there were no significant associations between individual VT characteristics and mortality, patients with longer runs of VT tended to have a higher mortality rate, and both patients with sustained VT died in the first month after the index infarct.

Ventricular tachycardia had a strong and statistically significant association with all-cause and arrhythmic mortality independent of other risk variables that were associated with VT. When adjusted for other risk indicators, VT nearly doubled the risk of dying during an average follow-up of 31 months.

▶ While these careful studies clearly provide evidence for ventricular tachycardia as an independent predictor of mortality following myocardial infarction, the need for testing therapy to control ventricular tachycardia in properly designed randomized trials is emphasized. The Multicenter Post-Infarction Study Program has provided important insights to our management of patients following myocardial infarction.—R.L. Frye, M.D.

Prognostic Significance of the Treadmill Exercise Test Performance 6 Months After Myocardial Infarction

Peter H. Stone, Zoltan G. Turi, James E. Muller, Corette Parker, Tyler Hartwell, John D. Rutherford, Allan S. Jaffe, Daniel S. Raabe, Eugene R. Passamani, James T. Willerson, Burton E. Sobel, Thomas L. Robertson, Eugene Braunwald, and the MILIS Study Group (Harvard Univ., Boston, and cooperating institutions of the Multicenter Investigation of the Limitation of Infarct Size)

J. Am. Coll. Cardiol. 8:1007–1017, November 1986 4–17

The results of a predischarge treadmill exercise test are often used as a prognostic indicator for patients suffering uncomplicated myocardial infarctions. However, little information is available regarding the value of a maximal exercise test performed at least 6 months after the myocardial infarction to identify prognosis later in the convalescent period. The authors examined the results of a 6-month postinfarction treadmill exercise test and morbidity and mortality during the following year, as well as the prognostic value of this test compared with the predischarge exercise test.

A subgroup of patients at the Multicenter Investigation of the Limitation of Infarct Size were studied. A 6-month postinfarction visit included interval history review, physical examination, and an exercise test performed according to a modification of the Bruce protocol if the patient consented and did not have any cardiac or physical limitations preventing the test. Patients were followed up over the next year by telephone interview. End points for the study were mortality, development of nonfatal recurrent infarction, and the need for coronary artery bypass surgery.

Of 719 patients available for 6-month follow-up, 473 performed the exercise test and 246 did not. The mortality rate 6–18 months post infarction was significantly higher among patients who were unable to perform the exercise test owing to cardiac limitations compared with those who could. Among the 473 patients who performed the exercise test, exercise-induced ST segment elevation, inadequate arterial blood pressure response during exercise, development of ventricular premature depolarizations during exercise, and failure to exercise past stage I of the protocol were identified as significant risk factors for mortality. A 1% incidence rate of death was found among patients with none of these factors compared with a rate of 17% in patients manifesting three or four factors. A significantly increased incidence of recurrent nonfatal infarction was found in patients whose cardiac limitations prevented performance of the exercise test compared with those who performed the test.

There was a significant relationship between the development of ST segment depression of at least 1 mm during the test and the need for coronary bypass surgery. The presence of heart failure or angina at the 6-month visit were strong predictors of increased mortality among all 719 patients evaluated. However, the exercise test results were much more useful prognostic indicators than the clinical information among the 473 low-risk patients who performed the test.

Unique prognostic information can be obtained from a maximal effort treadmill test performed 6 months after acute myocardial infarction. This may be useful in identifying survivors without clinical complications who are at high risk in the subsequent 12 months.

▶ An interesting study from the MILIS Trial regarding the utility of exercise testing 6 months after myocardial infarction to identify patients at high risk. Again, one of the most important variables is the ability to perform the test, and at 6 months it seems to clearly add to the predictive value of testing, in contrast to the previously noted study early after myocardial infarction (Abstract 4–15).—R.L. Frye, M.D.

PTCA

Aspirin and Dipyridamole in the Prevention of Acute Coronary Thrombosis Complicating Coronary Angioplasty

Elliot S. Barnathan, J. Sanford Schwartz, Lynne Taylor, Warren K. Laskey, J. Patrick Kleaveland, William G. Kussmaul, and John W. Hirshfeld, Jr. (Univ. of Pennsylvania)

Circulation 76:125–134, July 1987 4–18

Pretreatment with antiplatelet agents may reduce the risk of acute coronary thrombosis which complicates percutaneous transluminal coronary angioplasty (PTCA). Data on 300 consecutive angioplasties that were initially successful were studied for evidence of thrombus at the PTCA site immediately after the procedure and at least 30 minutes after the last balloon inflation. The antiplatelet drugs were aspirin and dipyridamole. Heparin was routinely used in conjunction with angioplasty.

Definite thrombus was found at 39 (15%) of 263 evaluable dilated sites. Fifteen of the thrombi were clinically significant, representing 6% of all sites that were dilated. Six were treated with intracoronary streptokinase alone, but 8 required emergency bypass surgery. In 1 case no immediate intervention was used. A lack of antiplatelet therapy was the most powerful predictor of acute thrombosis, and it was an even better predictor of clinically significant thrombosis at the angioplasty site. Smoking, greater stenosis, and dissection also were markers of thrombosis.

Administration of aspirin and dipyridamole may lower the risk of thrombosis at the site of PTCA, but prospective controlled trials are needed. Antiplatelet therapy is especially helpful in decreasing the occurrence of clinically significant thrombosis.

▶ This study certainly does seem to show the importance of adequate antiplatelet therapy in prevention of thrombi at the time of coronary angioplasty. The authors are appropriately cautious in interpretation of their data and point out the limitations of the study, particularly the angiographic end point, and heterogeneity of the treatment groups. The need for appropriately designed prospective randomized trials is emphasized.—R.L. Frye, M.D.

Percutaneous Transluminal Angioplasty of Stenotic Coronary Artery Bypass Grafts: 5 Years' Experience

Gilles Cote, Richard K. Myler, Simon H. Stertzer, David A. Clark, Jodi Fishman-Rosen, Mary Murphy, and Richard E. Shaw (Seton Med. Ctr., Daly City, Calif.)

J. Am. Coll. Cardiol. 9:8–17, January 1987 4–19

Transluminal angioplasty was performed to dilate 101 stenotic sites in 82 patients in 1981–1985. Eighty-three saphenous vein grafts and five internal mammary artery grafts were dilated. Angioplasty was performed a mean of 51 months after bypass surgery. About 75% of patients were in functional class III and IV at the time of angioplasty.

The procedure was technically successful in 85% of patients, in whom all graft and lesion sites were dilated without serious complications. Eighty-five percent of all treated sites were successfully dilated. Three patients had distal coronary embolization or abrupt closure after angioplasty and evidence of myocardial infarction. One of them had emergency bypass surgery. There were no hospital deaths. Ten of 26 evaluable patients had evidence of recurrence in at least one site on postangioplasty angiography, a mean of 8 months after angioplasty. The degree of stenosis just after dilation was a good predictor of stenosis at follow-up. One of two late deaths was related to graft occlusion. More than two thirds of patients were in angina class I at follow-up.

Angioplasty is an effective approach to both saphenous vein graft and internal mammary artery graft stenoses. Recurrences might be reduced by using higher pressure balloons and by achieving slightly greater balloon/graft ratios.

Percutaneous Transluminal Coronary Angioplasty in Patients With Prior Coronary Artery Bypass Grafting: Long-Term Results

Sjef M.P.G. Ernst, Taco A. van der Feltz, Carl A.P.L. Ascoop, Egbert T. Bal, Freddy E.E. Vermeulen, Paul J. Knaepen, Leo van Bogerijen, Eduard J.M. van den Berg, and H.W. Thijs Plokker (St. Antonius Hosp., Nieuwegein, Utrecht, The Netherlands)

J. Thorac. Cardiovasc. Surg. 93:268–275, February 1987 4–20

Percutaneous transluminal coronary angioplasty (PTCA) is an attractive alternative to reoperation in patients with prior coronary artery bypass grafting (CABG) and severe angina pectoris resulting from stenoses either in the vein graft or in the native coronary arteries. However, the long-term effect of this procedure is not known. The authors evaluated this procedure as a long-term effective method of treatment of patients with prior CABG and return of disabling symptoms.

The study group included 83 patients with previous coronary artery bypass grafting in whom 92 percutaneous transluminal coronary angioplasty attempts were performed. Of these 92 PTCA attempts, 33 were in a venous bypass graft (success rate, 97%) and 59 were in a native coronary artery (success rate, 86.4%). There were no procedural-related deaths, although there were 2 myocardial infarctions. Of the patients with successful angioplasty after previous bypass grafting, 46% remain symptom free after 5 years (79% of the patients without previous bypass grafting). Long-term success rates for native vessel angioplasty compared with bypass graft angioplasty were similar. The patients with a short interval between the recurrence of angina after bypass grafting and the angioplasty attempt had a better chance of long-term success. Repeat angiography indicated that a restenosis occurs after angioplasty of a venous graft in 31% and in the native system in 28.6%, and that signs of progression of coronary artery disease elsewhere could be demonstrated in 30%. Eleven of the 83 patients eventually underwent reoperation.

Percutaneous transluminal coronary angioplasty after coronary bypass grafting gives less satisfactory results than a primary procedure. In addition, angioplasty provides symptomatic relief in a smaller number of patients than in those with primary angioplasty; however, symptomatic relief is often sufficient to further postpone or prevent bypass grafting and can be achieved with low mortality and complication rates.

▶ These two articles (Abstracts 4–19 and 4–20) reporting experience of PTCA in patients with prior coronary bypass grafting are important observational studies. They document success rates and subsequent course of such patients. With the increasing number of patients with prior coronary bypass surgery, these observations will be of interest to all clinicians and surgeons.—R.L. Frye, M.D.

Angiographic Patterns of Restenosis After Angioplasty of Multiple Coronary Arteries

Germano DiSciascio, Michael J. Cowley, and George W. Vetrovec (Med. College of Virginia, Richmond)

Am. J. Cardiol. 58:922–925, November 1986 4–21

Although percutaneous transluminal coronary angioplasty (PTCA) is a widely used revascularization technique, the angiographic presentation of patients with clinical recurrence of ischemia after PTCA of multiple arteries has not been characterized. The authors analyzed angiographic patterns of restenosis in patients with clinical recurrence after PTCA of multiple arteries and investigated factors that may be predictive of recurrence of individual narrowings.

The angiograms of 40 patients with clinical recurrence after PTCA of multiple arteries were reviewed. Clinical recurrence was defined as return of signs or symptoms after successful PTCA of more than one major artery or branch and angiographic evidence of restenosis of one or more lesions. In these 40 patients, 83 arteries and 103 narrowings were successfully dilated. Restenosis developed in 57 (69%) of 83 arteries at risk; 23 patients (58%) had restenosis in only one artery, and 17 patients (42%) had restenosis in two arteries. Restenosis occurred in 63 (61%) of 103 lesions at risk; 20 patients (50%) had restenosis of one narrowing, 17 (43%) patients had restenosis of two narrowings; and 3 (7%) having restenosis of three narrowings. Only 13 patients (33%) had restenosis of all narrowings dilated. Predictors of restenosis of individual narrowings included higher pre-PTCA percent stenosis and higher degree of residual stenosis after PTCA. Balloon size or inflation pressure did not predict recurrence of narrowings. Repeat PTCA was successful in 97% (33 of 34) of cases attempted; 3 patients underwent elective bypass surgery, and 3 were managed with medical therapy.

Most patients with clinical recurrence of multiple arteries after PTCA do not have restenosis of multiple arteries or narrowings, and only one third will have recurrence of all narrowings. A higher degree of pre- and post-PTCA stenosis was associated with recurrence of individual narrowings.

▶ An interesting observational study of the patterns of restenosis following angioplasty of multiple coronary arteries. It is a complicated set of data to analyze since one needs to consider not only patients dilated but numbers of lesions as well as perhaps numbers of arteries. The authors reflect that "only one third will have recurrence of all narrowings." It would actually seem to this reviewer that the restenosis rate is rather high based on that figure, as well as the fact that restenosis developed in 69% of the 83 arteries at risk and in 61% of 103 lesions at risk. Thus, clinical recurrence, a requirement for entry into this study, seems to be associated with a significant degree of incomplete revascularization based on these restenosis rates.—R.L. Frye, M.D.

Percutaneous Transluminal Coronary Angioplasty: A Growing Surgical Problem

U. Scott Page, J. Edward Okies, Leon Q. Colburn, John C. Bigelow, Neal W. Salomon, and Albert H. Krause (Good Samaritan Hosp. and Med. Ctr., Portland, Ore.)

J. Thorac. Cardiovasc. Surg. 92:847–852, November 1986 4–22

In 1985, 11.4% of the authors' patients undergoing pure revascularization had undergone a prior percutaneous transluminal angioplasty (PTCA). The yearly increase in the PCTA rate is nearly doubling; most of these patients were low-risk surgical candidates before PTCA. Higher perioperative infarction and mortality rates prompted the authors to compare the mortality rates for patients undergoing a coronary artery bypass grafting procedure who had undergone prior PTCA with those who had not undergone PCTA before surgery.

One hundred thirty-five patients with prior PTCA were compared with 2,205 patients without PTCA. The mortality was 3.2 times higher in the angioplasty patients than in the control patients, and the perioperative infarction rate was 2.5 times higher. There were 44 patients who were taken directly to the operating room from the catheterization laboratory; 50 patients were operated on within 10 days, and 41 patients underwent operation more than 10 days after angioplasty. All of these late failures were of the lesion previously dilated. The infarction rate was lower in patients taken immediately to the operating room on an emergency basis compared with those whose operation was delayed up to 10 days (30% vs. 70%). All of the patients who died had undergone angioplasty of the anterior descending coronary artery.

Angioplasty of the anterior descending coronary artery increases operative mortality in patients in whom treatment becomes acutely necessary. Patients should be informed before angioplasty of the increased surgical risks after a failed angioplasty procedure.

▶ This is a provocative article documenting the experience of these investigators, an increased risk of coronary bypass surgery and perioperative myocardial infarction in patients with prior PTCA, particularly of the left anterior descending coronary artery. As might be expected, this was most obvious in the emergent patients, but when compared with the patients undergoing coronary bypass surgery not previously dilated, there were differences noted. This study emphasizes the need for a carefully controlled prospective randomized trial to test the impact of an initial strategy of PTCA compared with coronary bypass surgery and the penalty paid in trying to delay surgery by the initial PTCA.—R.L. Frye, M.D.

Percutaneous Transluminal Coronary Angioplasty for Chronic Total Coronary Arterial Occlusion

Jean Paul Melchior, Bernhard Meier, Philippe Urban, Leo Finci, Giuseppe Steffenino, Jacques Noble, and Wilhem Rutishauser (Univ. Hosp., Geneva, Switzerland)

Am. J. Cardiol. 59:535–538, March 1, 1987 4–23

Percutaneous transluminal coronary angioplasty (PTCA) is used to treat a wide range of coronary lesions. The authors determined the initial and long-term success rate of PTCA for total occlusion and its impact on anginal symptoms, defined the factors associated with good immediate and long-term results, and analyzed the nature and frequency of complications.

The study group included 100 consecutive patients in whom PTCA was attempted on chronically occluded coronary arteries that had no visible anterograde flow. Ninety-eight patients had angina, and all had collateral vessels to the occluded artery on angiography. The overall initial PTCA success rate was 56% and was related to duration of occlusion (69% success rate for 1–6 months, and 11% after 6 months). There were only minor complications; none of the patients died or required emergency bypass operation. There were 44 patients in whom PTCA failed, 20 of whom underwent elective bypass surgery for relief of angina; the other 24 were treated medically.

Follow-up data (mean, 8 months) were available for 49 of the 56 patients in whom PTCA was successful. Forty of these patients had subjective improvement, 6 experienced no change, and 3 felt worse. Control angiography was performed in 40 of the 56 patients with primary success and demonstrated long-term success in 18, and reocclusion or marked restenosis in 22. Of these 22 patients, 11 were successfully treated by a second PTCA, 2 underwent operation, and 9 were treated medically.

Recanalization of totally occluded coronary arteries with no forward flow has a lower initial success rate (56%) than PTCA for stenoses and the recurrence rate is higher (55%); however, effective relief of angina is achieved in successful cases. The risk of serious complications appears to be low.

▶ An interesting additional bit of data regarding the use of transluminal coronary angioplasty in patients with total coronary artery occlusion. It seems clear from this and other studies that the success rate is highly dependent on the time from the complete occlusion until the attempted angioplasty.—R.L. Frye, M.D.

Unstable Angina

Comparison of Medical and Surgical Treatment for Unstable Angina Pectoris: Results of a Veterans Administration Cooperative Study

Robert J. Luchi, Stewart M. Scott, and Robert H. Deupree (VA Med. Ctr., Houston, VA Med. Ctr., Asheville, N.C., and VA Med. Ctr., West Haven, Conn.)

N. Engl. J. Med. 316:977–984, April 16, 1987 4–24

A prospective multicenter VA study comparing medical therapy plus coronary bypass surgery with medical treatment alone enrolled 468 men younger than 70 years who had unstable angina pectoris. Treatment was randomly assigned. Medical treatment included short-acting and long-acting nitrates, β-blockers, and aspirin, as well as measures designed to reduce risk factors.

Survival after 2 years did not differ significantly according to assigned treatment except in patients with depressed left ventricular ejection fractions. Total operative mortality was 4.1%. One third of patients crossed over from medical to surgical treatment in the first 2 years. Operative mortality was about 10% in this group. Nonfatal myocardial infarction occurred in about 12% of both treatment groups.

Coronary bypass surgery improves survival in patients with unstable angina who have an abnormal left ventricular ejection fraction at rest.

▶ This is an important comparision of a *strategy* of initial medical therapy versus CABG. It is not a comparison of medical therapy alone versus surgery alone, since the high crossover rates from medicine to surgery reflect realities of clinical practice and research. In dealing with the high crossover rates, the investigators have analyzed the data not only by intention to treat but by other approaches. The results are all comparable. Of particular concern is the high perioperative death rate at the time of crossover (10.3% vs. 4.1%).—R.L. Frye, M.D.

Early Treatment of Unstable Angina in the Coronary Care Unit: A Randomised, Double Blind, Placebo Controlled Comparison of Recurrent Ischaemia in Patients Treated With Nifedipine or Metoprolol or Both

Holland Interuniversity Nifedipine/Metoprolol Trial (HINT) Research Group (Netherlands Interuniv. Cardiology Inst., Utrecht)

Br. Heart J. 56:400–413, November 1986 4–25

The goals of treating unstable angina, after initial relief of pain, are to prevent recurrent ischemia or infarction and restore stability. A multicenter, double-blind trial of nifedipine, metoprolol, and both agents was carried out in 338 patients with unstable angina who were not pretreated with a β-blocker. Nifedipine was given to 177 patients pretreated with a β-blocker. Nifedipine was administered in six 10-mg doses per 24 hours, and metoprolol was administered in two 100-mg doses per 24 hours.

Event rate ratios, considering recurrent ischemia and myocardial infarction within 48 hours as even, were 1.15 for nifedipine, 0.76 for metoprolol, and 0.80 for both drugs in patients not pretreated with a β-blocker. In pretreated patients, addition of nifedipine was beneficial, yielding a rate ratio of 0.68. Most infarctions occurred within 6 hours of randomization into the trial. The nifedipine rate ratio for infarction only in nonpretreated patients was 1.51.

Metoprolol appears to have a beneficial short-term effect on unstable angina in patients not previously given a β-blocker. Nifedipine alone is not of use in this setting, and may have an adverse effect, but patients already receiving β-blockade may benefit from the addition of nifedipine if their condition becomes unstable.

▶ An important study that had to be stopped because of high infarction rates in the nifedipine-alone group. Unfortunately, small treatment groups with an important baseline imbalance as regards a high-risk variable (time between last episode of angina and therapy) and a large number of protocol violations complicate the interpretation of this important trial.—R.L. Frye, M.D.

Stress Testing and Silent Ischemia

The Changing Role of the Exercise Electrocardiogram as a Diagnostic and Prognostic Test for Chronic Ischemic Heart Disease

Bernard R. Chaitman (St. Louis Univ.)

J. Am. Coll. Cardiol. 8:1195–1210, November 1986 4–26

The exercise ECG has been researched intensely in the past 50 years, as both a diagnostic and prognostic method to evaluate patients with chronic ischemic heart disease. The strengths and limitations of this method to predict coronary and multivessel disease in clinical patient subsets are understood. The changing role of the exercise ECG was reviewed, with emphasis on the strengths and limitations of the technique.

The diagnostic accuracy of the exercise ECG is improved by consideration of the Bayesian theory (the concept of a continuum of posttest risk based on the pretest risk of coronary disease and likelihood ratio, explaining how conditional probability should be used to report exercise test results); multivariate models, whereby the posttest risk of disease can be estimated; and new non-ST segment criteria. Posttest coronary disease risk estimates should be reported in terms of a conditional probability, rather than as positive or negative. Recent reports of long-term follow-up data in asymptomatic and symptomatic patients have considerably enhanced the value of exercise testing in prognostic risk stratification. Powerful prognostic data can be obtained when the clinical, electrocardiographic, and physiologic information from the test are used in formulating the posttest risk of a cardiac event, even in patients whose coronary anatomy is known.

The main indications for performing an exercise test in patients with typical angina are to determine functional capacity and a baseline for repeated measures in future years, to assess antianginal drug therapy and revascularization procedures, and to obtain a prognostic risk estimate to use in deciding indications for coronary angiography and revascularization procedures. In most asymptomatic, apparently clinically healthy patients, an abnormal exercise ECG does not indicate obstructive coronary disease. Studies show that the cardiac event rate in patients with known coronary disease is relatively low when patients are able to achieve a high exercise work load.

Asymptomatic patients with high clinical pretest risk and marked ECG changes at low exercise work loads require further assessment. The greatest diagnostic value of exercise testing may be in patients with atypical angina and intermediate pretest risk, in whom ECG changes can help in formulating a decision for coronary angiography.

▶ This is an excellent review of the evolution of exercise ECG testing in diagnosis and prognosis of patients with coronary artery disease. The appraisal for exercise testing is a critical one with excellent reproductions from the important studies accomplished in the field. It is worth a review by all those utilizing exercise ECG testing in their practice.—R.L. Frye, M.D.

Value of Exercise Testing in Determining the Risk Classification and the Response to Coronary Artery Bypass Grafting in Three-Vessel Coronary Artery Disease: A Report From the Coronary Artery Surgery Study (CASS) Registry

Donald A. Weiner, Thomas J. Ryan, Carolyn H. McCabe, Bernard R. Chaitman, L. Thomas Sheffield, Lloyd D. Fisher, and Felix Tristani (University Hosp., Boston, St. Louis Univ., Univ. of Alabama, Univ. of Washington, and Med. College of Wisconsin)

Am. J. Cardiol. 60:262–266, Aug. 1, 1987 4–27

Data from 1,249 nonrandomized patients with triple-vessel coronary artery disease from the Coronary Artery Surgery Study (CASS) registry were analyzed to determine whether exercise testing can identify higher risk patients who might live longer after coronary artery bypass grafting. Patients were followed up for 5 years or longer. There were 470 medically treated and 779 surgically treated patients in the series. The former patients had more severe heart failure and poorer left ventricular (LV) function. Surgically treated patients had more abnormal responses to exercise testing.

The LV score, final exercise stage, and treatment had independent effects on survival. Among patients who had normal LV function, those with at least 1 mm of ischemic ST depression or low exercise capacity had better 7-year survival if they were operated on. No such difference was found for patients without ischemic ST depression or those with good exercise capacity, but among patients with impaired LV function surgery improved the outlook in most subsets of patients as long as exercise capacity was impaired.

Exercise testing is relevant when planning treatment for patients with triple-vessel coronary artery disease. Surgery appears to be helpful to patients who have ischemic ST-segment depression on exercise and impaired exercise tolerance, whether LV function is normal or abnormal.

▶ There are several consistent themes when one analyzes the CASS data. In the randomized trial, left ventricular function and exercise-induced ischemia as evidenced by angina identify patients with a compromised survival that was improved with surgical therapy, particularly in patients with triple vessel coronary artery disease. The observations in the nonrandomized patients are consistent with the above, but emphasize the prognostic value of stress testing in patients with normal LV function and, again, the benefits of surgery in improving survival in patients with triple vessel disease and the described features on exercise testing. ST segment shifts were predictive in the nonrandomized patients.—R.L. Frye, M.D.

Anatomic and Functional Significance of a Hypotensive Response During Supine Exercise Radionuclide Ventriculography

Raymond J. Gibbons, David C. Hu, Ian P. Clements, Harold T. Mankin, Alan R. Zinsmeister, and Manuel L. Brown (Mayo Clinic and Found.)

Am. J. Cardiol. 60:1–4, July 1, 1987 4–28

The significance of a decline in systolic blood pressure during supine exercise is uncertain. Both supine exercise gated equilibrium radionuclide ventriculography and coronary angiography were performed in 820 patients within a 3-month period. Twenty-seven patients (3%) developed systolic hypotension, with a mean fall in blood pressure of 24 mm Hg.

Patients with systolic hypotension were older than the others and more likely to have abnormal findings on resting ECG. Past infarction was not significantly more frequent. Patients with systolic hypotension had poor exercise tolerance. Angina was present on exercise in 56% of these patients, and 74% had at least 1 mm of ST depression on the exercise ECG. Mean resting ejection fraction was 47% and mean exercise value was 41%. Coronary angiography nearly always showed severe disease. All but 5 of 27 patients had triple-vessel disease.

Systolic hypotension that occurs during supine exercise is a marker of severe coronary artery disease, even when other indicators are not suggestive of severe ischemia. Abnormal global and regional left ventricular function may not be noted in some cases because of the marked change in left ventricular loading conditions that are associated with systolic hypotension.

▶ While differences in physiologic response to supine versus upright exercise have been well documented, these studies reflect a remarkable similarity of the clinical significance of a drop in blood pressure during supine exercise, compared with other studies previously reported by other investigators in patients undergoing stress testing in the upright position. The lack of ST segment shifts and angina at the time of exercise even in patients with critical high-risk anatomy is noteworthy as described by the authors.—R.L. Frye, M.D.

Incremental Prognostic Power of Clinical History, Exercise Electrocardiography and Myocardial Perfusion Scintigraphy in Suspected Coronary Artery Disease

Marc L. Ladenheim, Todd S. Kotler, Brad H. Pollack, Daniel S. Berman, and George A. Diamond (Cedars-Sinai Med. Ctr., Los Angeles, and Univ. of California, Los Angeles)

Am. J. Cardiol. 59:270–277, Feb. 1, 1987 4–29

An attempt was made to develop a rational scheme of prognostic evaluation in a series of 3,155 patients undergoing exercise perfusion scintigraphy in 1979–1982 who were followed up for at least 1 year. The final study group included 1,659 patients without documented coronary artery disease. The total coronary event rate in this group was 5%, with 11 deaths, 24 nonfatal infarctions, and 41 late surgical referrals.

The event rate was 4% in patients with normal ECG findings and 7% in the 208 patients with abnormal ECG. Analysis using ROC curves derived from logistic regression indicated that the clinical history alone provided the most prognostic power. The history was less predictive in patients with an abnormal resting ECG, but each test significantly improved predictions.

The probability of coronary disease is the most useful prognostic descriptor in patients referred for stress testing with suspected coronary artery disease. Intermediate probability calls for exercise ECG testing, and those with positive findings are referred for scintigraphy. All patients with a high probability of disease and a normal resting ECG are referred for exercise ECG study. The overall costs of testing are substantially reduced by this approach. Each physician should choose thresholds for acceptable and unacceptable risk and cost.

▶ This excellent study from the group at Cedars-Sinai, which has contributed so importantly to our understanding of test selection, is a further enhancement of knowledge. It emphasizes the critical analysis of the incremental value of additional testing over and above the more simply obtained prognostic variables such as clinical history and resting ECG, as noted in this and other studies. Establishing one's own level of risk acceptance in terms of being wrong is one of the challenges to all physicians.—R.L. Frye, M.D.

Safety of Intravenous Dipyridamole for Stress Testing With Thallium Imaging

Shunichi Homnma, Yvonne Gilliland, Timothy E. Guiney, H. William Strauss, and Charles A. Boucher (Massachusetts Gen. Hosp., Boston)
Am. J. Cardiol. 59:152–154, Jan. 1, 1987 4–30

Intravenous (IV) dipyridamole is an effective adjunct to thallium imaging when exercise is inappropriate. Side effects were examined in 1985 in a series of 293 consecutive patients having dipyridamole-thallium imaging. The indications included claudication, stroke, arthritis, amputation, and a previous nondiagnostic submaximal stress test. Sixty-two patients had coronary angiography within 6 months of dipyridamole imaging. The dose of dipyridamole was 0.56 mg/kg, totalling 20–78 mg, and was infused over 4 minutes, 10 minutes before thallium-201 injection. A bolus of 50 mg of aminophylline was injected after the anterior myocardial image was acquired.

The peak rise in mean heart rate was 9 beats per minute, and the mean fall in systolic blood pressure was 12 mm Hg 6 minutes after dipyridamole. Side effects occurred in 55% of patients. The most frequent noncardiac effects were headache, lightheadedness/dizziness, and nausea. Chest pain developed in 26% of patients, and 10% had ST segment depression as well. A single injection of aminophylline usually sufficed. No patient had myocardial infarction or sustained severe arrhythmia. Arrhythmias were more common in patients with multivessel or left main coronary disease.

Dipyridamole infusion in conjunction with thallium imaging can produce myocardial ischemia, presumably through "coronary steal" of blood from the least adequately perfused part of the myocardium. Close cardiac monitoring is indicated when this test is performed. Aminophylline is useful in patients with side-effects from dipyridamole, but there is no evidence that its routine use prevents late side effects.

▶ The technique of thallium imaging with dipyridamole stress is being used with increasing frequency in patients with peripheral vascular disease who are unable to exercise. As noted in this article, however, while it does appear to be safe, a clear knowledge of the potential problems with intravenous dipyridamole is essential for those conducting these studies. An appropriate pharmacologic therapy available to counteract the effects of dipyridamole must be immediately at hand. It has recently been brought to my attention that several patients have been observed to have cerebral transient ischemic attacks during intravenous administration of dipyridamole. This will have to be added to the list of potential complications in considering the use of this test in patients with vascular disease.—R.L. Frye, M.D.

Circadian Variation of Transient Myocardial Ischemia in Patients With Coronary Artery Disease

Michael B. Rocco, Joan Barry, Stephen Campbell, Elizabeth Nabel, E. Francis Cook, Lee Goldman, and Andrew P. Selwyn (Brigham and Women's Hosp. and Harvard Univ., Boston)

Circulation 75:395–400, February 1987 4–31

Patients with coronary artery disease suffer symptoms and damage to left ventricular myocardium through the development of active myocardial ischemia. The authors studied the character of ischemic heart disease activity by evaluating whether there is a significant circadian variation of transient myocardial ischemia during daily life.

The study group included 32 patients with chronic stable symptoms of coronary artery disease who underwent 1 or more days of ambulatory monitoring of ischemic ST segment changes during daily life. A total of 251 episodes of ischemic ST segment depression occurred in 24 (75%) patients with a median duration of 5 minutes. There was a significant circadian increase in ischemic activity, with 39% of episodes and 46% of total ischemic time occurring between 6 A.M. and 12 P.M. In 21 patients with ST segment depression during the 6 hours after waking and the 6 hours before sleep, 68% of episodes occurred in the morning compared with 32% in the evening. There were no significant differences in heart rate at onset, heart rate at 1 minute before onset, and activity score associated with ST segment depression. The proportion of minutes with ST segment depression when the heart rate was above the lowest rate associated with ST segment depression was markedly greater in the morning compared with the evening.

The early morning increase in ST segment depression does not appear to be explained by differences in extrinsic activity and/or stress measured by physical activity score and heart rate response. The authors stress that this phenomenon is usually ignored by the usual patterns of drug administration for treatment of angina. They argue that this may have clinical relevance, because the observed circadian variation coincides with that reported for onset of acute myocardial infarction and sudden death.

Clinical Significance of Exercise-Induced Silent Myocardial Ischemia in Patients With Coronary Artery Disease

Colomba Falcone, Stefano de Servi, Ercole Poma, Carlo Campana, Aldo Sciré, Carlo Montemartini, and Giuseppe Specchia (Instituto di Ricovero e Cura a Carattere, Scientifico, Pavia, Italy)

J. Am. Coll. Cardiol. 9:295–299, February 1987 4–32

Although it is known that asymptomatic myocardial ischemia may occur during exercise stress testing in some patients with coronary artery disease, the significance of ST segment changes in the absence of angina is still controversial. The authors analyzed the subjective and objective responses to exercise testing in a large series of patients with angiographically proved coronary artery disease and compared the clinical and angiographic features of patients who complained of angina during the exercise test with those of patients who developed exercise-induced asymptomatic myocardial ischemia.

The study group included 269 patients who complained of chest pain during an exercise test (group I) and 204 patients who developed exercise-induced silent myocardial ischemia (group II). Group I patients more frequently had anginal symptoms of class III and IV of the Canadian Cardiovascular Society than did group II patients, who had milder symptoms. The only angiographic difference noted between the two groups was a slight, but significantly higher, left ventricular end-diastolic pressure in group II patients, who also demonstrated a longer exercise duration with a higher heart rate-systolic pressure product and more pronounced ST segment depression at peak exercise. Furthermore, ventricular ectopic beats during exercise were more frequently observed in group II patients. Of the patients in group I, 45% underwent coronary bypass surgery, compared with 24% of patients in group II. Survival curves of medically treated patients did not show any statistically significant difference between the two groups.

Although patients with a defective anginal warning system may have more pronounced signs of myocardial ischemia and a greater incidence of ventricular arrhythmias during exercise, their long-term prognosis is not different from that of patients who are stopped by angina from the activity that is inducing the myocardial ischemia.

Silent Myocardial Ischemia During Daily Activities in Asymptomatic Men With Positive Exercise Test Responses

Kevin M. Coy, Greg M. Imperi, Charles R. Lambert, and Carl J. Pepine (Univ. of Florida and VA Med. Ctr., Gainesville, Fla.)

Am. J. Cardiol. 59:45–49, January 1987 4–33

Silent ischemia appears to occur frequently in patients with the usual symptomatic phases of coronary artery disease (CAD). Studies of patients in the asymptomatic phase of CAD are difficult. Studies have suggested that some asymptomatic patients may also have silent myocardial ischemia during ambulatory electrocardiographic monitoring (AEM). The authors investigated the presence, extent, and characteristics of "ischemic-type" ST depression using AEM in 17 asymptomatic men with positive treadmill response and determined whether the occurrence of ST depression in these patients identifies a subgroup with severe CAD.

A total of 1,154 hours (64–72 hours per patient) of high-quality AEM recordings were obtained. None of the men took anti-ischemic medications, and all underwent coronary angiography. Silent ischemia (episodes of asymptomatic ischemic-type ST depression of at least 60 seconds) occurred in 11 patients during daily activity detected by AEM. No myocardial ischemic episodes were seen in the other 6 patients; however, 1 of these men withdrew after 24 hours of AEM. The 11 patients with silent ischemia had significant CAD of at least 50% stenosis on angiography. Wide intrapatient variability in the frequency of silent ischemic episodes was noted. Silent ischemia was identified in 6 patients after 24 hours of AEM, in 2 after 48 hours, and in 3 after 72 hours.

Asymptomatic men with positive exercise test responses and CAD had silent ischemic episodes during daily activity detected by AEM. Ambulatory electrocardiographic monitoring may be useful in predicting which patients with asymptomatic positive exercise test responses have CAD; however, extended AEM periods are necessary.

Silent Ischemia Predicts Infarction and Death During 2 Year Follow-up of Unstable Angina

Sidney O. Gottlieb, Myron L. Weisfeldt, Pamela Ouyang, E. David Mellits, and Gary Gerstenblith (Johns Hopkins Hosp.)
J. Am. Coll. Cardiol. 10:756–760, October 1987 4–34

Seventy patients with unstable angina underwent Holter monitoring for 2 days in coronary care and were followed up for 2 years during com-

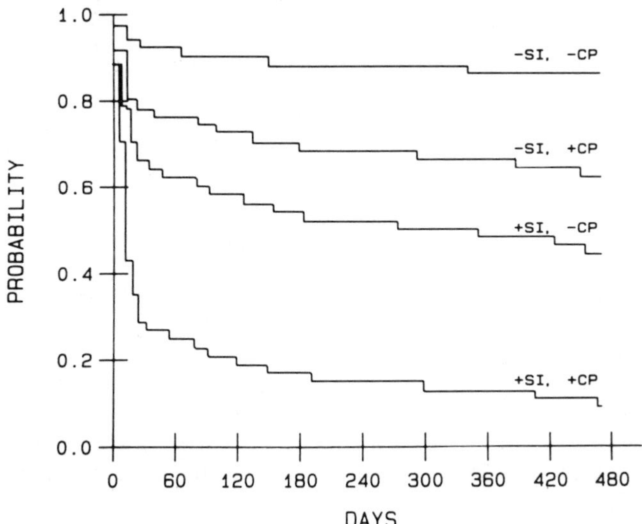

Fig 4–7.—Relative risk curve derived from Cox's hazard function analysis demonstrating the risk for death, myocardial infarction, or revascularization for recurrent symptoms and illustrating the effects of silent ischemia *(SI)* and recurrent chest pain *(CP)* variables on adverse outcome. There is a fivefold relative risk for outcomes associated with SI and a threefold relative risk associated with CP during first 2 days. When both variables are present, the relative risk for experiencing adverse outcome is increased by factor of 15. (Courtesy of Gottlieb, S.O., et al.: J. Am. Coll. Cardiol. 10:756–760, October 1987.)

bination drug treatment that included nitrates, β-blockers, and calcium channel antagonists. All patients had at least one episode of resting chest pain with ischemic ECG changes.

Thirty-seven of the 70 patients had silent ischemic ST changes on Holter monitoring. Cardiovascular risk factors and medical treatment were similar in the patients with and those without silent ischemia, as was the extent of fixed coronary artery disease.

Ten patients with silent ischemia had myocardial infarction during the next 2 years and 2 died. Only 1 of those without silent ischemia had infarction. Eleven patients with silent ischemia and 5 without required angioplasty or bypass surgery for medically refractory symptoms. Silent ischemia was the most important predictor of an unfavorable outcome (Fig 4–7).

The findings on Holter monitoring should be incorporated into the management plan for patients with unstable angina. Patients who fail to respond to intensive medical care should have cardiac catheterization and early coronary revascularization. The ambulatory ECG findings will be helpful, along with low-level exercise testing, in deciding on the management of patients whose chest pain is controlled medically.

▶ The place for ambulatory ECG monitoring in assessing coronary artery disease patients for silent ischemia is not settled in my view. We need to know the degree to which such studies improve our classification of high-risk patients over and above other clinical and laboratory data. Such data will need to be obtained in large numbers of patients. Until such data are available, despite results of these carefully performed studies (Abstracts 4–31 to 4–34) in small groups of patients, widespread routine application of ambulatory ST segment does not seem justified. Furthermore, attention to details of technical requirements for ST segment monitoring versus rhythm analysis needs emphasis.—R.L. Frye, M.D.

Miscellaneous Topics

Beneficial Effects of Combined Colestipol-Niacin Therapy on Coronary Atherosclerosis and Coronary Venous Bypass Grafts

David H. Blankenhorn, Sharon A. Nessim, Ruth L. Johnson, Miguel E. Sanmarco, Stanley P. Azen, and Linda Cashin-Hemphill (Univ. of Southern California, Los Angeles)

JAMA 257:3233–3240, June 19, 1987 4–35

It has been hypothesized that aggressive lowering of low-density lipoprotein (LDL) cholesterol with concomitant increase in high-density protein (HDL) will reverse or retard the growth of atherosclerotic lesions. The Cholesterol-Lowering Atherosclerosis Study (CLAS), a randomized, placebo-controlled, selectively blinded angiographic trial, was designed to test this hypothesis.

Subjects were 162 nonsmoking men, aged 40–59 years, who had had previous bypass surgery. Angiography to obtain baseline data on the atherosclerotic disease of the carotid, femoral, coronary arteries, and coronary bypass grafts was performed. Subjects were then randomized to receive either 30 gm of colestipol hydrochloride plus 3–12 gm of niacin daily or placebo. Niacin was taken three times a day in the middle of a meal. Subjects were seen monthly for 6 months, then at 2-month intervals for 2 years.

During the 2 years of treatment, a 26% reduction in total plasma cholesterol, a 43% reduction in LDL cholesterol, and a 37% elevation in HDL cholesterol were noted in men in the drug group. This resulted in a significant reduction in the average number of lesions per subject who progressed as well as in the percentage with new atheroma formation in native coronary arteries. The percentage of subjects exhibiting new lesions or any adverse changes in bypass grafts was also significantly decreased. Deterioration in overall coronary status was noted to be significantly less in the drug-treated subjects than in the placebo-treated subjects. Atherosclerosis regression, determined by perceptible improvement in overall coronary status, was seen in 16.2% of the drug-treated subjects and in 2.4% of the placebo-treated subjects.

It appears that aggressive lowering of LDL cholesterol levels with concomitant increase in HDL cholesterol levels produces significant benefit for both native coronary arteries and venous bypass grafts. Deterioration of average global coronary change scores was significantly reduced in subjects treated with drugs when compared with those treated with placebo, and atherosclerosis regression occurred in significantly more drug-treated subjects than placebo-treated subjects.

▶ This study by Blankenhorn and colleagues has had a major impact on the attitudes toward aggressive lipid lowering therapy. Unfortunately, the main end point of the study—namely, an angiographic scoring process to judge changes in severity of coronary arterial or vein graft lesions—is poorly described in the article. It is difficult for this reviewer to fully accept the conclusion of the paper without more details regarding the absolute findings at the time of coronary angiography. We are actually presented with no data of the estimates of luminal diameter narrowing in the groups studied. If one accurately interprets the data presented in the paper, the major changes seem to occur in those patients with mild to moderate disease where we know the interobserver and intraobserver variability is the greatest. There is no statistically significant difference in progression to complete occlusion between the treated and untreated groups. The possibility that regression observed may relate to spontaneous lysis of thrombus has also not been fully addressed. In my opinion, the whole situation would be greatly enhanced if the absolute lesion estimates in terms of severity of disease were presented rather than a rather vague sliding scale of categories of lesions.—R.L. Frye, M.D.

Long-Term Prognosis of Patients With Acute Myocardial Infarction: Is Mortality and Morbidity as Low as the Incidence of Ischemic Heart Disease in Japan?

Muneyasu Saito, Ken-ichi Fukami, Katsuhiko Hiramori, Kazuo Haze, Tetsuya Sumiyoshi, Humiyoshi Kasagi, and Hiroshi Horibe (Natl. Cardiovascular Ctr., Osaka, Japan)

Am. Heart J. 113:891–897, April 1987 4–36

The incidence of ischemic heart disease in Japan is much lower than in Western countries. The authors examined the long-term prognosis of hospital survivors with acute myocardial infarction (MI) to determine whether the incidence of ischemic heart disease in Japan is low, and analyzed the factors that influence the long-term prognosis for these patients.

Of the 686 patients with acute MI, there were 563 hospital survivors. The cumulative mortality rate of these patients was 6.2% in the first year, 12.0% in the third year, and 19.1% in the fifth year, with cardiac death accounting for 63% of the deaths. The cumulative rates for recurrent MI were 4.4% in the first year, 11.0% in the third year, and 13.2% in the fifth year. The parameters that influenced long-term mortality rates included arteriosclerosis-related factors, presence of congestive heart failure at admission, age, and presence of previous MI. The parameters that influenced the recurrence of MI were congestive heart failure, arteriosclerosis-related factors, and ischemic factors at discharge.

The prognosis for patients with MI is far better in Japan than in Western countries, and these findings support the previous claims about the low incidence of ischemic heart disease in Japan. Factors influencing the prognosis are similar to those previously reported.

▶ This is an interesting observational study. Why the postmyocardial infarction mortality should be so much lower in the Japanese sample of patient study is not clear to me. While the investigators emphasize risk factor relationships, other unknown or unrecognized variables may well be at work. It would be of interest to study intra-arterial pathology of infarct-related arteries in Japan and compare the findings with those reported by Davies in a Western population. (Davis, M.J., Thomas, A.C.: Plaque fissuring: The cause of acute myocardial infarction, sudden ischemic death, and crescendo angina. *Br. Heart J.* 53:363, 1985).—R.L. Frye, M.D.

How Coronary Angiography Is Used: Clinical Determinants of Appropriateness

Mark R. Chassin, Jacqueline Kosecoff, David H. Solomon, and Robert H. Brook (Rand Corp. and Fink and Kosecoff, Inc., Santa Monica, Calif., and Univ. of California, Los Angeles)

JAMA 258:2543–2547, Nov. 13, 1987 4–37

Ratings of appropriateness derived from a panel of expert physicians were used to determine how appropriately physicians performed coronary angiography in a community-based sample of Medicare cases in 1981. Areas of high and low use in three states were surveyed.

For the high-use site 72% of procedures were classed as appropriate, compared with 77% and 81% for two low-use sites. Overall, 17% of procedures at all sites were considered to be inappropriate. Patients in the high-use site were older than those in either low-use site, had less marked angina, and were less intensively treated medically. Inappropriate studies most often were done in patients without angina who had not had exercise testing. There were no significant differences among sites in the severity of coronary artery disease at angiography.

The finding that 17% of coronary angiograms were done inappropriately may be cause for concern. Increased professional efforts may be needed to improve the appropriateness with which this procedure is used. The data should be confirmed for more recent years and in younger populations.

Does Inappropriate Use Explain Geographic Variations in the Use of Health Care Services? A Study of Three Procedures

Mark R. Chassin, Jacqueline Kosecoff, R.E. Park, Constance M. Winslow, Katherine L. Kahn, Nancy J. Merrick, Joan Keesey, Arlene Fink, David H. Solomon, and Robert H. Brook (Rand Corp. and Fink and Kosecoff, Inc., Santa Monica, Calif., and Univ. of California, Los Angeles)

JAMA 258:2533–2537, Nov. 13, 1987 4–38

The authors attempted to determine whether geographic variations in the use of health care services are explained by differences in the appropriateness with which physicians use medical and surgical procedures.

The use of coronary angiography, carotid endarterectomy, and endoscopy of the upper gastrointestinal (GI) tract was studied in elderly Medicare populations in 1981 in areas of the United States that are characterized by high, average, and low use of these procedures. Medicare beneficiaries who received one of the procedures were randomly sampled, and the indications for the procedure were determined.

Small but significant differences in appropriateness were found among the three sites that were examined for each procedure. For coronary angiography the highest use site had the lowest rate of appropriateness and the lowest use site had the highest. For endoscopy of the GI tract the low-use site had the lowest rate of inappropriate procedures.

Coronary angiography was done appropriately 74% of the time at all sites combined; indications were equivocal in 9% of cases. The respective figures for carotid endarterectomy were 35% and 32% and for endoscopy of the upper GI tract they were 72% and 11%.

Differences in appropriateness of use do not explain geographic variations in the use of coronary angiography, carotid endarterectomy, or endoscopy of the upper GI tract. This study should, however, be repeated for other procedures, for nonelderly populations, and for more recent periods.

▶ These two articles (Abstracts 4–37 and 4–38) are included for a perspective of current studies in quality of care assessments. The Rand Corporation has contributed importantly in this effort. The first article focuses in more detail on coronary arteriography while the second includes coronary arteriography, upper gastrointestinal tract endoscopy, and carotid endarterectomy in terms of the appropriateness of use of these procedures. Geographic variations do not appear to explain the differences observed. It should be noted, as the authors point out, that the differences are actually quite small in terms of the percentage of appropriate use of coronary arteriography. One might quibble with the subjectivity of the end point of appropriateness, but the investigators have identified the limitations of this approach. However, these studies are essential since we must critically and objectively evaluate the appropriate use of high-cost procedures and therapies in the current environment of cost containment.

The variations in use of coronary arteriography are interesting, but with the small differences, it seems hard to resolve with certainty the mechanisms involved. The authors point out the need for more extensive investigation of the potential problems associated with *underuse* of these procedures. This is an important point and should be included in further analyses. Particularly disturbing are the data on carotid endarterectomy, a commonly applied surgical procedure with continuing debate regarding indications. There are randomized trials in progress attempting to provide better data in making decisions in these patients. The results of these trials will be awaited with great interest. Both studies are thought provoking and should be read carefully by all physicians.—R.L. Frye, M.D.

Coronary Heart Disease in Residents of Rochester, Minnesota: VII: Incidence, 1950 Through 1982

Lila R. Elveback, Daniel C. Connolly, and L. Joseph Melton III (Mayo Clinic)

Mayo Clin. Proc. 61:896–900, November 1986 4–39

An earlier study reported the incidence of coronary heart disease in adult residents of Rochester, Minn., from 1950 to 1975. The authors updated these incidence rates through 1982, and evaluated trends since 1956 through 1969, when national and local mortality for coronary heart disease began to decline.

The study was population-based; all residents whose initial manifestation of coronary heart disease was angina pectoris, myocardial infarction, or sudden unexpected death were identified. Results showed that between the time that mortality began to decrease in the late 1960s through 1982, the age-adjusted incidence of all types of coronary heart disease in Rochester residents decreased by 11% in men and increased by 9% in women. This difference was accounted for mainly by changes in the incidence of myocardial infarction as the initial manifestation of coronary heart disease: the rates declined by 20% in men and increased by 17% in women. These changes were greatest among people aged 50–69 years.

The earlier decline in overall age-adjusted rates for sudden unexpected death continued through 1978, then increased slightly in the last period of study. Between the periods 1965–1969 and 1979–1982, the sudden unexpected death rate decreased 33% in men and 14% in women. The age-adjusted rates of angina pectoris in men and women increased since the late 1960s by 7% and 10%, respectively. The 24-hour and 30-day case fatality rates for myocardial infarction and the incidence rates for sudden unexpected death stabilized.

Mortality for coronary heart disease in white population in the United States has continued to decline in men and women. Additional studies are needed to investigate the reasons for the striking divergence in secular trends in coronary heart disease for men compared with those for women.

▶ The continued studies of the Rochester population by Drs. Elveback, Connolly, and Melton provide an important perspective of the clinical epidemiology of coronary heart disease. The changes in women as described in the current study are most intriguing. There are a number of other studies reflecting the unique risk of coronary disease associated with postmenopausal women. This is an important topic that needs considerably more study.—R.L. Frye, M.D.

Frequency of Hypokalemia After Successfully Resuscitated Out-of-Hospital Cardiac Arrest Compared With That in Transmural Acute Myocardial Infarction

David M. Salerno, Richard W. Asinger, Joseph Elsperger, Ernest Ruiz, and Morrison Hodges (Univ. of Minnesota, Minneapolis)

Am. J. Cardiol. 59:84–88, January 1987 4–40

Cardiac arrest outside a hospital setting is a major health problem in the United States. Although many risk factors are known, the triggering event has not yet been elucidated. This study evaluated the prevalence of hypokalemia in 138 cardiac arrests occurring outside the hospital that were successfully resuscitated. The initial serum potassium and arterial pH values were reviewed and compared with those of 62 patients with 62 transmural acute myocardial infarction (AMI) who did not experience cardiac arrest.

After resuscitation from cardiac arrest, the mean serum potassium level of these patients was 3.6 ± 0.6 mEq/L, significantly lower than that recorded during AMI, 3.9 ± 0.5 mEq/L. The incidence of hypokalemia, serum potassium less than 3.5 mEq/L, was 41% in the cardiac arrest patients. This was significantly greater than the 11% of AMI patients with hypokalemia.

Hypokalemia was common after cardiac arrest whether AMI was present or not. The presence of hypokalemia was independent of arterial pH; epinephrine or bicarbonate therapy; or prior therapy with diuretics, digoxin, or propranolol. The serum potassium level rapidly returned to normal without the predicted amount of potassium replenishment therapy.

Hypokalemia is common immediately after cardiac arrest but is uncommon in AMI alone. The cause and electrophysiologic consequences are unknown. Whether this hypokalemia should be treated with potassium infusions is unknown, as it appears to result from a recompartmentalization rather than a whole body depletion of potassium.

▶ An important study of potassium levels in patients with out-of-hospital cardiac arrest. The apparent abruptness of these shifts in potassium as pointed out by the authors is intriguing and of uncertain clinical importance in terms of need for specific potassium replacement therapy. The contribution of chronic diuretic therapy to the problem of cardiac arrest is still not clear, but most would agree to the importance of maintaining normal potassium levels.—R.L. Frye, M.D.

Histologic Evidence for Small-Vessel Coronary Artery Disease in Patients With Angina Pectoris and Patent Large Coronary Arteries

Morris Mossieri, Rena Yarom, Mervyn S. Gotsman, and Yonathan Hasin (Hadassah Univ. Hosp., Jerusalem, Israel)

Circulation 74:964–972, November 1986 4–41

Although angina pectoris associated with widely patent epicardial coronary arteries is a well-recognized clinical entity, it is poorly understood. The authors describe 6 patients with angina pectoris and widely patent large coronary arteries in whom endomyocardial biopsy revealed histologically and electron microscopically evident disease in the small coronary arteries.

Coronary angiography was performed in the investigation of chest pain in 769 patients; 54 patients did not have disease of the major epicardial arteries; 9 of these had slow flow of contrast medium in the coronary arteries. When biopsy specimens were obtained from 6 patients, 4 showed changes in the small arteries and capillaries. Two of the patients suffered also from congestive heart failure; 3 had supraventricular tachyarrhythmias; and 3 had conduction disturbances. Echocardiographic and Doppler flow studies showed a tendency for symmetrical thickening of the left ventricular wall, enlargement of the right ventricle, and reduced compliance of both ventricles. Right ventricular endomyocardial biopsy demonstrated pathologic small coronary arteries with fibromuscular hyperplasia, hypertrophy of the media, myointimal proliferation, and endothelial degeneration. The capillaries had swollen endothelial cells encroaching on the lumen. Myocardial hypertrophy, lipofuscin deposition, and patchy fibrosis were also noted.

These cases demonstrate that small-vessel coronary artery disease can cause classic angina pectoris. The diagnosis can be suspected when the coronary angiogram shows large patent arteries with slow flow of the angiographic contrast medium, and it can be confirmed by endomyocardial biopsy.

▶ A fascinating article with additional evidence in support of the occurrence of small vessel disease as a basis for angina pectoris in the presence of no arteriographic evidence of significant lesions in the epicardial coronary arteries, but with slow velocity of contrast flow through the coronary arteries. Of interest is the fact that half the patients did have AV conduction disturbances.—R.L. Frye, M.D.

Myocardial Perfusion Changes Following 1 Year of Exercise Training Assessed by Thallium-201 Circumferential Count Profiles

Christopher P. Sebrechts, J. Larry Klein, Staffan Ahnve, Victor F. Froelicher, and William L. Ashburn (Univ. of California, San Diego, and Long Beach VA Med. Ctr.)

Am. Heart J. 112:1217–1226, December 1986 4–42

The ability of patients with coronary artery disease (CAD) to exercise has been shown to increase with exercise training. Computer analysis of scintigraphic data in 56 CAD patients was used to evaluate the effect on myocardial perfusion of 1 year of exercise training thrice weekly. Nine regions of the heart in three projections based on computer-analyzed circumferential count profiles were used to quantitate thallium-201 (TI-201) initial distribution and 4-hour washout.

There was improvement in the count distribution profiles of 77.8% of the trained and 31.0% of the untrained control subjects. This difference was significant. The mean interval change in the initial global distribution over the course of the year was 5 ± 13 in the trained and −6 ± 14 in the control group. The mean initial distribution improved in all nine regions and was significantly improved in three in the trained group, while the control group showed improvement in one region. The trained group showed improvement in mean washout in five regions, and significant improvement was seen in three regions. No mean regional washout improvement occurred in the control group.

One year of exercise training significantly improved myocardial perfusion as measured by TI-201 distribution in patients with stable CAD. Exercise appears to have a direct cardiac training effect. The exact mechanism of this effect requires further study.

▶ This is a beautiful study of myocardial perfusion and the influence of exercise training. The data have been awaited for some time for those interested in critical evaluation of the influence of increasing cardiovascular fitness on myocardial perfusion. The results are quite convincing and should provide objective support for emphasizing cardiovascular fitness in our patients with coronary disease, obviously with appropriate safeguards in terms of safety.—R.L. Frye, M.D.

Intraoperative Doppler Echocardiography in Hypertrophic Cardiomyopathy: Correlations With the Obstructive Gradient

William J. Stewart, William A. Schiavone, Ernesto E. Salcedo, Harry M. Lever, Delos M. Cosgrove, and Carl C. Gill (Cleveland Clinic Found.)

J. Am. Coll. Cardiol. 10:327–335, August 1987 4–43

There is controversy as to whether there is true obstruction to left ventricular outflow in severe hypertrophic cardiomyopathy. At the time of septal myectomy, ten patients with hypertrophic cardiomyopathy were studied with Doppler echocardiography to evaluate the presence or absence of true obstruction.

A continuous-wave Doppler transducer placed on the ascending aorta was directed toward the left ventricular outflow tract to measure velocity. Simultaneous measurement of invasive gradient was taken by direct puncture of the left ventricle and aorta using solid-state hub transducers. Both measurements were taken at rest, before and after myectomy, and during interventions with isoproterenol, volume loading, and phenylephrine.

In patients with a significant gradient, high-velocity flow with a characteristic contour was recorded. There was good correlation between the Doppler-derived gradient and the peak instantaneous gradient as measured by transducers. Correlations between the two procedures were maintained during changes in gradient and velocity due to interventions.

Results support the hypothesis that there is true obstruction in patients with hypertrophic cardiomyopathy who have a significant outflow tract pressure gradient. Continuous-wave Doppler echocardiography can accurately estimate the outflow tract gradient.

▶ The debate continues regarding obstruction in hypertrophic cardiomyopathy. These studies seem to clearly support the obstruction theory, but there is still no concensus on the topic.—R.L. Frye, M.D.

Economic Consequences of Postinfarction Prophylaxis With β-Blockers: Cost Effectiveness of Metoprolol

Gunnar Olsson, Lars-Åke Levin, and Nina Rehnquist (Karolinska Inst., Stockholm)

Br. Med. J. 294:339–342, Feb. 7, 1987 4–44

Ischemic heart disease is the most common cause of death in the Western world, and substantial resources have been spent on improving the prognosis of these patients. Among the interventions studied to date, only stopping smoking and treatment with certain β-blockers have been shown to be effective. The authors examined the economic consequences of prophylactic treatment with a β-blocker after an acute myocardial infarction in patients younger than 70 years.

Data from a randomized placebo controlled study of the β_1-selective blocker metoprolol given as secondary prophylaxis were analyzed for the possible cost-effectiveness of extending this treatment to the general population of patients with myocardial infarction. Metoprolol, 100 mg twice daily, and matching placebo were given to 154 and 147 patients, respectively, for 3 years. During this period, drug costs for the β-blocker, digitalis, and diuretics were analyzed, as well as costs for readmission for cardiac problems and indirect costs arising from sick leave or early retirement. Active treatment with metoprolol markedly reduced costs of readmission, as well as indirect costs.

It is concluded that β-blocker treatment given as a secondary prophylaxis after myocardial infarction is highly cost-effective.

▶ This economic analysis of β-blocker therapy after myocardial infarction demonstrates a clear reduction of costs primarily based on a reduction in readmissions for cardiac events. Cost-effectiveness of diagnostic and therapeutic procedure is of growing concern as health care costs continue to escalate. The large randomized trials provide a unique opportunity to address not only medical but economic issues.—R.L. Frye, M.D.

Body Composition, Not Body Weight, Is Related to Cardiovascular Disease Risk Factors and Sex Hormone Levels in Men

Karen R. Segal, Andrea Dunaif, Bernard Gutin, Janine Albu, Asa Nyman, and F. Xavier Pi-Sunyer (Mount Sinai School of Medicine and Columbia Univ.)

J. Clin. Invest. 80:1050–1055, October 1987 4–45

Obesity is a significant independent predictor of cardiovascular disease, but the relation of obesity and being overweight to risk of disease is unclear. The roles of body composition, levels of sex steroids, and cardiovascular risk factors were studied in 8 men of normal weight; 16 overweight, obese men with greater than 25% body fat; and 8 overweight, lean men with less than 15% body fat. Both overweight groups were 135% to 160% of ideal weight. All subjects were healthy, and the groups were matched for age and height.

Diastolic blood pressure was greater in obese men than in the other groups. Levels of low-density lipoprotein and fasting plasma insulin, high-density lipoprotein-total cholesterol ratio, and estradiol-testosterone ratio all were higher in the obese group. Levels of estradiol were 25% greater in the overweight lean group than in the other groups. Total level of testosterone was lower in obese men than in normal or overweight, lean subjects. Risk factors did not differ significantly in the normal and overweight lean groups.

Total body weight itself is not independently related to cardiovascular risk factors. Instead, body composition is the important factor. Changes in sex steroids relate to body composition and are not an independent cardiovascular risk factor. The hyperestrogenemia of obesity may reflect an increased lean body mass and the increase in adipose tissue. Extragonadal aromatization of androgens to estrogens in both muscle and fat tissue may be responsible.

▶ These studies provide a unique perspective on the relation of obesity and overweight and sex steroid levels as independent risk factors for cardiovascular disease. Phillips' provocative paper in 1978 had identified hyperestrogenism in males with myocardial infarction. It appears from the studies by Segal et al. that these changes are related to body composition. Analysis of data in the

Multiple Risk Factor Intervention Trial showed no relationship between sex hormones and risk for heart attacks in men (Cauley, J.A., et al.: *Am. J. Cardiol.* 60:771, 1987). The problem in distinguishing obesity from overweight still seems difficult.—R.L. Frye, M.D.

Incidence of Early Tolerance to Hemodynamic Effects of Continuous Infusion of Nitroglycerin in Patients With Coronary Artery Disease and Heart Failure

Uri Elkayam, Daniel Kulick, Nancy McIntosh, Arie Roth, Willa Hsueh, and Shahbudin H. Rahimtoola (Univ. of California, Los Angeles)

Circulation 76:577–584, September 1987 4–46

Recent experience with transdermal nitroglycerin (NTG) in patients with ischemic heart disease suggests that the cardiocirculatory effects may be substantially attenuated over time. Tolerance to continuous intravenous NTG was studied in 40 patients who have coronary artery disease and a mean pulmonary arterial wedge pressure of at least 15 mm Hg, thus reflecting left ventricular failure. Nineteen patients were randomly assigned to continue receiving NTG intravenously or placebo, after responding initially to NTG by a lowering of the mean wedge pressure by 10 mm Hg or by 30%. Twenty-one received placebo.

In NTG-treated patients, wedge pressure continued to be significantly below baseline for 8 hours of infusion, but values at 12 hours and subsequently did not differ significantly from baseline or from values in placebo-treated patients. The effect of NTG persisted in 8 patients, but 7 developed tolerance. The only difference between these groups was a higher baseline systemic vascular resistance in patients who continued to respond to infusion of NTG.

About half the patients in this study became tolerant to infusions of NTG. Nitrate tolerance can be reversed or even prevented by intermittent dosing, and an intermittent regimen seems preferable in patients who receive prolonged organic nitrate therapy.

▶ Nitroglycerin tolerance has received increasing attention, and this excellent study adds important new information. It is particularly important for those managing patients in the coronary care unit setting. While IV nitroglycerin for relief of pain associated with myocardial ischemia represents a different clinical setting than that studied in this article, the case for intermittent dosing seems clear. The question of cross-tolerance with nitroprusside needs resolution. —R.L. Frye, M.D.

5 Cardiac Surgery

Introduction

As cardiac surgery evolves to meet the challenge of applying improved technology and art to needs of an ever older and ever sicker population, analysis of progress becomes increasingly complicated. The contents of this section well illustrates not only advances in cardiac surgical techniques but also describes problems encountered as a result of wider application of surgical therapy to patients with more severe degrees of illness and advancing age.

In the section on surgery for coronary heart disease an interesting argument is made to advance the hypothesis that the success of coronary surgery explains, at least in part, observed improvement in the overall prognosis for patients with coronary artery obstructive disease. While the precise contribution of myocardial revascularization is impossible to calculate, it does seem reasonable that revascularization has had some positive impact on the epidemiology of this disease. The particular problem of young patients with premature arteriosclerotic disease of the coronary arteries is also reviewed. Once again, the internal mammary artery graft seems superior to vein grafts. In the area of rehabilitation following coronary surgery, there has been a renewed interest in psychological and intellectual dysfunction after cardiac surgery and especially after coronary bypass surgery. Thus far, the approach to measurement of intellectual dysfunction has been remarkably diverse and conclusions are extremely difficult and often controversial.

Other reports of advances in coronary surgery emphasize a variety of clinical factors important in particular groups for determination of prognosis. The initial clinical application of "dynamic cardiomyoplasty" for left ventricular assist is reviewed. The future for this procedure is uncertain, but earliest results give reason for some optimism. Introduction of coronary angioscopy once again may perhaps be an example of technology in search of application. With further development of laser techniques, application may be closer than we think.

The principal developments in surgery for the cardiac valves continues to revolve around comparison of prosthetic and tissue valves. During the first 10 years after surgery there appears to be little advantage of the one over the other except in specific instances where anticoagulation is particularly hazardous or undesirable. During the interval after 10 years the probability of mechanical failure of tissue valves is substantially greater. Utilization of thrombolytic treatment for thrombosed cardiac valves has been occasionally utilized. Favorable results thus far suggest that wider application of this technique may be justified.

In the area of congenital heart disease, advances in noninvasive diagnostic studies have made it possible to avoid cardiac catheterization in many patients. This truly represents a remarkable advance in technology. Similar advances in postoperative monitoring are being made and the overall effect will be to eventually simplify both preoperative and postoperative evaluation.

Cardiac transplantation, now a well-established procedure for the treatment of end-stage cardiac failure, has not only been utilized for a somewhat older population, but there is some evidence that persons beyond the age of 50 years may actually have an improved prognosis by virtue of an attenuated immunologic response. It is interesting, and a reminder that organ transplantation remains in its infancy and that no specific relationship between HLA compatibility as currently measured and cardiac transplant recipient survival has yet been identified. In a variety of other aspects of cardiac surgery there has been some progress (although not perhaps significant) in the areas where greatest effort is being expended. For example, there seems to be no striking progress in the development of cardioplegic solutions. The questions of whether particular attention should be paid to free radicals or whether the passive provision of high energy phosphates may be helpful has not been solved but seem interesting avenues for investigation.

While these many technological changes and clinical advances drive the perfection of cardiac surgical techniques, there are other considerations that at times seem to threaten the very structure of our discipline. The increasing hazard of the acquired immunodeficiency syndrome (AIDS) has received a great deal of publicity, and many surgeons are concerned that possible transmission in the course of cardiac surgical operations may represent a major risk. There are many unanswered questions as to definition of the hazard but there seems little doubt that at least some hazard does exist. Screening studies have greatly reduced the risk of transmission of AIDS by blood transfusion. Only careful technique seems to stand in the way of transmission from patients with known infection to those involved in handling contaminated blood. It is hoped that the risk of transmission of untreatable infectious disease will not become a significant limiting factor for the treatment of patients requiring cardiac surgery.

John J. Collins, Jr., M.D.

Surgery for Coronary Disease and Complications

What Contribution Has Cardiac Surgery Made to the Decline in Mortality From Coronary Heart Disease?

John M. Neutze and Harvey D. White (Green Lane Hosp., Auckland, New Zealand, and Natl. Heart Found. of New Zealand)
Br. Med. J. 294:405–409, Feb. 14, 1987 5–1

Mortality from coronary heart disease is declining in some Western countries. In the United States, 40% of this decline, including a 4% contribution from cardiac surgery, is attributed to medical management. Similar percentages are reported for New Zealand. However, the authors contend that the actual contribution made by heart surgery is substantially higher and that, because previous studies used patients with few symptoms, data were unsuitable to assess improvement in mortality from cardiac surgery.

This study evaluates the number of patients undergoing surgery, the survival after surgery, and the predicted mortality had the patients not undergone surgery. Predicted mortality without surgical intervention was based on past reports of patients with similar symptoms, exercise data, studies of unstable angina, and the coronary artery surgical study register.

Using this method, the contribution of coronary surgery to lower mortality is estimated to be from 26% to 42%. Although this method emphasizes symptoms rather than the extent of the disease, these findings correlate well with a Cleveland Clinic study that predicted mortality based on the extent of coronary artery disease.

▶ This provocative study from New Zealand makes an excellent point. The prospective randomized controlled studies in both the United States and Europe have tended to concentrate on persons for whom continued medical treatment was a not unreasonable alternative at the time of selection. The New Zealand study, on the other hand, deals with a cohort of patients who were more severely threatened. Because of referral patterns and the characteristically long wait for coronary bypass surgery in New Zealand, most patients operated upon were more symptomatic then might be the case especially in the United States. Whether the low estimate (26%) or the high estimate (42%) is more nearly correct, the fact remains that coronary bypass surgery, as most surgeons suspect, may well have a more substantial impact on the declining death rate from coronary heart disease than most previous studies indicate.

As more and more patients with relatively uncomplicated coronary obstructive disease, mild to moderate angina, and intact left ventricular function are treated by balloon angioplasty or improved medical management techniques, the proportion of patients subjected to coronary bypass surgery shows ever worsening left ventricular function and increasingly severe diffuse or left main coronary obstruction. As Vigilante and associates point out (1), surgical intervention in this group may serve, at least for more than 5 years, to produce substantial improvement in life expectancy by surgical as compared to medical treatment. Thus, the New Zealand data may not only be applicable to the United States but perhaps are more so now than in previous years.—J.J. Collins, Jr., M.D.

Reference

1. Vigilante, G.J., Weintraub, W.S., Klein, L.W., et al.: Improved survival with coronary bypass surgery in patients with three-vessel coronary disease and abnormal left ventricular function. *Am. J. Med.* 82:697–702, 1987.

Coronary Artery Disease and Coronary Bypass Grafting in Young Men: Experience With 138 Subjects 39 Years of Age and Younger

Gerald M. Fitzgibbons, Mark G. Hamilton, Alan J. Leach, Henryk P. Kafka, Herbert V. Markle, and Wilbert J. Keon (Natl. Defence Med. Ctr., Ottawa, and Ottawa Heart Inst., Canada)

J. Am. Coll. Cardiol. 9:977–988, May 1987 5–2

A retrospective study was undertaken of 138 men, aged 39 years and younger, who underwent coronary bypass grafting during a 13-year period.

In 77% of patients, angina was the presenting symptom; 33% of patients had unstable angina. At least one myocardial infarct had been experienced by more than half the patients. There was a high prevalence of smoking and other coronary risk factors. More than 60% of patients had triple-vessel disease; 25% and 14% had double- and single-vessel disease, respectively. Nearly half the patients had serious functional impairment. Almost all the 461 coronary bypass grafts were vein grafts. No operative deaths occurred.

Patency rates for bypass grafts were satisfactory, but patency decreased with time. After 1 year, bypass grafts showed evidence of atherosclerosis that increased, especially after 5 years. Of 23 patients who were reoperated on, 2 died, and 44% had perioperoperative transmural myocardial infarction. The survival rate at 12 years was 76%.

Coronary bypass grafting appeared to be successful in managing coronary artery disease in these young men in the short term. However, patency of the graft steadily decreased with the passage of time, and graft atherosclerosis became an increasing difficulty.

▶ Severe coronary obstructive disease in persons younger than 40 years may be considered a premature, and therefore more severe, variant of coronary atherosclerosis. The experience reported above by Fitzgibbons et al. is similar to that previously reported by Lytle and associates from the Cleveland Clinic. Both long-term survival and event-free survival are compromised in these young persons as compared to results expected in older groups of patients having similar disease at the time of revascularization surgery. (1) Documented progression of arteriosclerosis at postoperative intervals at 5 or more years also seems to show a higher proportion of arteriosclerotic involvement or occlusion of vein grafts in this younger population. Perhaps younger patients may be better candidates for complex internal mammary artery grafting. (2–5) As observed by Cosgrove, exclusive or preponderant use of internal mammary arteries as conduits may substantially lower the high rate of reoperation that has been observed in younger patients undergoing coronary bypass, as described in the following report.—J.J. Collins, Jr., M.D.

References

1. Lytle, W.B., Kramer, J.R., Golding, L.R., et al.: Young adults with coronary atherosclerosis: 10-year results of surgical myocardial revascularization. *J. Am. Coll. Cardiol.* 4:445–453, 1984.

2. Rankin, J.S., Newman, G.E., Bashore, T.M., et al.: Clinical and angiographic assessment of complex mammary artery bypass grafting. *J. Thorac. Cardiovasc. Surg.* 92:832–846, 1986.
3. Olearchyk. A.S., Magovern, G.J.: Internal mammary artery grafting. *J. Thorac. Cardiovasc. Surg.* 92:1082–1087, 1986.
4. Loop, F.D., Lytle, B.W., Cosgrove, D.M., et al.: Free (aorta-coronary) internal mammary artery graft. *J. Thorac. Cardiovasc. Surg.* 92:827–831, 1986.
5. Jones, E.L., Lattouf, O., Lutz, J.F., et al.: Important anatomical and physiological considerations in performance of complex mammary-coronary artery operations. *Ann. Thorac. Surg.* 43:469–477, 1987.

Predictors of Reoperation After Myocardial Revascularization

Delos M. Cosgrove, Floyd D. Loop, Bruce W. Lytle, Carl C. Gill, Leonard A.R. Golding, Christopher Gibson, Robert W. Stewart, Paul C. Taylor, and Marlene Goormastic (Cleveland Clinic Found.)

J. Thorac. Cardiovasc. Surg. 92:811–821, November 1986 5–3

Although reoperation accounts for most nonfatal morbidity following coronary bypass surgery, there have been few studies to asses the incidence and predictors of reoperation. A retrospective study of 8,000 patients who had undergone primary elective myocardial revascularization during a 7-year period was undertaken to define these factors.

There were 25 patient predictors analyzed for reoperation and reoperation-free survival. Mean follow-up was 8.8 years.

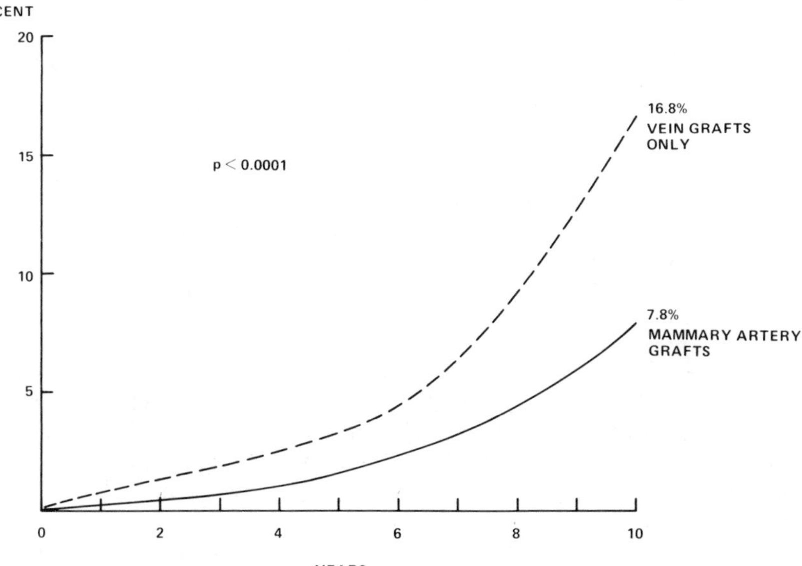

Fig 5–1.—The cumulative percent of reoperations is higher in patients with only vein grafts than in patients with an internal mammary artery graft. (Courtesy of Cosgrove, D.M., et al.: J. Thorac. Cardiovasc. Surg. 92:811–821, November 1986.)

Cumulative reoperation rate was 2.7% at 5 years, 11.4% at 10 years, and 17.3% at 12 years. The most important predictor for reoperation was young age. Patients with only vein grafts were more than twice as likely to have reoperation than those with internal mammary artery (IMA) grafts (Fig 5–1). Other risk factors were incomplete revascularization, New York Heart Association class III or IV, and single- or double-vessel disease. Absence of an IMA graft and incomplete revascularization were the only surgical variables to influence reoperation-free survival. Other factors influencing reoperation-free survival included smoking and moderate to severe left ventricular impairment. However, presence of an IMA neutralized other coronary risk factors.

Results show that complete revascularization and use of IMAs are the only surgical variables influencing late results. To improve reoperation-free survival, cardiac surgeons should use IMAs wherever possible and should strive for complete revascularization.

▶ This detailed analysis of a very large series of patients adds further weight to the argument that internal mammary artery grafting is clinically advantageous for most patients with coronary heart disease undergoing bypass surgery. It may possibly be a corollary, therefore, that progression of disease in vein grafts is more likely to cause early return of symptoms than is progression of disease in the native coronary arteries.—J.J. Collins, Jr., M.D.

Long-Term Intellectual Dysfunction Following Coronary Artery Bypass Graft Surgery: A Six Month Follow-up Study

Pamela J. Shaw, David Bates, Niall E.F. Cartlidge, Joyce M. French, David Heaviside, Desmond G. Julian, and David A. Shaw (Freeman Hosp. and Univ. of Newcastle upon Tyne, England)

Q. J. Med. 62:259–268, March 1987 5–4

Psychometric assessments were carried out before coronary bypass surgery and 1 week and 6 months afterward in 259 patients operated on electively in 1983–1984. Ten standard tests were utilized.

Mean neuropsychological scores for the group were unchanged or improved in a majority of tests. Nevertheless, 57% of patients showed deterioration on at least one test at 6 months. Impairment usually was mild. Only 17 patients exhibited moderate or severe cognitive dysfunction, with deterioration in scores on three or more tests. The impairment frequently was not important to the patient functionally. Only 2% of patients were seriously disabled. Intellectual impairment prevented return to work in only one instance. The only factors significantly related to long-term cognitive dysfunction were preoperative heart failure and global impairment of left ventricular function.

Neuropsychological functioning tends to improve 6 months after cardiopulmonary bypass surgery, but many patients do exhibit impaired cognitive function at this time. Preoperative cardiac dysfunction appears to dispose to long-term cognitive impairment. Persistent disabling dysfunction is rare. Patients and relatives may be told that, while some impairment may occur for months after operation, this usually will not interfere with normal activities.

▶ Rehabilitation of patients after cardiac surgery demands not only recovery of physical capability but return to a satisfactory intellectual capacity and personality profile. During the past year there has been an increase in the number of publications pertaining to intellectual and personality dysfunction following cardiac surgery and especially following coronary bypass surgery. While every surgeon has observed gross disturbances in psychological function in occasional patients, few have systematically investigated the incidence or significance of those deviations which are only discovered by close questioning or intellectual testing.

The publication of P.J. Shaw and associates emphasizes that some degree of intellectual change is measurable in many patients after coronary bypass surgery. What is not established is whether this deviation is specifically related to cardiopulmonary bypass, to the stress of this life-threatening situation, to changes in the perception of self-image, or to some other as yet undefined factors. Because of the large numbers of patients undergoing cardiac surgical operations, definition of the types of dysfunction and specific causes is a matter of significant impact. The design of the various studies intended to better define neuropsychological aberrations following surgery has been remarkably heterogenous.

The study by Calabrese et al. (1) from the Cleveland Clinic examined the incidence of postoperative delirium. It has been our experience in the past that postoperative confusion may be substantially reduced by careful preoperative teaching and education. No doubt this represents a functional effect rather than a physiologic one. Other authors have examined the possible affect of low blood flow (2,3) and prostacyclin (4) on cerebral integrity following cardiopulmonary bypass. Measurement of CSF enzymes has demonstrated abnormalities which may have some promise as indicators of the degree of cerebral damage and possibly even prognosis. This is obviously too complex for routine utilization, but in a study environment could provide useful information on the incidence and expected natural history of organic brain changes following cardiac surgery.—J.J. Collins, Jr., M.D.

References

1. Calabrese, J.R., et al.: Incidence of postoperative delirium following myocardial revascularization. *Cleve. Clin. J. Med.* 54:29–32, 1987.
2. Rebeyka, I.M., et al.: The effect of low-flow cardiopulmonary bypass on cerebral function: An experimental and clinical study. *Ann. Thorac. Surg.* 43:391–396, 1987.
3. Johnsson, P., et al.: Cerebral blood flow and autoregulation during hypothermic cardiopulmonary bypass. *Ann. Thorac. Surg.* 43:386–390, 1987.
4. Fish, K.J., et al.: A prospective, randomized study of the effects of prostacyclin on neuropsychologic dysfunction after coronary artery operation. *J. Thorac. Cardiovasc. Surg.* 93:609–615, 1987.
5. Vaagenes, P., Kjekshus, J., Sivertsen, E., et al.: Temporal pattern of en-

zyme changes in cerebrospinal fluid in patients with neurologic complications after open heart surgery. *Crit. Care Med.* 15:726–731, 1987.

Coronary Artery Bypass Surgery in Patients Aged 80 Years or Older

Keith S. Naunheim, Morton J. Kern, Lawrence R. McBride, D. Glenn Pennington, Hendrick B. Barner, Kirk R. Kanter, Andrew C. Fiore, Vallee L. Willman, and George C. Kaiser (St. Louis Univ.)

Am. J. Cardiol. 59:804–807, April 1, 1987 5–5

Recent reports have countered an early tendency to avoid coronary bypass surgery in aged patients. The outcome of bypass surgery was reviewed in 23 patients at least age 80 years (mean, 82 years) who were operated on from 1980 to 1986; this group represented 0.5% of all cardiac surgical patients treated in this period. Triple-vessel disease, severe left main coronary disease, and significant left ventricular dysfunction all were more prominent than in the Coronary Artery Surgery Study patients who were older than age 65. Overall, 74% of the patients had unstable and postinfarction angina and 61% had significant congestive heart failure.

None of 14 patients died after elective simple coronary bypass surgery. Of all 19 patients undergoing elective surgery, 2 (11%) died. Three of 4 patients died after emergency surgery, as did 4 of the 6 who required intra-aortic balloon counterpulsation. Half of the survivors had significant complications, but all improved by at least one New York Heart Association (NYHA) class. Thirteen of 16 long-term survivors were in NYHA functional class I or II at follow-up. The actuarial survival was 82% at 2 years.

This experience shows that coronary bypass surgery can be done electively in octogenarians, with acceptable mortality and morbidity resulting. Survivors experience excellent functional improvement.

▶ This very interesting report documents that "carefully selected" patients older than 80 years may be returned to a reasonable life-style albeit with a higher-than-average early mortality and a greater-than-average probability of significant complications. While experienced surgeons would certainly agree with this observation, the critical determinant of the impact of operation depends on the criteria for "careful selection." Frustration with frequent or prolonged hospitalization in elderly patients is not necessarily an indication for surgery. The widespread application of coronary bypass to patients over the age of 80 has extremely serious implications for the overall cost of myocardial revascularization in the United States.—J.J. Collins, Jr., M.D.

Aorta-Coronary Bypass Grafting With Polytetrafluoroethylene Conduits: Early and Late Outcome in Eight Patients

Richard B. Chard, David C. Johnson, Graham R. Nunn, and Timothy B. Cartmill (Westmead Hosp., Sydney, Australia)

J. Thorac. Cardiovasc. Surg. 94:132–134, July 1987 5–6

Synthetic grafts of polytetrafluoroethylene (PTFE) might serve for aorta-coronary bypass surgery where no suitable long or short saphenous veins are present. Eight such patients received grafts of 4-mm PTFE, using predominantly multiple sequential grafting methods. Multiple sequential grafts alone were used in six patients. Two patients had a sequential graft.

Seven of the eight patients were alive 45 months after operation. One patient died after 16 months following reoperation. Twenty-four of 28 anastomoses were patent at 1 week. At 1 year, 18 of 28 anastomoses were patent, and five patients were free of angina. At 45 months, only 4 anastomoses were patent and only one patient was free of angina. In the latter patient, 3 of 4 anastomoses on a sequential graft were patent.

It appears that, when PTFE grafts fail, the distal anastomoses become obstructed by pseudointimal thickening and bridging and, with reduced runoff, the aorta-graft anastomosis then is obstructed. The present results are unacceptable. The problem of what to do when the optimal conduits for aorta-coronary bypass grafting are unavailable remains to be solved.

▶ The temptation to use prosthetic materials for coronary bypass conduits surfaces from time to time. This short report documents once again the very short patency span to be expected from the present generation of polytetrafluoroethylene conduits. The authors' observation that PTFE graft failure seems to be dependent on pseudointimal thickening at the distal anastomosis may possibly be true. Perhaps this defect might be remedied by utilization of a short cuff of vein for the distal anastomosis.—J.J. Collins, Jr., M.D.

Coronary-Coronary Artery Bypass: An Alternative

Paul E. Rowland and Ronald K. Grooters (Iowa Methodist Med. Ctr., Des Moines)

Ann. Thorac. Surg. 43:326–328, March 1987 5–7

A patient with calcification of the ascending aorta will occasionally be unsuited for conventional saphenous vein aortocoronary bypass as will a patient with saphenous vein or internal mammary artery of inadequate quality or insufficient diameter. Two cases of coronary-coronary artery bypass illustrate an alternative method of revascularization.

In one patient, the aortic arch and innominate arteries were too calcified for cannulation or proximal anastomosis. The proximal right coronary was nondiseased, and coronary-coronary artery bypass was performed (Fig 5–2) by sequentially anastomosing a single segment of saphenous vein end to side from the right coronary artery, side to side to the circumflex and obtuse marginal arteries, and end to side to the left anterior descending coronary artery.

There were postoperative complications, and the patient died 2 months postoperatively of noncardiac complications. The second patient, who received a similar procedure, was free of chest pain and had no acute changes in ECG 4 months postoperatively.

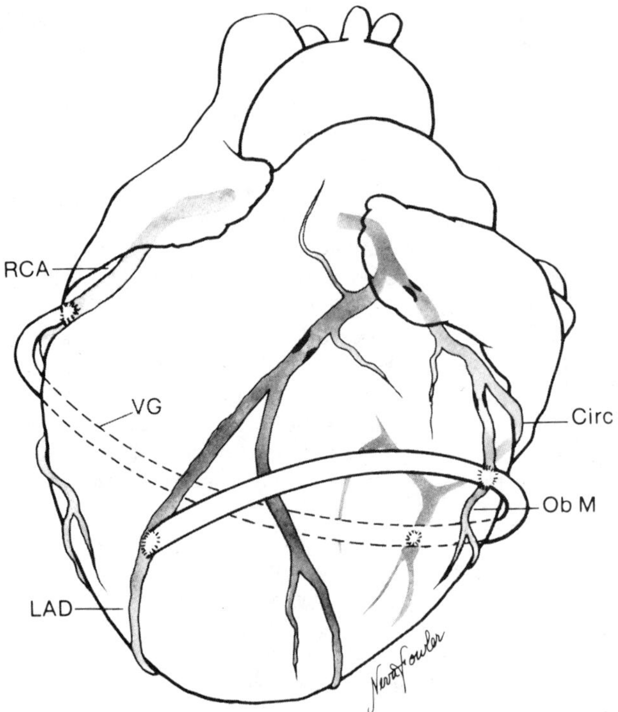

Fig 5–2.—Left anterior oblique projection demonstrating sequential vein graft (VG) between the right coronary artery (RCA), circumflex artery (Circ), obtuse marginal branch (Ob M), and left anterior descending artery (LAD). (Courtesy of Rowland, P.E., and Grooters, R.K.: Ann. Thorac. Surg. 43:326–328, March 1987.)

Coronary-coronary bypass appears to be an acceptable alternative when more conventional bypass is precluded.

▶ Probably all surgeons with substantial experience in coronary artery revascularization will have used novel techniques from time to time to achieve revascularization that would be impossible by more mundane means. While some disadvantages of the coronary-coronary bypass include the possibility of proximal occlusion of the feeding vessel and possible competitive flow inducing ischemia in the distribution of the feeding vessel, the technique may have occasional utility.—J.J. Collins, Jr., M.D.

Coronary Artery Bypass Graft Failure—An Autoimmune Phenomenon

Karen E. Morton, Thomas P. Gavaghan, Steven A. Krilis, Grant E. Daggard, David W. Baron, John B. Hickie, and Colin N. Chesterman (Univ. of New South Wales School of Medicine and St. George and St. Vincent's Hosps., Sydney, Australia)

Lancet 2:1353–1357, Dec. 13, 1986 5–8

High levels of anticardiolipin antibody (ACA) in young survivors of myocardial infarction are a marker of high risk for subsequent cardiovascular events. The course of ACA was studied in 83 patients having coronary bypass surgery. The findings were related to graft patency or occlusion, as judged angiographically, 1–2 weeks and 12 months after operation.

The preoperative ACA titer was related to late graft occlusion, but the number of patients affected and the number of distal anastomoses occluded. Eight of 15 patients whose peak plasma ACA values exceeded 4 SD of the control mean had late graft occlusion. When the titer was 2–4 SD above the control mean, 23% of patients had late occlusion. A postoperative increase in ACA was more frequent in patients having past myocardial infarction than in those with angina only.

Patients with high ACA titers might be considered for prophylactic measures designed to avoid graft occlusion, such as anticoagulation, antiplatelet therapy, or steroids to suppress circulating antibody. Monitoring of antibody levels after coronary bypass surgery would allow effective measures to be instituted in a timely manner. If antibody production is stimulated at the time of acute infarction, administration of ACA immediately after infarction might prevent sensitization.

▶ This interesting article raises the possibility that some patients may have a definable predilection to early thrombosis of bypass grafts. If this indeed could be demonstrated to be a frequent or even universal phenomenon, the authors' suggestion of special precautions in such patients is undoubtedly reasonable and perhaps even wise.—J.J. Collins, Jr., M.D.

A Reappraisal of Surgical Intervention for Acute Myocardial Infarction

C.L. Athanasuleas, D.A. Geer, J.G. Arciniegas, T.B. Cooper, R.G. Hess, W.A.H. MacLean, S.E. Papapietro, A.W.H. Stanley, and M. McEachern (Norwood Clinic and Carraway Methodist Med. Ctr., Birmingham, Ala.)

J. Thorac. Cardiovasc. Surg. 93:405–414, March 1987 5–9

Several methods of myocardial reperfusion are possible during acute evolving myocardial infarction. The authors compared surgical and nonsurgical reperfusion techniques, defined predictors of operative mortality, and described follow-up ventricular function data.

A group of 215 patients underwent either intracoronary thrombolysis, angioplasty, or both. Coronary artery bypass was performed in another 83 patients.

In the surgical group, predictors of mortality were 84% accurate. Predictors were cardiogenic shock, age older than 65 years, initial global left ventricular ejection fraction below .30, initial cardiac index below 2.0 L/min/sq m, and absent collateral flow. Time to reperfusion was not significant, nor was the infarct-related artery. The overall hospital mortality was 15.6%, but only 5.9% in the low-risk group. The graft patency rate was 94%, and ventricular performance was improved. In the nonsurgical group, reperfusion was successful in 67% of patients; the infarct artery was patent in 82% of patients.

It is recommended that choice of treatment of acute evolving infarction be determined on the basis of preoperative variables. Surgical intervention is warranted in low-risk patients.

▶ This article from a community hospital emphasizes that early mortality after emergency or urgent coronary bypass for evolving myocardial infarction compares favorably with early mortality risk for combined thrombolysis and angioplasty. Furthermore, the authors point out that certain variables are accurate predictors of mortality risk in patients subjected to coronary bypass surgery. Patients not showing high mortality risk factors had an early mortality of only about 6%, which may actually be safer than combined thrombolysis and angioplasty in similarly selected patients.—J.J. Collins, Jr., M.D.

Surgical Repair of Acquired Ventricular Septal Defect: Determinants of Early and Late Outcome

M.T. Jones, P.M. Schofield, J.F. Dark, H. Moussalli, A.K. Deiraniya, R.A.M. Lawson, C. Ward, and C.L. Bray (Wythenshawe Hosp., Manchester, England)
J. Thorac. Cardiovasc. Surg. 93:680–686, May 1987 5–10

Because of the high incidence of preoperative death when repair of ventricular septal defect (VSD) is delayed, this procedure is generally considered a surgical emergency. The early and long-term results of surgical repair of postinfarction VSD is investigated and outcome is related to preoperative right and left ventricular function in a group of patients operated between 1970 and 1985.

Data on a group of 60 patients who underwent surgery for repair of postinfarction VSD were reviewed. Preoperative cineangiograms were studied to measure left ventricular ejection fraction and assess right ven-

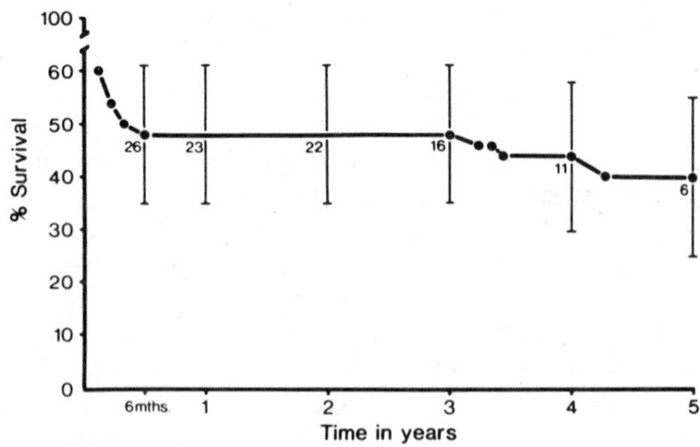

Fig 5–3.—Actuarial survival curve of the 60 patients who underwent surgical repair of postinfarction ventricular septal defect. (Courtesy of Jones, M.T., et al.: J. Thorac. Cardiovasc. Surg. 93:680–686, May 1987.)

tricular function by determining the percentage reduction in right ventricular midcavity diameter.

There were 23 early deaths; in 7 patients death was caused by failure to wean from cardiopulmonary bypass; in 4, death resulted from failed VSD procedure; 8 patients died of myocardial failure; and the others died of renal failure, reinfarction, or cerebrovascular accident. There were also 14 late deaths (Fig 5–3). Early mortality was more than twice as high for inferior infarction than for anterior infarction. The time interval between infarction and operation also influenced survival. Early survival was improved by good preoperative right ventricular function, but was unaffected by left ventricular function before operation. However, long-term survival was enhanced by preserved preoperative left ventricular function and unaffected by preoperative right ventricular function. Of the 23 long-term survivors, 87% are in the New York Heart Association class I or II.

To date, this is the largest study of surgical repair of postinfarction VSD. Results have improved between two successive time frames in this series.

▶ Even with the possibility of reparative surgery the occurrence of postinfarction ventricular septal rupture is an extremely serious complication of myocardial infarction. The early mortality of more than 35% in this series is probably typical of the experience in most centers throughout the world. Experienced surgeons would undoubtedly agree that the best prognosis in this defect is seen in those patients having an anteroapical septal perforation, good residual myocardial function, and intact or graftable vessels in the lateral and posterior myocardial distribution.—J.J. Collins, Jr., M.D.

Left Ventricular Aneurysm With Predominating Congestive Heart Failure: A Comparative Study of Medical and Surgical Treatment

Yves Louagie, Taoufik Alouini, Jacques Lespérance, and L. Conrad Pelletier
(Montreal Heart Inst. and Univ. of Montreal)

J. Thorac. Cardiovasc. Surg. 94:571–581, October 1987 5–11

In patients with congestive heart failure caused by a left ventricular aneurysm, surgery is associated with high operative mortality, and the long-term outlook is poor. A review was made of experience with 109 patients treated between 1979 and 1985 for congestive failure secondary to postinfarction left ventricular aneurysm. Of these, 73% were in functional class III or IV at the time of diagnosis. The total ejection fraction averaged 30%, and the mean telediastolic volume of the aneurysm was 76 ml.

Aneurysmectomy was performed in 49 patients and 60 clinically similar patients were managed medically. The surgical patients had more extensive coronary disease. Survival was similar in the two groups after an average follow-up of 4 years. Surgical patients, however, experienced significantly fewer complications. Surgery independently lowered the risks of both cardiac complications and death, as did a shorter interval between initial infarction and the diagnosis of aneurysm, and the absence of right ventricular failure. Functional improvement was directly related to surgical treatment.

Aneurysmectomy improves the quality of life in patients with left ventricular aneurysm and predominant congestive failure. Patients who have a proximal left anterior descending artery lesion and a contractile segment ejection fraction of 41% or more have an excellent long-term outlook after surgical treatment.

▶ The report of Louagie and associates represents yet another publication in which no difference in survival (with an average follow-up of 4 years) was observed in patients treated with aneurysm resection as compared to those managed medically. However, the substantially better rehabilitation of patients after surgery is also consistent with many previous reports and continues to justify aneurysm resection for patients disabled by congestive heart failure produced by localized aneurysms in the presence of adequate residual contractile myocardium.—J.J. Collins, Jr., M.D.

Resorbable Suture Support for Ventricular Aneurysmectomy

Josef G. Vincent, Stefan H. Skotnicki, Jaap J. van der Meer, and Karel Kubat (St. Radboud Univ., Nijmegen, The Netherlands)

J. Thorac. Cardiovasc. Surg. 94:430–433, September 1987 5–12

Great care is needed for the edge of tissue remaining after ventricular aneurysmectomy. Teflon felt support can redistribute pressure, preventing the sutures from cutting through vulnerable tissue. Teflon felt reinforcement often is preferable to direct unsupported closure, but full immobilization of the sutured area, foreign body infection, and adhesion formation are possible complications.

Polydioxine resorbable pledgets and strips were used for suture support in closing 29 ventricular aneurysmectomies and 4 ischemic ventricular septal defects in a 2-year period. All procedures but one were done in conjunction with coronary bypass grafting. The polydioxine material was easy to apply and caused no complications. The closure was with 3–0 Prolene monofilament mattress sutures, which were supported on both sides by a polydioxine fabric strip. A running over-and-over suture spread the fabric strip wider to distribute pressure on the sutured region. Reoperation after 18 months in one patient showed that the polydioxine material was fully resorbed. This fabric appears to be a suitable alternative to Teflon felt in ventricular aneurysmectomy. Resorption of the material may improve the prognosis in patients with postoperative infection.

▶ The utilization of Teflon felt for suture reinforcement has become extremely common in cardiac surgery. Not only is it routinely used for closure of muscular defects by many surgeons but it has become popular to utilize felt pledgets for the implantation of valves. No doubt, many surgeons feel more secure when using pledgets; unfortunately, the consequences may be undesirable or even hazardous. Adhesion of the pericardium to the massive felt buttressing often used for aneurysm repair usually results in tight adhesion of the ventricle to the pericardium beneath the phrenic nerve. In the event of reoperation dissection in this area may often result in division of that nerve. The use of absorbable buttressing would presumably obviate that hazard.

In commenting on this publication, Borst points out that pledgets are a major problem in the event of postoperative infection (1). In our experience, pledgets are also a serious nuisance when it is necessary to replace a prosthetic or bioprosthetic valve which has been previously implanted with the use of multiple pledgets. Chasing these bits of felt around inside the heart can be unpleasant even when they are not actively infected. In the event of infection, it is extremely difficult to be sure that all of the felt has been removed.

It is quite possible and often relatively simple to use strips of pericardium for pledget material and, as Vincent et al. point out, the polydioxine material seems to perform quite adequately also.—J.J. Collins, Jr., M.D.

Reference

1. Borst, H.G.: Dire consequences of the indiscriminate use of Teflon felt pledgets. *J. Thorac. Cardiovasc. Surg.* 94:442–443, 1987.

Paced Latissimus Dorsi Used for Dynamic Cardiomyoplasty of Left Ventricular Aneurysms

George J. Magovern, Fredrick R. Heckler, Sang B. Park, Ignacio Y. Christlieb, George J. Magovern, Jr., Race L. Kao, Daniel H. Benckart, Gene Tullis, Ed Rozar, George A. Liebler, John A. Burkholder, and Thomas D. Maher (Allegheny Gen. Hosp. and Allegheny-Singer Research Inst., Pittsburgh)

Ann. Thorac. Surg. 44:379–388, October 1987 5–13

Unsatisfactory results with artificial heart devices prompted use of the latissimus dorsi muscle to repair large ventricular aneurysms in two patients. It was hoped that a dynamic cardiomyoplasty procedure, using the left latissimus dorsi muscle with its neurovascular bundle, would increase the ejection fraction through stimulation with a programmed dual-chamber cardiac pacemaker. The goal was to train the muscle to contract synchronously with ventricular systole and convert to mostly fatigue-resistant, metabolically oxidative slow-twitch fibers.

Both patients had a large left ventricular aneurysm and severe coronary artery disease. Congestive failure was present; the ejection fraction was less than 30%. Resection of the entire aneurysm probably would seriously impair residual ventricular capacity in these patients. Postoperatively (Figs 5–4 and 5–5), the transposed muscle was trained electrically to contract with each systole. Both patients improved steadily and returned to normal activities. The ejection fraction improved with synchronous contraction of the skeletal muscle.

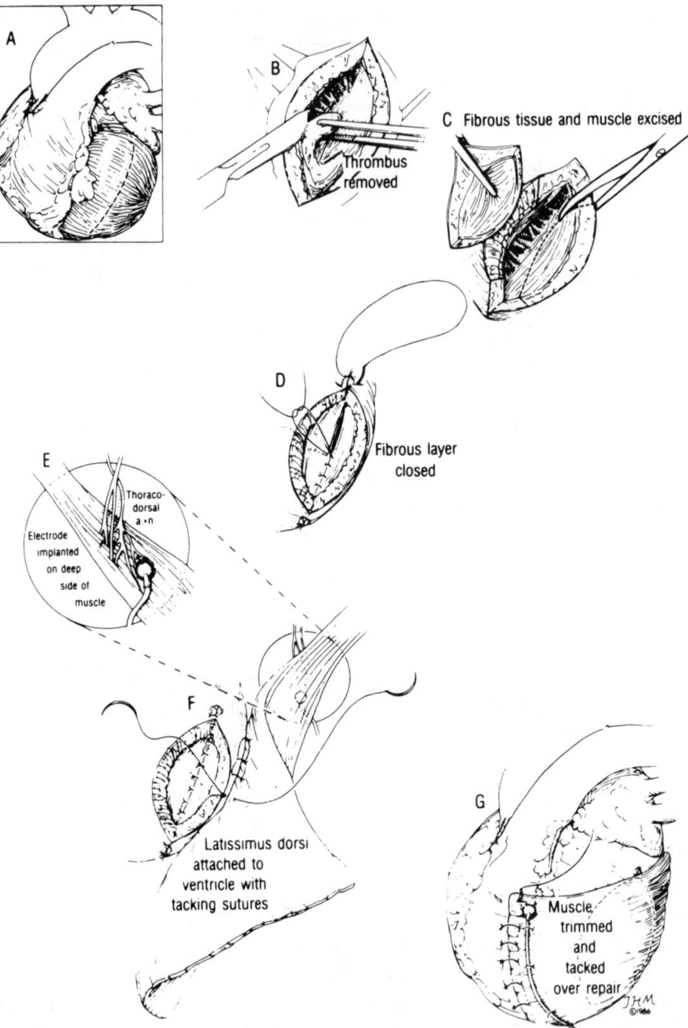

Fig 5–4.—**A,** incision line in the aneurysm. **B,** removal of intracavitary thrombus. **C,** excision of fibrous wall of the aneurysmal sac sparing useful endocardial and subendocardial tissue. **D,** suture of the inner fibrous layer. A myocardial defect is left over which the latissimus dorsi (LD) flap will be sewn. **E,** proximal electrode implanted where the thoracodorsal nerve branches down. **F,** LD flap tacked to ventricular wall to cover the myocardial defect. **G,** final position of the LD flap overlapping the myocardial defect at the site of ventricular repair. *a,* artery; *n,* nerve. (Courtesy of Magovern, G.J., et al.: Ann. Thorac. Surg. 44:379–388, October 1987.)

Much more experience is needed with this approach, and a way must be found to determine geometrically how to wrap the muscle flap around the heart. In time it might prove easier and safer to use a thin-walled dyskinetic anterolateral ventricle for cardiomyoplasty rather than risk the complications of bypass and anticoagulation.

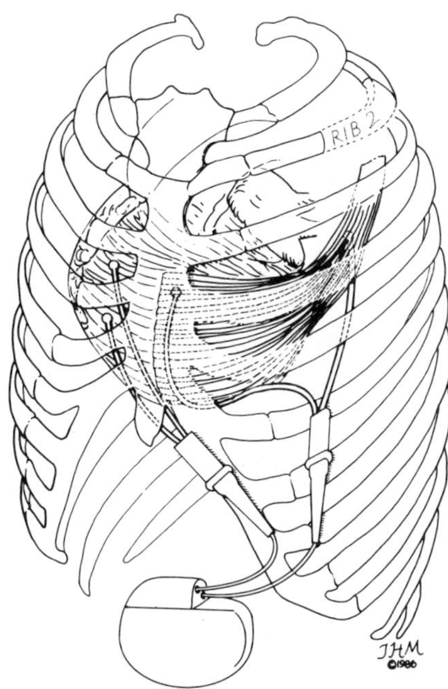

Fig 5–5.—Latissimus dorsi (LD) flap in place partially wrapping the ventricles. Two sensing leads are connected to the right side (atrial or ventricular) of the heart, and two pacing leads, one proximal (—) and one distal (+) are connected to the LD flap as in a dual-chamber bipolar system. (Courtesy of Magovern, G.J., et al.: Ann. Thorac. Surg. 44:379–388, October 1987.)

Canine Diaphragm Muscle After 1 Yr of Continuous Electrical Stimulation: Its Potential as a Myocardial Substitute

Michael A. Acker, John D. Mannion, Wendy E. Brown, Stanley Salmons, Jan Henriksson, Terremun Bitto, Dennis R. Gale, Robert Hammond, and Larry W. Stephenson (Univ. of Pennsylvania, Univ. of Birmingham, England, and Karolinska Inst., Stockholm)

J. Appl. Physiol. 62:1264–1270, March 1987 5–14

A muscle's susceptibility to fatigue is not a fixed characteristic; it depends on properties that can change in adaptive response to a long-term increase in functional demand. Skeletal muscle has been rendered fatigue resistant by chronic stimulation and thus may be an active substitute for damaged myocardium. A study was done to determine whether stimulation produces any deleterious effects in the long term.

Hemidiaphragm muscles of four dogs were examined after chronic stimulation at 2 or 4 Hz for 1 year. On gross inspection, the stimulated hemidiaphragms appeared normal and were still vigorously contracting. On histochemical and immunohistochemical assessment, the muscles had acquired a uniformly type I character, in contrast to the mixed fiber type composition of the unstimulated hemidiaphragms. This transformation was also evident in the muscles' complement of myosin isozymes. Enzymatic evidence suggested an associated shift towards aerobic pathways of energy generation. No evidence of degenerative changes were seen on histologic examination. Trends observed at 6–8 weeks toward a decrease in fiber area and an increase in connective tissue showed no further progression at 1 year.

Indirect electrical stimulation at frequencies at or exceeding the dog's heart rate caused the diaphragm to acquire a histochemical, immunohistochemical, and biochemical profile similar to that of a slow-twitch muscle. Under constant stimulation, this state was maintained for as long as 1 year without evidence of damage.

▶ During the past few years, there have been reports of the utilization of skeletal muscle for strengthening or reconstructing the cardiac ventricles. The report by Magovern and associates (Abstract 5–13) represents the initial clinical experience with an operation they have termed "dynamic cardiomyoplasty." The observation of an improved ejection fraction using noninvasive study techniques, with exercise in one patient and at rest in another, is exciting news for those investigators who have doggedly pursued the basic research necessary to the clinical application of this concept. In particular, the group led by Stephenson, Acker, and associates from Philadelphia (Abstract 5–14) must be congratulated for providing a large portion of the basic physiologic studies essential for eventual clinical application (1).

Whether this concept of dynamic cardiomyoplasty eventually becomes an accepted technique for myocardial contractile enhancement, the evolution of the technique represents a remarkable accomplishment of cooperation between basic animal research and human therapeutic application. In particular, this illustration should serve as a cautionary note to those who would abolish animal experimentation.—J.J. Collins, Jr., M.D.

Reference

1. Acker, M.A., Anderson, W.A., Hammond, R.L., et al.: Skeletal muscle ventricles in circulation. *J. Thorac. Cardiovasc. Surg.* 94:163–174, 1987.

Intraoperative Coronary Angioscopy: Technique and Results in the Initial 58 Patients

Aurelio Chaux, Myles E. Lee, Carlos Blanche, Robert M. Kass, Todd C. Sherman, Ann E. Hickey, Frank Litvack, Warren Grundfest, James Forrester, and Jack Matloff (Cedars-Sinai Med. Ctr., Los Angeles)

J. Thorac. Cardiovasc. Surg. 92:972–976, December 1986 5–15

Angioscopes may be used to directly visualize the intraluminal coronary arteries and to detect plaques and thrombus. Angioscopes ranging from 1.25–1.8 mm in external diameter were utilized. A total of 124 studies were done in 58 patients. Forty-three were to inspect coronary grafts and anastomoses.

Lesions were visualized by angioscopy in 86% of patients. Atheromatous lesions of varying severity were seen in 24 of 28 patients with stable angina. Eight of 9 patients with progressive angina had complex lesions with ulcerated surfaces. Angioscopic findings were abnormal in 12 of 15 patients with unstable rest angina, showing thrombus at the level of atheromatous disease. Venous valves and anastomotic suture lines were readily visualized. No significant complications resulted from angioscopy.

Coronary angioscopy can provide useful information more safely than can other study methods. Changes in the arterial intima can be correlated with the clinical manifestations of atherosclerotic disease. Unstable angina is associated with ulcerated plaque or with associated thrombus, or both. Most failures have been due to lack of steerability of the angioscope or inadequate irrigation. The possible therapeutic applications of this technology are exciting.

▶ Cardiac surgeons have long dreamed of the possibility of visualization of the interior of blood vessels and the heart but have been unable to develop the necessary instrumentation. A combination of modern fiberoptic technology and the utilization of blood-free perfusion fluids during cardiopulmonary bypass allows observation of the intimal surface of intact blood vessels with sufficient definition that important observations may be made. While this may be interpreted as technology in search of application at the present time, the report by Chaux and associates suggests that useful data concerning the adequacy of coronary grafts may already be available by angioscopy. With the increased incidence of reoperations and with the possible inclusion of angioplasty more frequently during coronary bypass surgery, angioscopy may become a practical necessity for the cardiac surgeon. For the moment, however, it remains under investigation.—J.J. Collins, Jr., M.D.

Valvular Surgery

Long-Term Follow-up of Patients With the Antibiotic-Sterilized Aortic Homograft Valve Inserted Freehand in the Aortic Position

Brian G. Barratt-Boyes, A.H.G. Roche, R. Subramanyan, J.R. Pemberton, and R.M.L. Whitlock (Green Lane Hosp., Auckland, New Zealand, and Univ. of Auckland)

Circulation 75:768–777, April 1987 5–16

The antibiotic sterilized aortic homograft valve (ASAHV) has provided superior results to chemical sterilization in the short- and midterm. This study reports long-term follow-up results of the ASAHV and analyzes the incidence and causes of homograft failure.

In 248 patients, a series of 252 aortic homograft valves have been followed for a mean period of 10.8 years. All valves were nonvital and were sterilized in antibiotic solution and maintained in a nutrient medium at 4 C.

There were 15 hospital deaths; of these, most were class V patients. In patients undergoing elective first operation, the death rate was 2.7%. Reoperation death rate was 13%, and overall for class V patients, the death rate was 50%. Most patients died of myocardial failure and cerebral damage. Survival rate was 57% at 10 years and 38% at 14 years with the valve in situ (Fig 5–6). Homograft valve failure was responsible for only

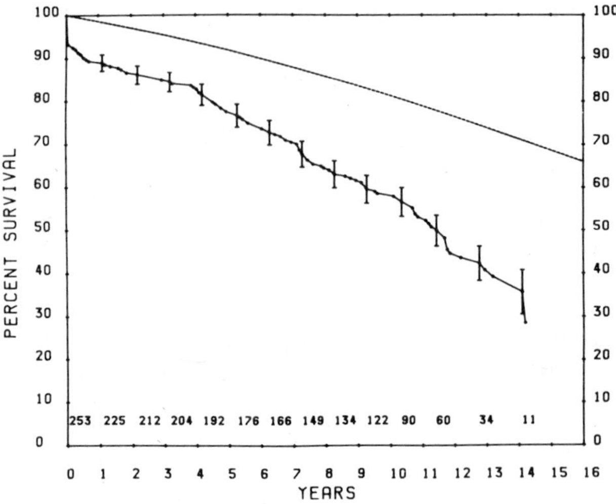

Fig 5–6.—Actuarial survival curve for aortic valve replacement with an ASAHV with the study valve in situ. The bars represent 1 SE (70% confidence limits). The dashed line is survival of an age- and sex-matched population. The numbers at risk are noted. (Courtesy of Barratt-Boyes, B.G., et al.: Circulation 75:768–777, April 1987.)

8.4% of late deaths. Valve failure was caused solely by incompetence, either from valve wear or endocarditis. Valves were 95% free from significant incompetence at 5 years, 78% at 10 years, and 42% at 14 years (Fig 5–7). The incidence of significant incompetence was significantly lower than for chemically treated valves (Fig 5–8). Increasing donor

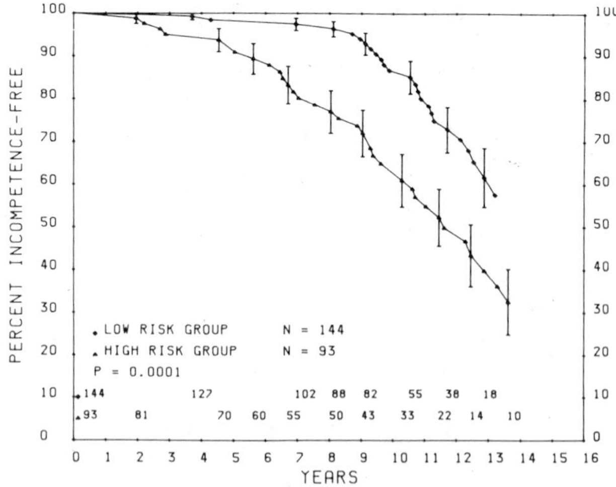

Fig 5–7.—Actuarial incidence of freedom from significant incompetence in patients in the low-risk group (>15 years of age + donor valve <50 years + aortic root size ≤30 mm) and high-risk group (<15 years of age or donor valve ≥ 50 years or aortic size ≥ 30 mm). Bars represent 1 SE (70% confidence limits). (Courtesy of Barratt-Boyes, B.G., et al.: Circulation 75:768–777, April 1987.)

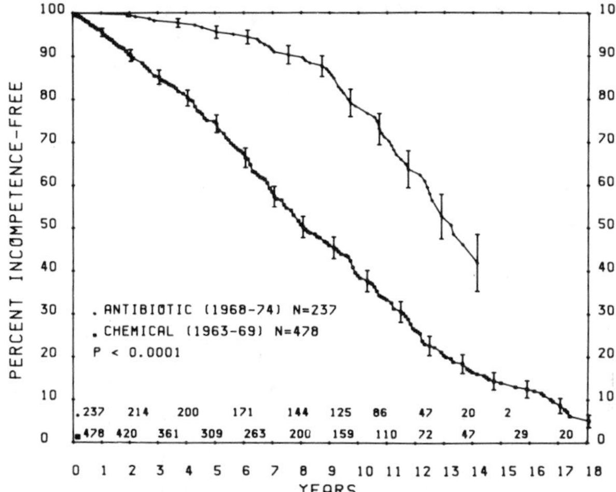

Fig 5–8.—Actuarial incidence of freedom from significant incompetence in ASAHVs and valves chemically sterilized and stored either in Hanks' solution at 4 C or by freeze-drying. The bars represent 1 SE (70% confidence limits). The numbers at risk and the *P* value are noted. (Courtesy of Barratt- Boyes, B.G., et al.: Circulation 75:768–777, April 1987.)

valve age, recipient age younger than 14 years, and aortic root diameter over 30 mm increased the risk of significant incompetence.

The ASAHV was demonstrated to be a satisfactory device for aortic valve replacement and is recommended over other valves in almost all patients. The results may be less satisfactory in children, but the ASAHV is still preferred in this age group.

Performance of a Fabricated Trileaflet Porcine Bioprosthesis: Midterm Follow-up of the Hancock Modified-Orifice Valve

Verdi J. DiSesa, Elizabeth N. Allred, Wendy Kowalker, Richard J. Shemin, John J. Collins, Jr., and Lawrence H. Cohn (Harvard Med. School, Brigham and Women's Hosp., and Harvard School of Public Health, Boston)
J. Thorac. Cardiovasc. Surg. 94:220–224, August 1987 5–17

In the Hancock modified-orifice porcine valve, the muscle bar at the base of the noncoronary cusp of a native valve is replaced by a muscle-free cusp from a second valve to reduce inherent functional stenosis. A total of 315 patients had undergone aortic valve replacement with Hancock modified-orifice valves since 1976. Most had aortic stenosis as the predominant lesion. The mean age was 63 years. Anulus-enlarging procedures were avoided, but other cardiac surgery was done at the same time in 127 patients, most of whom underwent coronary bypass grafting.

Hospital mortality was 1.6% (5 of 315 patients). Of the survivors, 222 were in New York Heart Association functional classes I and II a mean of 53 months postoperatively. Only patients with documented thromboembolism received long-term anticoagulation. Forty-three patients had

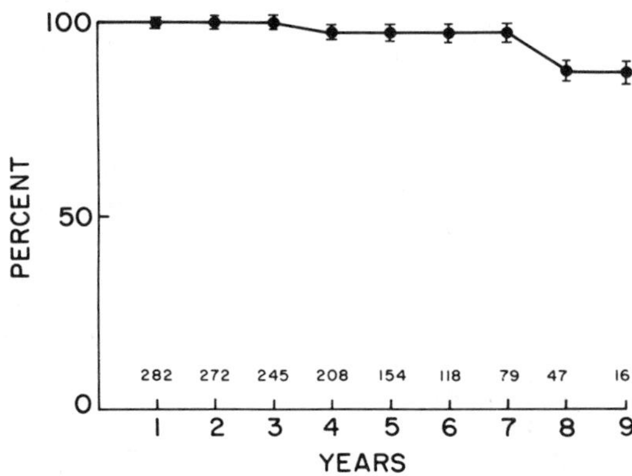

Fig 5–9.—Actuarial probability of freedom from primary valve dysfunction. (Courtesy of Di Sesa, V.J., et al.: J. Thorac. Cardiovasc. Surg. 94:220–224, August 1987.)

valve-related complications; 25 had nonfatal thromboembolism; and 11 had endocarditis. Twelve patients required reoperation. Primary valve dysfunction has occurred at a rate of 0.6% per patient-year (Fig 5–9).

The Hancock modified-orifice bioprosthesis is acceptably durable. Thromboembolic complications are infrequent without routine anticoagulation. These valves perform well clinically. Primary valve dysfunction is no more frequent than with unmodified porcine valves or fabricated pericardial valves. The modified-orifice porcine valve effectively relieves severe aortic valve disease in patients who have a small aortic anulus.

Comparison of Outcome After Valve Replacement With a Bioprosthesis Versus a Mechanical Prosthesis: Initial 5 Year Results of a Randomized Trial

Karl E. Hammermeister, William G. Henderson, Cecil M. Burchfiel, Gulshan K. Sethi, Julianne Souchek, Charles Oprian, Alan B. Cantor, Edward Folland, Shukri Khuri, Shahbudin Rahimtoola, and other participants in the VA Cooperative Study of Valvular Heart Disease (VA Med. Ctr., Denver, and elsewhere)
J. Am. Coll. Cardiol. 10:719–732, October 1987 5–18

In all, 575 patients requiring mitral or aortic valve replacement were assigned to receive a Hancock porcine heterograft or the Björk-Shiley mechanical spherical disk valve. More than one third of the patients had concomitant coronary bypass grafting. Patients given a bioprosthesis received anticoagulant therapy for 4–8 weeks in the absence of clinical indications. The average follow-up was 5 years.

Overall operative mortality was 7.7%. Survival was comparable in both groups after aortic replacement (Fig 5–10). Valve-related complications were significantly more frequent in those with the mechanical prosthesis. Clinically significant bleeding constituted 58% of all complications. Systemic embolism was somewhat more frequent in patients given a bioprosthesis, but life-table analysis showed the risk to be similar in the

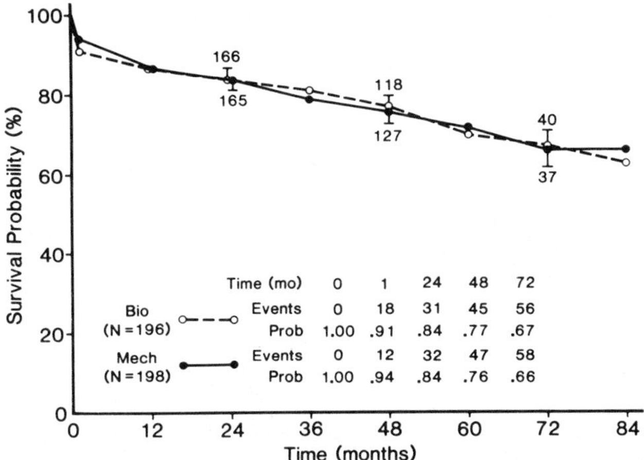

Fig 5–10.—Actuarial analysis of survival using death from any cause as the end point. Comparison of patients undergoing aortic valve replacement with a bioprosthesis (Bio) versus patients receiving a mechanical (Mech) prosthesis. One standard error of the survival probability (Prob) is shown at 2, 4, and 6 years by the *vertical bars*. The numbers adjacent to the points at 2, 4, and 6 years are the numbers of patients available for observation at that time. (Courtesy of Hammermeister, K.E., et al.: J. Am. Coll. Cardiol. 10:719–732, October 1987.)

two treatment groups. Reoperation was necessary in similar numbers of patients. After mitral replacement, the survival rate was somewhat better in patients given a bioprosthesis (Fig 5–11). Valve-related complications, chiefly bleeding, were more common in the mechanical valve group. Systemic embolism was similarly frequent in the two treatment groups. Twice as many patients with a mechanical valve required reoperation.

The clearest difference between the bioprosthesis and mechanical pros-

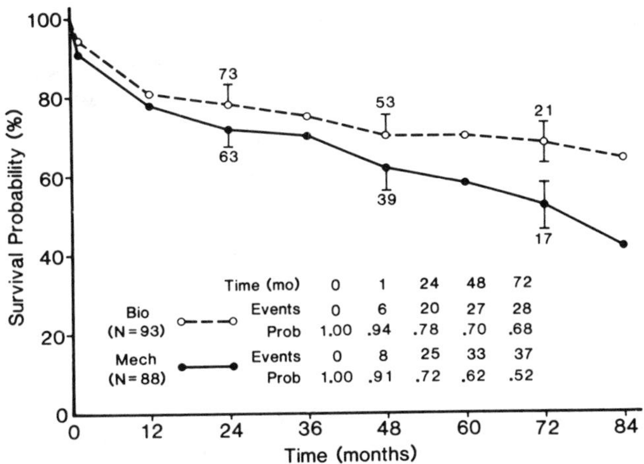

Fig 5–11.—Actuarial analysis of survival using death from any cause as the end point. Comparison of patients undergoing mitral valve replacement with a bioprosthesis vs. those receiving a mechanical prosthesis. Format and abbreviations as in Figure 5–10. (Courtesy of Hammermeister, K.E., et al.: J. Am. Coll. Cardiol. 10:719–732, October 1987.)

thesis is a greater frequency of nonfatal bleeding with the latter device. Obtaining a careful history to detect past bleeding problems is important when valve replacement is planned.

Comparative Clinical Experience With Porcine Bioprosthetic and St. Jude Valve Replacement

Lawrence S.C. Czer, Jack M. Matloff, Aurelio Chaux, Michele A. DeRobertis, and Richard J. Gray (Cedars-Sinai Med. Ctr., Los Angeles, and Univ. of California at Los Angeles)

Chest 91:503–514, April 1987 5–19

Various prosthetic valves are available for patients requiring valve replacement. A comparison is made between patients receiving either Hancock or Carpentier-Edwards porcine valves (POR) and those receiving St. Jude bileaflet valves (SJ).

A group of 293 patients received 316 porcine bioprostheses, whereas 363 patients received 415 St. Jude prostheses.

Patients who received the St. Jude valve were of more advanced New York Heart Association (NYHA) classification preoperatively, required smaller prostheses, and more frequently had associated coronary artery disease that required bypass grafting. However, POR and SJ recipients had similar 30-day mortality, 5-year absence of embolism, freedom from all valve-related complications (Fig 5–12), and survival (Fig 5–13). The only structural failures occurred in POR recipients (Fig 5–14). Endocarditis was also more common in POR recipients.

These two factors contributed to a three-times higher reoperation rate

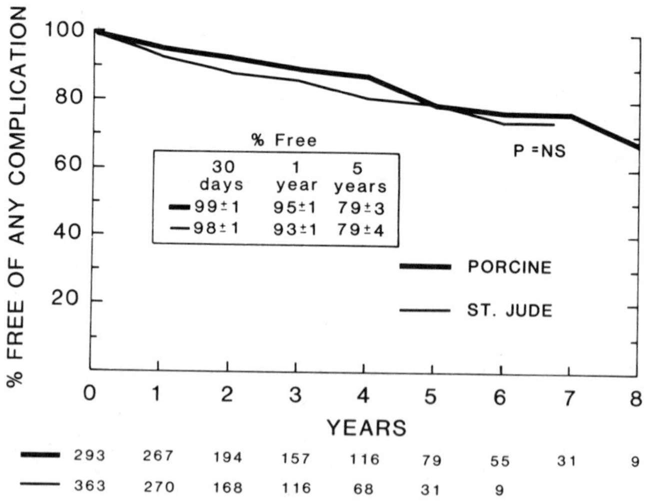

Fig 5–12.—Actuarial freedom from all valve related complications in porcine and St. Jude valve recipients. Valve related complications occurred equally frequently with both prostheses (P = NS). (Courtesy of Czer, L.S.C., et al.: Chest 91:503–514, April 1987.)

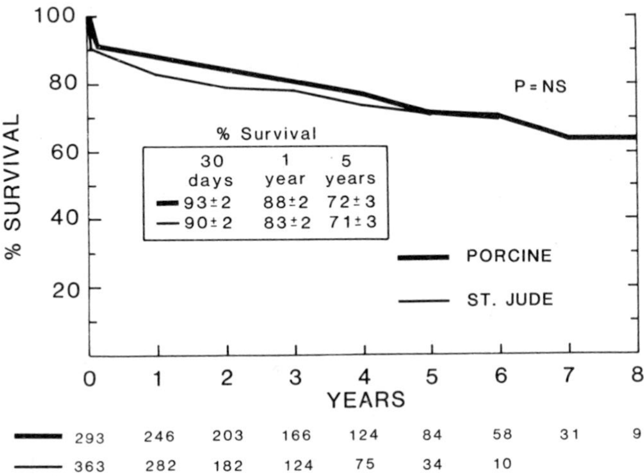

Fig 5–13.—Actuarial survival in porcine and St. Jude valve recipients. All mortalities (early and late) were included in the analysis. There was no difference in survival after 5–6 years of follow-up. (Courtesy of Czer, L.S.C., et al.: Chest 91:503–514, April 1987.)

in POR recipients than SJ recipients. Warfarin-related bleeding was the most usual complication in SJ recipients, but POR recipients requiring anticoagulation had this complication with equal frequency. Over 40% of 16 valve-related late deaths were warfarin-related. Possibly because of the better hemodynamic performance of the SJ valve, NYHA class I was achieved in 60% of SJ recipients, as opposed to 39% in POR recipients.

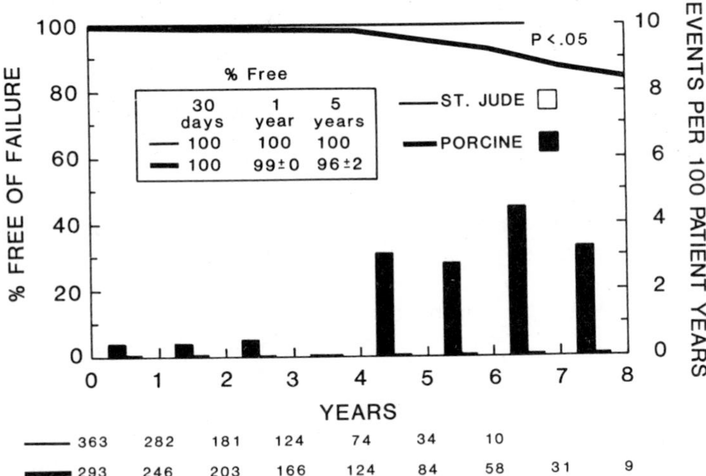

Fig 5–14.—Freedom from structural failure in porcine and St. Jude valve recipients, shown actuarially by the lines at the top of the figure, referenced to the scale at the left. The box insert depicts the percentage of patients free of failure at 30 days, 1 year, and 5 years. The yearly linearized event rates are depicted as bar graphs and are referenced to the scale at the right. No structural failures occurred in the St. Jude valve recipients. Numbers below the figure indicate patients at risk during follow-up. (Courtesy of Czer, L.S.C., et al.: Chest 91:503–514, April 1987.)

Although there were differences in patient selection and types of complications noted, both valves provided similar early and late survival, frequency of embolism, overall complication rate, and freedom from valve-related morbidity and mortality at 5-year follow-up. However, the POR bioprosthesis does have limited durability, susceptibility to infection, and inferior hemodynamics. Limitations of the SJ valve include the necessity of warfarin anticoagulation and the frequency of resultant bleeding.

▶ The above four publications (Abstracts 5–16 to 5–19) serve to summarize the continuing competition and controversy relating to the selection of a valve replacement device for any individual patient.

The report of Sir Brian Barratt-Boyes et al. (Abstract 5–16) emphasizes the excellent results that have been experienced by the group at Green Lane Hospital using "fresh" antibiotic sterilized homografts for aortic valve replacement. Whether these results may be improved in the future by techniques allowing better maintenance of graft viability remains to be seen. Certainly, survival over the short and medium term (5–10 years) has been excellent with homograft valves as well as with glutaraldehyde-preserved porcine valves, as indicated by the reports summarized by DiSesa, Hammermeister, and Czer and their associates (Abstracts 5–17 to 5–19). At least up to approximately 10 years after surgery, there does not seem to be a specific and major advantage in longevity for either tissue valves or modern prosthetic valves. The principal difference is the avoidance of anticoagulation in tissue valves (in the aortic position or, for patients, in sinus rhythm in the mitral position). Since no one wishes to have a second operation, and since the hazard of reoperation increases with age, the tendency for deterioration of tissue valves between 10 and 15 years after surgery is a substantial disadvantage.

It would appear that there are two general avenues where important improvements can be sought for valve replacement devices. For the tissue valves, an improvement in durability to allow an expected longevity of 20–30 years would appear to be an achievable objective. For prosthetic valves a more reasonable anticoagulation program that could effectively protect against thromboembolism while presenting a minimal risk of bleeding complications is also a theoretically obtainable objective. The concept that currently acceptable levels of warfarin anticoagulation (1½–2 times the control prothrombin time) is an absolute minimum for protection against thromboembolic events is inadequately supported by the available evidence in my opinion.

There seems little doubt that the propensity toward thromboembolism is to some extent predetermined by measurable variations in clotting factors. I wonder whether routine preoperative testing of multiple clotting factors may not produce a spectrum of thromboembolic risk, allowing selection of anticoagulant programs for patients having a special risk for the development of thromboembolic events. In the absence of such a special risk, a very low level of anticoagulation may be entirely adequate for the majority of persons.

At present there still is room for investigation for both tissue and prosthetic valves. The end is not yet in sight.—J.J. Collins, Jr., M.D.

References

1. Bortolotti, U., Milano, A., Thiene, G., et al.: Long-term durability of the Hancock porcine bioprosthesis following combined mitral and aortic valve replacement: An 11 year experience. *Ann. Thorac. Surg.* 44:139–144, 1987.
2. Hammond, G.L., Geha A.S., Kopf, G.S., et al.: Biological versus mechanical valves. *J. Thorac. Cardiovasc. Surg.* 93:182–198, 1987.
3. Borkon, A.M., Soule, L., Baughman, K.L., et al.: Ten-year analysis of the Bjork-Shiley standard aortic valve. *Ann. Thorac. Surg.* 43:39–51, 1987.
4. Hackett, D., Fessatidis, I., Sapsford, R., et al.: Ten-year clinical evaluation of Starr-Edwards 2400 and 1260 aortic valve prostheses. *Br. Heart J.* 57:356–363, 1987.

Mechanical Failure of the Björk-Shiley Valve: Incidence, Clinical Presentation, and Management

Dan Lindblom, Viking O. Björk, and Bjarne K.H. Semb (Karolinska Hosp., Stockholm)

J. Thorac. Cardiovasc. Surg. 92:894–907, November 1986 5–20

Mechanical disruption has been described in many mechanical heart valves. Even biologic valves may require emergency treatment. Recently, there has been an interest in the increased incidence of strut fractures among convexo-concave Björk-Shiley valves. The manufacturer has recalled these valves several times. The experience after implantation of 3334 Björk-Shiley valves in a 15-year period was described.

The follow-up rate was 99.2%, covering 17,511 patient year. The mean follow-up time was 6.3 years. The autopsy rate was 75% among all fatalities. A total of 19 cases of mechanical failure was documented. There were no mechanical failures among the 271 patients with standard Delrin Björk-Shiley valves, the 739 patients with the aortic standard Pyrolyte Björk-Shiley valves, or the 377 patients with the Monostrut Björk-Shiley valve. One of the 430 mitral standard Pyrolyte valves fractured. Eighteen of the 1,461 convexo-concave valves fractured, 6 of 884 with an opening angle of 60 degrees, and 12 of 577 with an opening angle of 70 degrees. The actuarial incidence of mechanical failure at 5 years for the 60-degree convexo-concave valve was 0.6%; for the 70-degree convexo-concave valve, it was 2.8% (Fig 5–15).

Two groups of valves were found to be especially affected by this complication: the 23-mm aortic 60-degree convexo-concave valve, with a 5-year actuarial incidence of 2.2%, and the 29- to 31-mm mitral 70-degree convexo-concave valve, with a 5-year actuarial incidence of 8.3%. The hazard function indicates a constant or decreasing tendency for mechanical failure in the 60-degree convexo-concave valve and the 70-degree convexo-concave valve, respectively.

The time interval between the first symptom of mechanical failure and circulatory collapse was found to be significantly shorter after aortic fail-

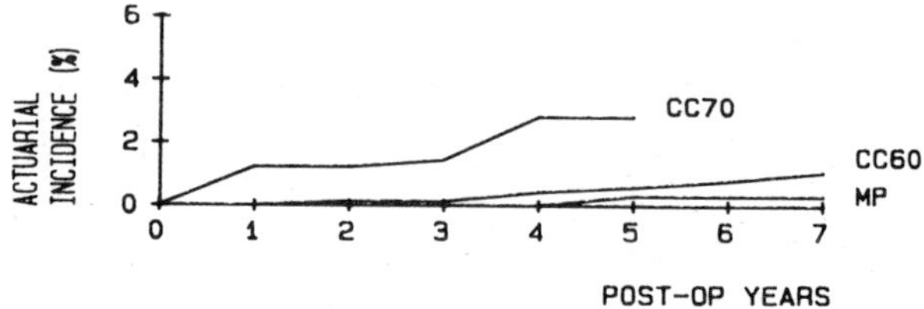

Fig 5–15.—Actuarial incidence of MF with different valve models. MP, mitral, standard Pyrolyte prosthesis. CC60/70, Convexo-concave valves with the disc opening to 60/70 degrees. (Courtesy of Lindblom, D., et al.: J. Thorac. Cardiovasc. Surg. 92:894–907, November 1986.)

ure than after mitral failure. No patient with a fractured aortic prosthesis survived long enough to undergo reoperation. The incidence of mechanical failure among patients dying suddenly who underwent autopsy was 9.6%. Most cases of sudden death were unrelated to the prosthesis.

These results confirm that the incidence of mechanical failure increased with the introduction of the convexo-concave valves. This increase was especially marked among the 70-degree valves, which is not used in the United States. Mechanical failure was found to be responsible for death in a minor fraction of patients dying suddenly after valve replacement. Aortic mechanical failure was associated with almost instantaneous death; mitral mechanical failure allows the patients to live long enough for repair. The diagnosis of patients with suspected mechanical failure must be based on plain chest x-ray films, invasive investigations should not be done. Prophylactic re-replacement was not recommended at this time.

▶ This analysis of a large number of Björk-Shiley valves in both the aortic and mitral positions followed over a long interval is a valuable contribution, particularly for those surgeons who have not had extensive experience with all the various types of Björk-Shiley valves that have been introduced. The close relationship between changes in the configuration of valves and the probability of mechanical failure urges extra caution in the design and fabrication of prosthetic cardiac valves.—J.J. Collins, Jr., M.D.

Thrombolytic Therapy for Prosthetic Cardiac Valve Thrombosis

Steven Kurzrok, Arun K. Singh, Albert S. Most, and David O. Williams (Brown Univ.)

J. Am. Coll. Cardiol. 9:592–598, March 1987 5–21

Surgery for prosthetic valve thrombosis is technically difficult, and often is done urgently. Mortality rates of up to 42% have been reported following valve replacement or debridement. Thrombolytic therapy was evaluated in 3 of the authors' patients and in 38 previously reported patients with prosthetic valve thrombosis. The mean age was 48 years. There were 18 mitral, 15 tricuspid, and 8 aortic prostheses in the series. Streptokinase was used in 28 patients, urokinase in 11, and both agents in 2.

Thirty-two patients (78%) had a successful outcome. Twenty-four of these patients remained asymptomatic and did not require surgery during follow-up for 2–60 months. One patient had elective valve replacement. Seven patients had recurrent thrombosis, and 4 again responded to thrombolytic treatment. Four of 26 patients with a mitral or aortic prosthesis had complications possibly due to embolization of thrombotic material from the prosthesis. No patient, however, had a permanent neurologic or circulatory deficit.

Thrombolytic treatment is an effective approach to prosthetic valve thrombosis. It may preclude the need for surgery in a substantial number of cases. In other cases elective surgery will be possible, at a lower risk. Embolism has been relatively infrequent and minor. Treatment for 48–72 hours might increase the chance of success without incurring added mortality.

▶ This report of published data on the utilization of thrombolytic therapy for prosthetic valve thrombosis suggests that, at least in patients with recent catastrophic valve failure, thrombolytic therapy may be an alternative to immediate open surgery. With modern techniques of echocardiographic assessment of prosthetic valve function, thrombolytic therapy may come to have a secure place in the management of prosthetic valve thrombosis. It is certainly simpler (on the surface) than reoperation valve replacement for many patients. Long-term results are awaited with some interest.—J.J. Collins, Jr., M.D.

Reoperations for Valve Surgery: Perioperative Mortality and Determinants of Risk for 1,000 Patients 1958–1984

Bruce W. Lytle, Delos M. Cosgrove, Paul C. Taylor, Carl C. Gill, Marlene Goormastic, Leonard R. Golding, Robert W. Stewart, and Floyd D. Loop (Cleveland Clinic Found.)

Ann. Thorac. Surg. 42:632–643, December 1986 5–22

There is a low perioperative risk for most primary cardiac surgical procedures. An increasing number of cardiac operations are being performed, and the outlook for late survival is favorable. Many patients who undergo valve operations survive to become candidates for reoperation to repair or replace valves. However, reoperation presents numerous problems. One thousand valve reoperations were studied in 897 patients to determine perioperative risks and to identify predictors of survival.

Patients were subgrouped according to the number of previous cardiac procedures performed and the type of valve or valves replaced/repaired (table). Other variables were examined for their relationships with inhospital deaths.

Most patients were undergoing either their first or second reoperation. Mortality increased from 11% at first reoperation to 44% at third reoperation. There were only 2 patients each in groups undergoing fourth and fifth reoperation; neither patient died after fourth reoperation, but both patients undergoing fifth surgeries died.

Cardiac Reoperations for Valve Surgery in 897 Patients*

	Aortic Valve	Mitral Valve	Tricuspid Valve	Multiple Valves	Total
Reoperation 1	26/239 (11%)	45/458 (10%)	2/10 (20%)	20/145 (14%)	93/852 (11%)
Reoperation 2	3/24 (13%)	9/77 (12%)	0/4 (0)	7/23 (30%)	19/128 (15%)
Reoperations 3–5	2/6 (33%)	5/10 (50%)	0/1 (0)	2/3 (67%)	9/20 (45%)

*One thousand consecutive cardiac operations for valve surgery were performed in 897 patients. Subgroups based on the number of previous cardiac procedures and the valve (s) replaced or repaired at reoperation included aortic valve, mitral valve, tricuspid valve, or multiple valves. Data are expressed as deaths/number of procedures (% mortality).

(Courtesy of Lytle, B.W., et al.: Ann. Thorac. Surg. 42:632–643, December 1986.)

Age was the most consistent predictor of increased risk at reoperation. Other predictors of increased risk for a first aortic valve reoperation were endocarditis, female sex, impaired left ventricular function, and total of coronary vessels obstructed by 70% or more. Preoperative shock or cardiac arrest, previous aortic or tricuspid valve operations, impaired left ventricular function, and type of mitral valve procedure were factors in increasing risk at first mitral valve reoperation. For a first multiple valve reoperation, diabetes and ascites were risk predictors. Patients undergoing mitral valve replacement and tricuspid valve surgery were at decreased risk. Risk increased for succeeding procedures except for aortic or mitral valve operations.

A variety of factors place patients at increased risk at reoperation for valve procedures; however, age had a major impact on mortality.

▶ Repeated valve replacement operations are difficult for the surgeon and dangerous for the patient. Hazards to the patients are remarkably variable, as detailed in the above presentation; but, to summarize most succinctly, age, myocardial failure, and magnitude of operation are probably the principal determinants of survival and rehabilitation. It is always well to remember when contemplating reoperation on persons of advanced age that the probability of rehabilitation is as important an indication for surgery as the seriousness of the disease.—J.J. Collins, Jr., M.D.

Combined Valve and Coronary Artery Bypass Procedures in Septuagenarians and Octogenarians: Results in 120 Patients

Tsung Po Tsai, Jack M. Matloff, Aurelio Chaux, Robert M. Kass, Myles E. Lee, Lawrence S.C. Czer, Michele A. DeRobertis, and Richard J. Gray (Cedars-Sinai Med. Ctr., Los Angeles)

Ann. Thorac. Surg. 42:681–684, December 1986 5–23

Although coronary artery bypass (CAB) procedures have substantially reduced morbidity and mortality in selected elderly patients, the risks from this procedure in this population are still high, especially when combined with valve replacement. A review was undertaken to define

MORTALITY BY TYPE OF PROCEDURE*

Procedures	Age 70–79	Age 80–89	Total Deaths/Patients (%)
	Deaths/Patients		
AVR + CAB	9/45	3/13	12/58 (21)
MVR + CAB	14/31	5/7	19/38 (50)
MV repair + CAB	1/8	1/3	2/11 (18)
DVR + CAB	1/8	1/1	2/9 (22)
MV repair + AVR + CAB	1/2	0	1/2 (50)
MV repair + CAB + ASD Repair	0/2	0	0/2
Total	26/96	10/24	36/120 (30)

*AVR = aortic valve replacement; MVR = mitral valve replacement; DVR = aortic and mitral valve replacements; CAB = coronary artery bypass; ASD = atrial septal defect.

(Courtesy of Tsai, T.P., et al.: Ann. Thorac. Surg. 42:681–684, December 1986.)

preoperative characteristics and postoperative outcomes in patients between 70 and 90 years old who underwent combined CAB and valve surgeries.

A group of 96 septuagenarians and 24 octogenarians underwent CAB and valve surgeries using hypothermia and hyperkalemic cardioplegia. Preoperatively, most patients were New York Heart Association (NYHA) class IV.

There were 19% early deaths for septuagenarians and 37% for octogenarians; late death rates were 9% and 6%, respectively. Of the survivors, most improved by at least one NYHA class postoperatively. In patients in whom CAB was combined with aortic valve replacement, 21% died; with mitral valve replacement, 50% died; with double valve replacement, 22% died; with mitral valve repair, 18% died (table). Overall patients who had valve replacement alone had lower death rates.

There is a significantly increased risk in elderly patients with combined valve procedures and bypass surgery. Surgical intervention should be carefully considered, especially where the mitral valve is involved.

▶ Several cautions are evident in this report. First is the observation, perhaps obvious, that advancing age is correlated with increased surgical risk. Furthermore, in the experience of nearly all surgeons, advanced age is also correlated with imperfect or absent rehabilitation. Another very important prognostic factor, particularly in aged patients, is the complexity of the operative procedure necessary to effect survival. Fine judgment may be necessary to avoid the pitfall of attempting an unnecessarily complicated repair.

A hidden hazard of this report may be increased enthusiasm for operating on older and older individuals. When does risk of mortality become unacceptable? When is convalescence too prolonged? The object of surgery is not to eradicate disease so much as to promote rehabilitation.—J.J. Collins, Jr., M.D.

Inoperable Aortic Stenosis in the Elderly: Benefit From Percutaneous Transluminal Valvuloplasty

Graham Jackson, Stephen Thomas, Mark Monaghan, Andrew Forsyth, and David Jewitt (King's College Hosp., London)

Br. Med. J. 294:83–86, Jan. 10, 1987 5–24

Without corrective surgery, the life expectancy for patients with symptomatic aortic stenosis ranges from 2–4 years. Nevertheless, surgery is not always appropriate, particularly for patients with life-threatening illnesses such as cancer or for those too old and infirm to undergo operations. Considerations of this nature prompted this trial of percutaneous transluminal aortic valvuloplasty.

Eight patients with severe symptomatic calcific aortic stenosis were judged to be unlikely subjects for valve replacement. Three of them were in cardiogenic shock, four had pulmonary edema, and one suffered from angina at rest. Percutaneous transluminal aortic valvuloplasty was performed with the use of echocardiographic and radiographic guidance. There was an average of 40% reduction in aortic gradients. Immediate improvement was noted in all four cardiac failure cases, and these patients remained well 6 months later. Two of the three patients who had been in cardiogenic shock also exprienced immediate improvement and remained well several months later; the other died 4 hours after treatment. The angina patient remained symptom free 9 months later. A slight initial increase in aortic incompetence was documented by Doppler echocardiography, but there was no worsening of the condition. Valvar gradients still showed improvement in follow-ups.

It appears that aortic valvuloplasty has a useful role in the treatment of symptomatic cases of aortic stenosis who seem to be poor risks for surgery. In some cases it affords symptomatic benefit, and in others valvuloplasty might provide stabilization of a poor hemodynamic state so that surgery could be performed later with lowered risk. The role of percutaneous transluminal balloon dilatation of the aortic valve as an alternative to surgery deserves investigation in controlled clinical trials.

▶ The natural history of most surgical operations includes initial attempts with patients for whom no alternative exists. Subsequently, presuming a favorable initial experience the procedure is extended to patients for whom established, albeit more complex or less effective measures, exist. While open surgery for valve replacement is undoubtedly complex and requires a certain systemic stamina for survival, the mechanical correction of aortic stenosis is virtually uniformly satisfactory.

The communication by Jackson and associates is typical of numerous publications attesting to the early clinical improvement observed after balloon valvuloplasty for severe calcific aortic stenosis. No doubt, some critically ill patients may be sufficiently improved that an elective valve replacement becomes possible. Whether balloon valvuloplasty for some patients may be a definitive procedure, or may be repeated from time to time to provide for long benefit, remains to be seen. A cautionary note by Robicsek and Harbold is based on direct observation of the effect of balloon valvuloplasty in patients undergoing aortic valve replacement. Their observation that the mechanical effect of balloon dilation in the orifice of a severely calcified valve is "minimal" does not necessarily mean that it is also "negligible."

In the presence of extremely tight aortic stenosis even a small improvement in the aperture during systole may provide a substantial hemodynamic benefit. The contention of Robicsek and Harbold (1) that the improvement will necessarily by short lived is probably true but remains to be demonstrated.—J.J. Collins, Jr., M.D.

Reference

1. Robicsek, F., Harbold, N., Limited value of balloon dilatation in calcified aortic stenosis in adults: Direct observations during open heart surgery. *Am. J. Cardiol.* 60:857–864, 1987.

Adjustable Annuloplasty for Tricuspid Insufficiency

Paul Kurlansky, Eric A. Rose, and James R. Malm (Columbia Univ.)

Ann. Thorac. Surg. 44:404–406, October 1987 5–25

A modified de Vega annuloplasty for functional tricuspid insufficiency individualizes the repair performed on the intact beating heart. Twelve patients underwent such repair for congenital or acquired valve conditions between 1981 and 1982.

TECHNIQUE.—A suture annuloplasty is carried out after correction of left-sided abnormalities. After aortic cross-clamping and institution of cold crystalloid cardioplegia, a transverse right atriotomy is made and a double suture line begun septally of the anteroseptal commissure, using a double-ended 2–0 polypropylene suture buttressed with a Teflon felt pledget. Two suture lines 2–3 mm apart are run about the annular insertions of the tricuspid leaflets to a point just beyond the posteroseptal commissure, where the orifice is tightened with an obturator. The annuloplasty is then adjusted over a tube snare to the minimum required to eliminate palpable regurgitation.

Hemodynamic improvement was confirmed intraoperatively. Long-term clinical improvement was obtained in all ten survivors as confirmed in a follow-up of 15–30 months. This reproducible repair is easily taught and normal valve function is preserved. The conduction system is not damaged. The efficacy of the repair may be confirmed with the patient off bypass without risking restenosis or residual insufficiency.

▶ This modification of the de Vega annuloplasty allows for adjustment of the degree of constriction of the tricuspid annulus under dynamic conditions, which is a substantial advantage over the originally described technique. Tying down an annuloplasty suture over a measured obturator or over the assistant's fingertips is uncertain at best when performed without hemodynamic control. This modification deserves thorough evaluation.—J.J. Collins, Jr., M.D.

Congenital Heart Surgery

Accuracy of Subcostal Two-Dimensional Echocardiography in Prospective Diagnosis of Total Anomalous Pulmonary Venous Connection

Alvin J. Chin, Stephen P. Sanders, Frederick Sherman, Peter Lang, William I. Norwood, and Aldo R. Castaneda (Children's Hosp. and Harvard Univ., Boston)
Am. Heart J. 113:1153–1159, May 1987 5–26

Reparative surgery without cardiac catheterization has been suggested for total anomalous pulmonary venous connection (TAPVC). Therefore, it is important to evaluate the accuracy of two-dimensional (2-D) echocardiography in the prospective diagnosis of this lesion to determine whether there is justification for abandoning invasive procedures.

A group of 2,444 infants aged younger than 2 years underwent subcostal 2-D echocardiography, first to discover a descending vein then to look for an ascending vein and, if neither was seen, to search for sites of direct connection of the pulmonary venous confluence to the right superior vena cava, coronary sinus, or right atrium.

In 38 patients, TAPVC was diagnosed as being the only major cardiac defect. There were neither false negative nor false positive results. Drainage sites were correctly diagnosed in 95% of patients. In 2 of 5 patients with mixed-type TAPVC, 2-D echocardiography missed the second drainage site.

In the absence of other cardiac abnormalities, 2-D echocardiography alone seems to be sufficient in diagnosis of TAPVC. Several echocardiographic windows are unnecessary; accurate diagnosis can be made by imaging from the subcostal window only.

Surgery Without Catheterization for Congenital Heart Defects: Management of 100 Patients

James C. Huhta, Patrick Glasgow, Daniel J. Murphy, Jr., Howard P. Gutgesell, David A. Ott, Dan G. McNamara, and E. O'Brian Smith (Baylor College, Houston, and other U.S. universities, medical centers, and research centers)
J. Am. Coll. Cardiol. 9:823–829, April 1987 5–27

Little is known about mortality in children with congenital heart disease who undergo operation using echocardiographic diagnosis without cardiac catheterization. This article reviews a study undertaken to determine whether omission of catheterization improves survival.

One hundred patients (group I) were diagnosed with echocardiography but did not have preoperative catheterization. These were compared with a diagnosis-matched control group (group II) who did have catheterization.

Echocardiographic diagnosis proved to be accurate in all but one case. Operative mortality in group I was 18%; in group II it was 9%. Nevertheless, patients in group I were younger, sicker, and required preoperative prostaglandin more often. Females had a higher survival rate than males. Correcting for age alone showed a probability of survival of 88% in group I as compared with 82% in group II. When other variables were adjusted, the trend continued, suggesting that odds for survival favored group I.

It appears that accurate preoperative diagnosis of pediatric patients with congenital heart defects can be achieved with echocardiography and without catheterization. Catheterization can be omitted in selected patients, and surgical mortality may be decreased in younger and sicker patients.

▶ The increased accuracy possible with advanced techniques of noninvasive diagnosis has particular application to congenital heart disease where knowledge of the coronary artery anatomy is not so important as with adult patients. In both these articles (Abstracts 5–26 and 5–27) there is good evidence for the adequacy of noninvasive studies prior to definitive corrective surgery. Avoidance of catheterization with its attendant complications, discomfort, and expense is certainly worthwhile when it can be accomplished safely.—J.J. Collins, Jr., M.D.

Constant Postoperative Monitoring of Cardiac Output After Correction of Congenital Heart Defects

Blair A. Keagy, Benson R. Wilcox, Carol L. Lucas, Henry S. Hsiao, G. William Henry, Michael Baudino, and Gene Bornzin (Univ. of North Carolina and Medtronic, Inc., Minneapolis)

J. Thorac. Cardiovasc. Surg. 93:658–664, May 1987 5–28

Several methods are available to monitor cardiac output following heart surgery, including the electromagnetic flow probe and thermodilution; however, these procedures have limitations. Recently, ultrasound has been used postoperatively to monitor mean and phasic cardiac output.

After surgery in 20 patients, a tiny ultrasound probe was attached to the adventitia of the ascending aorta and wired to the monitoring equipment through the chest wall (Fig 5–16). When the patient's condition was stable, the probe was easily removed by gentle traction. Cardiac output with ultrasound was correlated with output measured with a standard electromagnetic flow probe. Patients underwent surgery for atrial or ventricular septal defects, tetralogy of Fallot, stenotic valve defects, and Senning procedures.

There was one operative death, but there were no complications due to probe application or removal. Cardiac output measurements were nearly identical with ultrasound and the electromagnetic flow probe; there was a high linear correlation between the two techniques.

The extraluminal removable probe permits virtually continuous monitoring of postsurgical cardiac output after correction of congenital heart

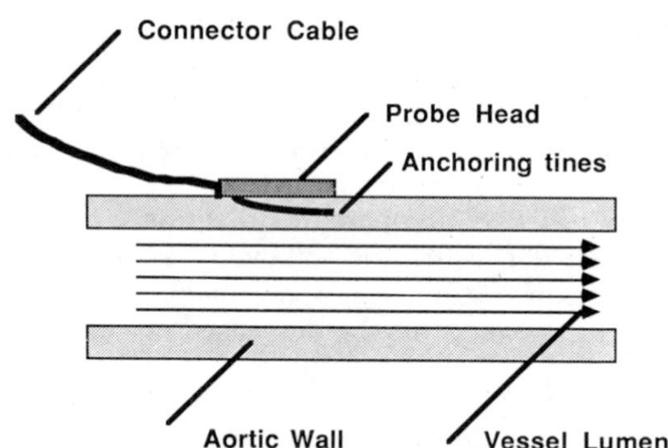

Fig 5–16.—Schematic representation of the probe anchored to the aortic wall with the metal tines. (Courtesy of Keagy, B.A., et al.: J. Thorac. Cardiovasc. Surg. 93:658–664, May 1987.)

defects. An additional advantage is that the monitor can display the output minute by minute, thus facilitating adjustments in fluid administration and intravenous drug therapy.

▶ The advantage of cardiac output monitoring without the necessity of repeated injections of iced saline is obvious, especially in infants and children. The technique described by Keagy and associates seems reasonably simple, safe, and effective, particularly when it is used for determination of trends during postoperative care.—J.J. Collins, Jr., M.D.

Results With the Mustard Operation in Simple Transposition of the Great Arteries: 1963–1985

George A. Trusler, William G. Williams, Kim F. Duncan, Peter S. Hesslein, Lee N. Benson, Robert M. Freedom, Teruo Izukawa, and Peter M. Olley (Hosp. for Sick Children and Univ. of Toronto)

Ann. Surg. 206:251–260, September 1987 5–29

The results of repair of simple transposition by the Mustard technique were compared in 106 children undergoing surgery between 1963 and 1973 (group I) and 223 operated on between 1974 and 1985 (group II).

Whereas operative mortality was 10% in group I, it was only 0.9% in group II. The 10-year actuarial survival rates were 73% and 94%, respectively (Fig 5–17). Baffle complications were similar in the two groups. The latest ECG showed 47% of group I patients, but 72% of group II patients, to be in normal sinus rhythm. Most patients, however, had sinus node dysfunction or other dysrhythmias detected on ambulatory ECG study. Right ventricular contractility was definitely reduced in 11% of the children studied. Further, 76% of the children were in New York Heart Association class I at late follow-up and the rest were in class II. About 20% of the patients were taking medication, chiefly for dysrhythmia.

Mortality associated with the Mustard operation has declined signifi-

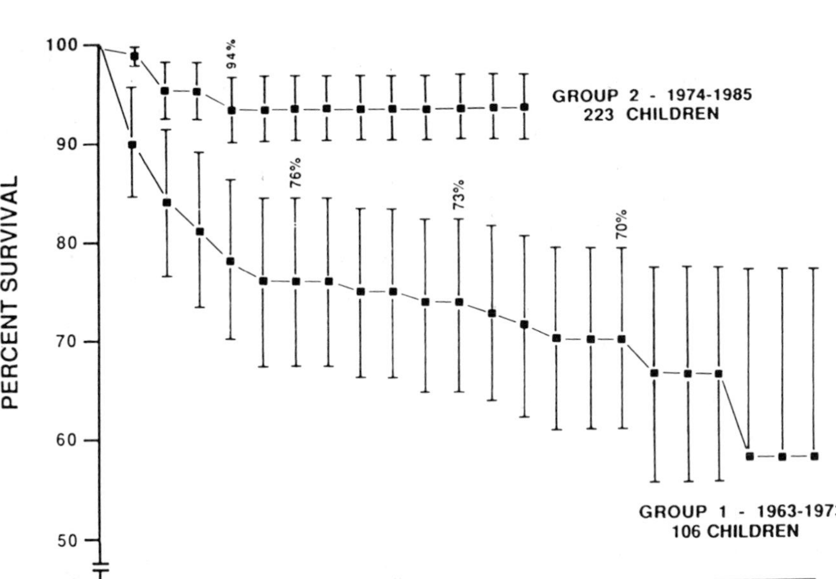

Fig 5–17.—Comparison of survival in group I and group II patients. Group II patients had a survival rate at 5 years and 10 years of 93.7% compared with 75.4% and 73.4%, respectively, in group I patients. (Courtesy of Trusler, G.A., et al.: Ann. Surg. 206:251–260, September 1987.)

cantly, and serious baffle-related complications are infrequent. However, dysrhythmia remains a major problem. Such complications are expected to be less frequent with arterial repair, but it remains to be learned whether the good early results obtained by a few surgeons can be reproduced without excessive risk.

▶ This very interesting article illustrates that, although the arterial switch operation has largely replaced the Mustard operation for operative correction of transposition, excellent results were obtained by some centers with the Mustard operation. The long-term survival rate of 94% (at 10 years) in patients operated on since 1974 is excellent indeed.—J.J. Collins, Jr., M.D.

Cerebral Infarction Complicating Fontan Surgery for Cyanotic Congenital Heart Disease

Katherine Mathews, James F. Bale, Jr., Edward B. Clark, William J. Marvin, Jr., and Donald B. Doty (Univ. of Iowa)

Pediatr. Cardiol. 7:161–166, 1986 5–30

There have been few reports of neurologic complications as a result of using the Fontan procedure in children with cyanotic congenital heart disease. The authors describe four children who had cerebral infarction within 3 months of Fontan surgery.

In all patients the surgical procedure successfully separated the pulmonary and systemic circuits. No patient was cyanotic after surgery, and none had residual right-left shunting. Two of four patients had platelet counts greater than 400,000/cu mm, and one patient with a normal platelet count had recurrent deep venous thrombosis.

The pathogenesis of stroke in these patients has not been completely determined, but it is suggested that children who undergo Fontan surgery may be at increased risk for stroke. Severe cyanosis, congestive heart failure, arrhythmias, and thrombocytosis may be contributing factors. Further study should be undertaken to determine the potential risk of neurologic complications following Fontan surgery.

▶ The increasing utilization of various modifications of the Fontan operation has significantly increased the number of patients who may have palliation in various types of cyanotic congenital heart disease. The report by Mathews and associates of cerebral vascular accidents in several children late after Fontan operations, and the absence of previously reported similar complications, raises the possibility that the incidence may be higher than expected. This report should serve to alert especially those pediatric cardiologists following groups of patients after Fontan operations to the necessity of reporting such complications until a proper estimate is made of the incidence and seriousness of this potential hazard.—J.J. Collins, Jr., M.D.

References

1. Mayer, J.E., Helgason, H., Jonas, R.A., et al.: Extending the limits for modified Fontan procedures. *J. Thorac. Cardiovasc. Surg.* 92:1021–1028, 1986.
2. DeLeon, S.Y., Ilbawi, M.N., Idriss F.S., et al.: Fontan type operation for complex lesions. *J. Thorac. Cardiovasc. Surg.* 92:1029–1037, 1986.

Current Risks and Protocols for Operations for Double-Outlet Right Ventricle: Derivation From an 18 Year Experience

John W. Kirklin, Albert D. Pacifico, Eugene H. Blackstone, James K. Kirklin, and L.M. Bargeron, Jr. (Univ. of Alabama at Birmingham)

J. Thorac. Cardiovasc. Surg. 92:913–930, November 1986 5–31

The authors reviewed 127 cases of patients having initial intracardiac repair of double-outlet right ventricle (DORV), which was defined as a ventriculoarterial connection where the aorta and pulmonary artery both arose more than 50% from the right ventricle. The median follow-up was 51 months.

Fifty-eight patients failed to survive the early and late postoperative periods. The actuarial survival at 12 years was 38%. Six deaths followed reoperation. Acute heart failure was responsible for nearly half the remaining deaths. Eight patients had complete heart block after repair. Most surviving patients were fully active and asymptomatic at follow-up. Reoperation was carried out in 17 patients. Operative mortality after reoperation at the authors' center was 31.

Double-outlet right ventricle should be repaired at age 6–12 months, or sooner if necessary. Preliminary pulmonary artery banding is not indicated. A DORV with subpulmonary ventricular septal defect is managed by closure of the septal defect and an arterial switch operation. Shunting may be indicated if pulmonary stenosis is present. The Fontan operation is technically feasible in DORV with noncommittee ventricular septal defect associated with pulmonary stenosis. The septal defect should be enlarged if it is restrictive, and the tricuspid valve closed.

▶ This review of a large series of patients having undergone reparative operations for double-outlet right ventricle emphasizes the improvement in early and projected late survival in recent years. The authors are highly experienced in congenital cardiac surgery, and their presentation and discussion of the development of optimal treatment protocols is both rational and practical.—J.J. Collins, Jr., M.D.

Transatrial-Transpulmonary Repair of Tetralogy of Fallot

Albert D. Pacifico, Mark E. Sand, Lionel M. Bargeron, Jr., and Edward C. Colvin (Univ. of Alabama at Birmingham)

J. Thorac. Cardiovasc. Surg. 93:919–924, June 1987 5–32

A transatrial-transpulmonary approach was used to repair classic tetralogy of Fallot in 61 of 70 patients operated on in 1981–1985. Sixteen patients had a shunt in place. The mean follow-up was 23 months.

No hospital or late deaths occurred, and no reoperations were necessary. The mean peak RV/LV pressure gradient was 0.50 in patients without transannular patching and 0.56 in those with a transannular patch. Postoperative complications included one reentry for bleeding, one case of chylothorax, and one sternal infection. All patients were in New York Heart Association functional class I without medication at follow-up. Nine repeated catheterizations, done 4–28 months postoperatively, showed no residual ventricular septal defects. The mean RV/LV pressure gradient was 0.42.

Transatrial-transpulmonary repair has been done successfully in nearly 90% of patients with classic tetralogy. The method is useful even in infants. This repair is not feasible if the infundibulum has a long, narrow configuration. The stenotic pulmonary valve probably is best exposed by a pulmonary arteriotomy. Longer-term studies are needed, but the present findings support the continued use of transatrial-transpulmonary repair for classic tetralogy of Fallot.

▶ Avoidance of right ventriculotomy in the repair of tetralogy of Fallot represents a major advance in the management of this relatively common congenital heart defect. Experience of the authors emphasizes the safety of the operation as well as its wide applicability and excellent long-term results.—J.J. Collins, Jr., M.D.

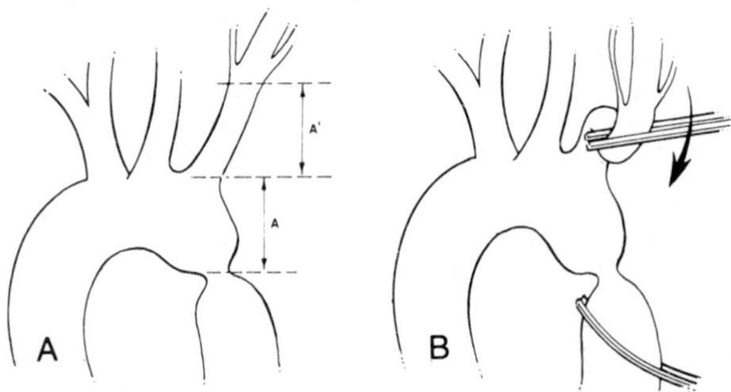

Fig 5–18.—**A,** once the LSCA is mobilized, the distance from its origin to the coarctation site determines the location of the LSCA clamp. **B,** the clamp is brought toward the level of origin of the LSCA to determine the feasibility of the operation before any incision is performed. (Courtesy of Meier, M.A., et al.: J. Thorac. Cardiovasc. Surg. 92:1005–1012, December 1986.)

A New Technique for Repair of Aortic Coarctation: Subclavian Flap Aortoplasty With Preservation of Arterial Blood Flow to the Left Arm

Milton A. Meier, Fernando A. Lucchese, Waldir Jazbik, Ivo A. Nesralla, and José Teles Mendonça (Univ. Hosp.-State Univ. of Rio de Janeiro and other Brazilian medical institutions)

J. Thorac. Cardiovasc. Surg. 92:1005–1012, December 1986 5–33

There is controversy as to the appropriate surgical technique for repair of coarctation of the aorta. A procedure is described that uses the subclavian artery as a flap and preserves arterial blood flow to the left arm.

The technique completely mobilizes the left subclavian artery (LSCA) to the origin of its first branches. At this point before any incision is made, the distance from the origin of the LSCA to the coarctation site should be determined to assess the feasibility of the operation (Fig 5–18). If the decision is made to proceed, it is not necessary to mobilize the

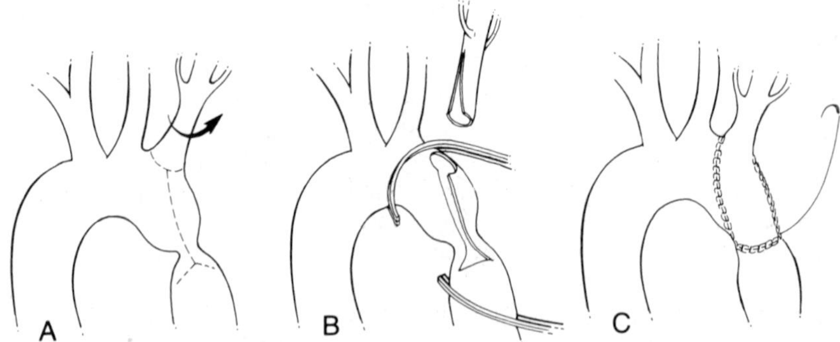

Fig 5–19.—**A,** the incisions to detach the LSCA and open the descending aorta are made according to the *interrupted lines*. **B,** the LSCA is opened in its posterior wall. The incision in the aorta goes 12 to 15 mm below the site of coarctation and is extended 3 to 4 mm laterally. **C,** the LSCA is sutured over the coarctation site, widening the obstruction and preserving the blood flow to the arm. (Courtesy of Meier, M.A., et al.: J. Thorac. Cardiovasc. Surg. 92:1005–1012, December 1986.)

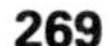

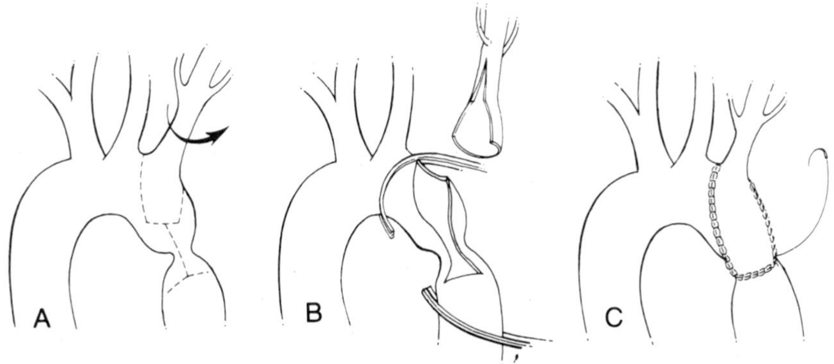

Fig 5–20.—**A,** when the narrowing of the isthmus is long, the LSCA is detached along with a portion of the anterior wall of the aorta to make the flap longer and wider. **B** and **C,** same as in Fig 5–19. (Courtesy of Meier, M.A., et al.: J. Thorac. Cardiovasc. Surg. 92:1005–1012, December 1986.)

aorta extensively; intercostal arteries are individually controlled with snares. The LSCA is detached from the aorta at its source and incised longitudinally on the posterior aspect.

Beginning with the opening at the origin of the LSCA, the anterior wall of the aorta is incised distally to the descending aorta past the coarctation, the coarctation membrane is excised, and the ductus is ligated and divided. The flap formed by the opened LSCA is sutured to the edges of the aorta, thus widening the coarctation site and preserving blood flow to the left arm (Fig 5–19). When there is a long narrowing of the isthmus, the LSCA is detached together with a portion of the anterior wall of the aorta to form a longer, wider flap (Fig 5–20).

In 28 patients, ranging in age from 2 months to 25 years, who were treated with this technique, there were no hospital deaths. At postoperative follow-up, patients showed satisfactory correction, normal blood flow through the LSCA, and no gradients through the isthmus area. Normal growth of the aorta at the coarctation site was strongly suggested.

Findings indicate that the procedure is feasible and preferable to other techniques in most cases of discrete isthmic coarctation, and in some cases of long narrowing of the isthmus, in patients ranging widely in age and weight.

▶ This ingenious technique for the repair of aortic coarctation has produced excellent results for the authors. Whether growth at the coarctation site is normal in all patients has not been proven and further follow-up is necessary.—J.J. Collins, Jr., M.D.

Evaluation of Long-Term Results of Homograft and Heterograft Valves in Extracardiac Conduits

Catherine Bull, Fergus J. Macartney, Pavel Horvath, Rui Almeida, Walter Merrill, John Douglas, James F.N. Taylor, Marc R. de Leval, and Jaroslav Stark (Hosp. for Sick Children, London)

J. Thorac. Cardiovasc. Surg. 94:12–19, July 1987 5–34

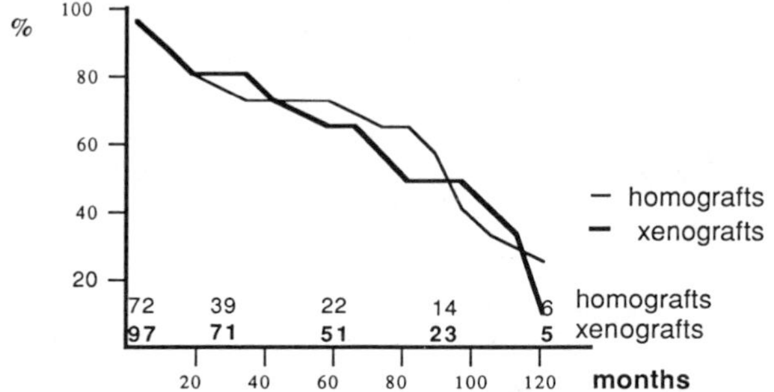

Fig 5–21.—Survival free of conduit obstruction of patients surviving 30 days with homograft and xenograft valved conduits. Early deaths are excluded. (Courtesy of Bull, C., et al.: J. Thorac. Cardiovasc. Surg. 94:12–19, July 1987.)

Because there are numerous problems associated with implantation of extracardiac conduits, including conduit compression, deterioration of conduit valves, and formation of an obstructive coating within Dacron carrying tubes, there has been a search for alternate procedures. This study evaluates the long-term results of conduit procedures and compares the durability of homografts and heterografts.

Data were reviewed on a group of 173 surviving children who received right heart extracardiac conduits. Of these, 72 had antibiotic-sterilized aortic homografts, 97 had various types of xenografts, and 4 had valveless tubes.

There were 45 reoperations, approximately half of which were for conduit replacement; there were also 6 second reoperations. Reoperation for conduit obstruction was necessitated as early as 13 months after initial operation. However, there was no difference in late deaths or survival free of conduit obstruction between the heterograft and the homograft conduit groups (Figs 5–21). The principal factors influencing late conduit complications or death were the original diagnosis (Fig 5–22), the severity of associated lesions, and the number of early postoperative complications. Conditions that required a long conduit were most prone risk

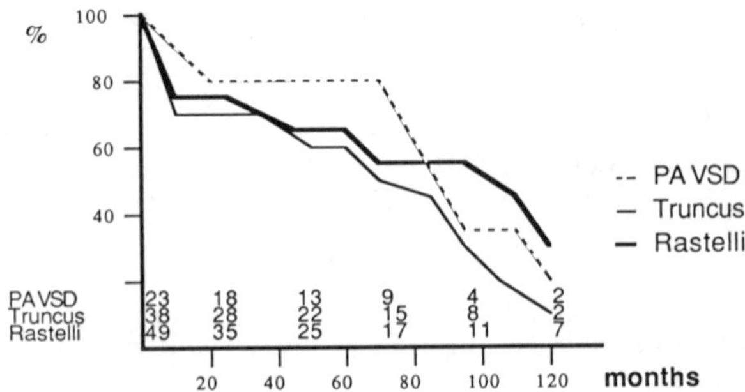

Fig 5–22.—Survival free of any reoperation for patients surviving 30 days after repair of PA VSD, truncus, or Rastelli operations. Early deaths are excluded. (Courtesy of Bull, C., et al.: J. Thorac. Cardiovasc. Surg. 94:12–19, July 1987.)

of late death or early conduit replacement. Obstruction was more commonly found in the Dacron carrying tube than at the valve level.

In most cases, extracardiac conduits fail to provide a permanent solution in children with complex congenital heart disease. In this study, the performance of conduits bearing homografts was disappointing, owing partially to complications within the Dacron carrying tubes. Alternatives that omit the use of conduits entirely should be explored.

▶ This series of extracardiac conduits details the reason for disappointment in the results with both homograft and heterograft valves in extracardiac conduits. More recent utilization of cryopreserved homografts may possibly offer a substantial improvement over what has previously been observed with nonviable homografts. Certainly, the utilization of prosthetic conduits has appeared uniformly unsatisfactory. Also, the possible obviation of conduits by some modifications of the Fontan operation may reduce the need for conduits altogether.—J.J. Collins, Jr., M.D.

Apicoaortic Conduits for Complex Left Ventricular Outflow Obstruction: 10-Year Experience

Michael S. Sweeney, William E. Walker, Denton A. Cooley, and George J. Reul (Univ. of Texas, Houston)

Ann. Thorac. Surg. 42:609–611, December 1986 5–35

Some patients with left ventricular outflow obstruction may be candidates for creation of a new outflow tract from the left ventricular apex to the aorta at the diaphragmatic level. Indications include fibrous tunnel obstruction of the LV outflow tract, severe hypoplasia of the aortic anulus, and tubular hypoplasia of the ascending aorta. Severe calcification of the ascending aorta was another indication. Valved conduits were placed in 38 such patients in a 10-year period. A porcine-valved Dacron conduit was used in each case. All operations but 2 were done under total cardiopulmonary bypass with cold cardioplegia.

Four hospital deaths occurred. Four of 8 late deaths were shunt-related, 3 resulting from disruption of the conduit from its left ventricular attachment. Three children have required replacement of the porcine valve 3–8 years after initial surgery. Two fatal infections occurred. All 26 long-term survivors are asymptomatic without cardiac medications. No thromboembolism has occurred, despite the omission of anticoagulation. None of the surviving patients is restricted physically.

The apicoaortic conduit operation is a useful approach to some patients having complex LV outflow tract obstruction. The operation seems most suited to patients having multiple attempts to open the aortic root; those with a failed Konno or Rastan procedure; and those with some major complication of a previous aortic root operation.

▶ Although most valved conduits are used for replacement of the pulmonary outflow tract, there are certain patients for whom deformities of the left ventricular outflow tract make necessary the utilization of valved conduits between the left ventricle and descending aorta. The series reported above is among the larger ones, and the results up to 10 years after operation have been reasonably good. Nevertheless, the utilization of porcine valves virtually ensures the necessity of repeated operations as these patients become older. Whether the use of a cryogenically preserved homograft would offer better long-term results remains to be demonstrated.—J.J. Collins, Jr., M.D.

Phrenic Nerve Paralysis After Pediatric Cardiac Surgery: Retrospective Study of 125 Cases

Takashi Watanabe, George A. Trusler, William G. Williams, John F. Edmonds, John G. Coles, and Yuhei Hosokawa (Hosp. for Sick Children and Univ. of Toronto)

J. Thorac. Cardiovasc. Surg. 94:383–388, September 1987 5–36

Phrenic nerve paralysis after cardiac surgery can cause severe respiratory distress to infants and children. Paralysis was diagnosed in 1.6% of 7,670 cardiac operations performed in pediatric patients from 1974 to 1985. The incidence was 1.9% after open heart surgery and 1.3% after closed heart operations. The most frequent open heart operations associated with phrenic paralysis were the Mustard procedure and right ventricular outflow tract reconstruction. Among closed heart operations, the Glenn anastomosis and Blalock-Hanlon atrial septectomy were most often implicated. Phrenic nerve paralysis occurred nearly twice as often after repeat surgery.

Seven patients with phrenic paralysis, or 5.6% of the total, died. Twelve patients survived diaphragmatic plication and were extubated after an average of 2.3 days. Patients younger than 2 years who were not operated on were intubated for 16 days on average, and older patients for an average of 7 days.

Phrenic nerve paralysis occurs most often after dissection near the nerve, or after secondary surgery when the phrenic nerve anatomy is obscured by adhesions. Initial treatment is ventilatory assistance, with continuous positive airway pressure to normalize lung volumes and stabilize the rib cage. If ventilatory assistance remains necessary after 2 weeks, diaphragmatic plication is considered, especially in children younger than 2 years.

▶ The authors report an incidence of nearly 2% for phrenic paralysis following open heart operations in infants and children and 1.3% after closed heart operations. This seems a remarkably high incidence, although quotation of other authors seems to indicate that this is not uncommon. Right-sided paralysis was significantly more common then left, suggesting that injury by cold secondary to topical hypothermia was not particularly common in this series. One has to suspect traction on the pericardium as perhaps a principal problem contributing to phrenic nerve paralysis. Since the great majority of patients eventually recovered phrenic nerve function, a stretch injury is perhaps the most likely. The substantial morbidity and a mortality rate of 5.6% makes caution mandatory.—J.J. Collins, Jr., M.D.

Cardiac Transplantation

HLA Compatibility and Cardiac Transplant Recipient Survival
William H. Frist, Philip E. Oyer, John C. Baldwin, Edward B. Stinson, and Norman E. Shumway (Stanford Univ.)
Ann. Thorac. Surg. 44:242–246, September 1987 5–37

The importance of the major histocompatibility complex to cardiac transplantation remains to be demonstrated. An attempt was made to relate survival to human lymphocyte antigen (HLA) compatibility in 164 consecutive cyclosporine-immunosuppressed patients undergoing orthotopic heart transplantation between 1980 and 1986. The mean recipient age was 36 years. All patients who were HLA-typed in this period were included.

Patients with fewer mismatches had better actuarial survival in the first 4.5 years postoperatively (Fig 5–23). Length of survival of those with three or four mismatches did not differ significantly. Infection was the most frequent cause of death, followed by atherosclerosis and rejection. Rejection rates did not differ significantly in the mismatch groups. The actuarial rates of infection were associated with the degree of HLA compatibility (Fig 5–24). Graft atherosclerosis could not be related to HLA compatibility.

It may not be easy to obtain donor-recipient pairs who are well matched for HLA-A and HLA-B on a prospective basis. When there is a long waiting list of recipients, however, the grade of HLA compatibility may be an important factor in selecting the appropriate recipient for an

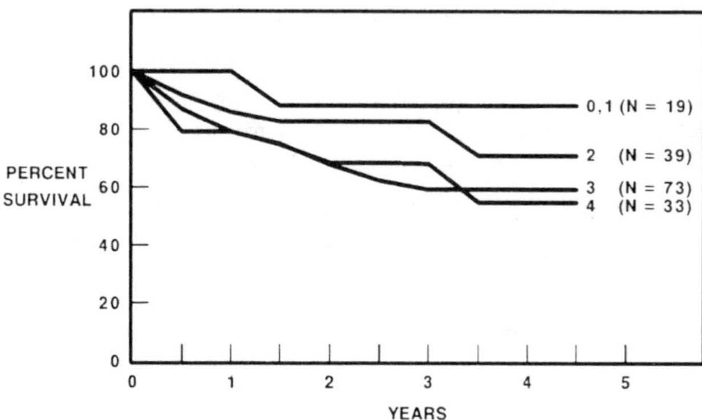

Fig 5–23.—Actuarial survival according to number of mismatches. (Courtesy of Frist, W.H., et al.: Ann. Thorac. Surg. 44:242–246, September 1987.)

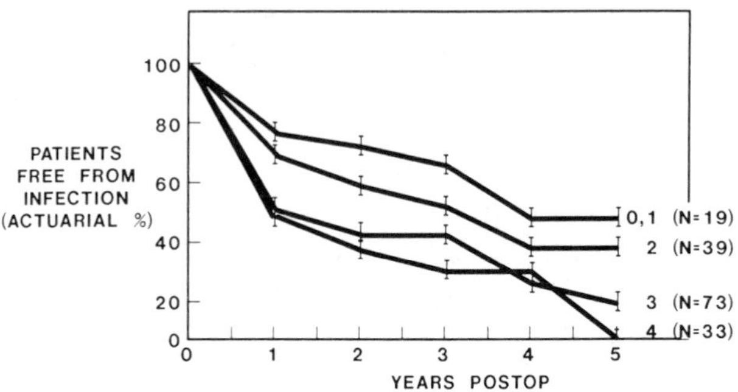

Fig 5–24.—Actuarial rate of infection according to number of mismatches. Data included bacterial, fungal, protozoan, and *Nocardia* infections. Viral infections are excluded. (Courtesy of Frist, W.H., et al.: Ann. Thorac. Surg. 44:242–246, September 1987.)

available donor. Well-matched grafts are related to better long-term survival and fewer infections in cardiac transplant recipients.

▶ It is axiomatic that probability of rejection is directly related to the degree of incompatibility between donor and recipient in organ transplantation. The fact that these authors in a relatively large series of cardiac transplant patients found no significant correlation between HLA mismatching and rejection reflects more upon the adequacy of our understanding of histocompatibility antigens then on anything else. There seems little doubt that specific antigen mismatches must be associated with a higher probability of rejection. We simply have not identified which mismatches are most important, and it is possible that the present techniques for determining compatibility using HLA matching are simply inadequate.—J.J. Collins, Jr., M.D.

Cyclosporine Serum Concentrations Soon After Heart or Heart-Lung Transplantation

Salim Aziz, Philip E. Oyer, and Robert E. Kates (Stanford Univ.)
J. Clin. Pharmacol. 26:652–657, November–December 1986 5–38

Cyclosporine effectively suppresses rejection of organ transplants, but the best dosage and means of administration remain uncertain. The authors used a specific high-performance liquid chromatographic (HPLC) method for cyclosporine to measure plasma concentrations in 11 patients after heart or heart-lung transplantation. Nine patients received cardiac transplants, and 2 received heart-lung transplants. Cyclosporine was given orally, usually starting 3 hours before surgery.

No consistent trend in plasma cyclosporine levels was noted, but levels estimated by HPLC were nearly always lower than those obtained by radioimmunoassay. No consistent trend in plasma profiles of antibody-reactive metabolites was evident. Early rejection, infection, and renal function could not be related to the mean plasma cyclosporin level or the level of antibody-reactive metabolites.

The use of radioimmunoassay to estimate cyclosporine levels requires review. It remains uncertain whether antibody-reactive metabolites contribute to the immunosuppressant properties of cyclosporine. If so, an assay for therapeutic monitoring must determine the accumulation of metabolites as well as unchanged drug.

▶ In this very interesting article comparing HPLC and RIA (radioimmunoassay) for determination of cyclosporine levels, the authors postulate that RIA provides a consistently higher measure of cyclosporine level because of accumulation of antibody-reactive metabolites of cyclosporine. One would expect a gradual rise in the level of these metabolites but such a consistent trend was not observed. The major (and most distressing) point of this report was the observation of no consistent relation between the levels of cyclosporine measured by either technique and the observed clinical outcome. In other words, either technique for measurement of cyclosporine levels is acceptable if the "therapeutic" levels are well appreciated, but neither level can be regarded as a standard for adequate immunosuppression. Kahan (1) has provided an extensive review of the promise and problems of immunosuppressive therapy using cyclosporine for heart transplantation.—J.J. Collins, Jr., M.D.

Reference

1. Kahan, B.D.: Immunosuppressive therapy with cyclosporine for cardiac transplantation. *Circulation* 75:40–65, 1987.

Histologic Predictors of Acute Cardiac Rejection in Human Endomyocardial Biopsies: A Multivariate Analysis

Ahvie Herskowitz, Lisa M. Soule, E. David Mellits, Thomas A. Traill, Stephen C. Achuff, Bruce A. Reitz, A. Michael Borkon, William A. Baumgartner, and Kenneth L. Baughman (Johns Hopkins Hosp.)

J. Am. Coll. Cardiol. 9:802–810, April 1987 5–39

A study was undertaken to determine whether histologic patterns of abnormalities could be seen in endomyocardial biopsy samples before the development of myocyte necrosis in cardiac transplant patients.

Specimens from 18 cardiac transplant recipients were studied retrospectively using 17 histologic variables frequently found in post-transplantation biopsy samples. Predictor samples were identified when immediate subsequent samples contained foci of myocyte necrosis. All samples that were neither predictors nor rejectors were classified as other.

Interstitial edema, perivascular karyorrhexis, and perivascular infiltrate with intermyocyte extension were predictors. However, because interstitial edema is difficult to define histologically, it was considered present only when there were both wide separation of individual muscle bundles or individual myocytes and wide separation and dispersion of interstitial collagen fibrils in more than one specimen. Diagnosis of interstitial edema was 84% reliable using these criteria. Other variables were nonspecific and did not necessarily reflect early rejection.

Biopsy samples with interstitial edema and foci of perivascular karyorrhexis or perivascular infiltrate can be considered evidence of early cardiac rejection and are an indication for the introduction of immunosuppressive therapy.

▶ Classification of rejection by the histology of endomyocardial biopsy samples has become the standard method for determination of immunologic status in cardiac transplant recipients. Every center has had some patients who, after having mild or moderate rejection (or absence of any rejection), have gone on within a very short period of time to severe symptomatic or even fatal rejection.

These authors have attempted to add a new category of early serious rejection to the well accepted criterion of widespread myocyte necrosis. Interstitial edema may be more difficult to diagnose then perivascular inflammatory change. Their observation that capillary or arteriolar inflammatory change is associated with a high probability of life-threatening rejection is consistent with other publications emphasizing the prognostic severity of coronary arteritis in transplant recipients (1,2).—J.J. Collins, Jr., M.D.

References

1. Frazier, O.H., McAllister, H.A., Jammal, C.T., et al.: Occlusive coronary arteritis: A cause of early death in a cardiac transplant patient. *Ann. Thorac. Surg.* 43:554–556, 1987.
2. Smith, S.H., Kirklin, J.K., Geer, J.C., et al.: Arteritis in cardiac rejection after transplantation. *Am. J. Cardiol.* 59:1171–1173, 1987.

Age-Associated Decline in Cardiac Allograft Rejection

Dale G. Renlund, Edward M. Gilbert, John B. O'Connell, William A. Gay, Jr., Kent W. Jones, Nelson A. Burton, Donald B. Doty, Shreekant V. Karwande, Charles W. Dewitt, Ronald L. Menlove, Colette M. Herrick, Michael R. Bristow, and the Utah Transplantation Affiliated Hospitals Cardiac Transplant Program (Univ. of Utah, L.D.S. Hosp, and VA Hosp., Salt Lake City)

Am. J. Med. 83:391–398, September 1987 5–40

Because T lymphocyte function is responsible for most cardiac allograft rejections and aging is associated with decreased T effector cell-mediated immunity, less allograft rejection may occur in older patients. The effect of age on rejection was examined in 57 consecutive cardiac allograft recipients, 21 of whom were at least 54 years of age (mean, 58 years). The other 38 younger patients had a mean age of 40 years. Immunosuppressive management, which was similar in the two groups, included administration of antithymocyte globulin or murine OKT3 monoclonal antibody as well as cyclosporine, azathioprine, and methylprednisolone.

The older recipients had fewer rejection episodes, both in the first 4 months and during total follow-up, and initial rejection episodes occurred later in this group. Multivariate analysis confirmed that younger age was a significant predictor of rejection. The rate of serious infection was 67% in both groups. Actuarial survival at 1 year was 100% in the older group and 94% in the younger patients.

The lower risk of cardiac graft rejection in older patients probably represents an age-related decrease in immune function. This may be an advantage of transplantation in carefully selected older patients. The overall risk of infection was not increased in older patients in the present series.

▶ This provocative report is based on a relatively small number of patients. Nevertheless, the concept that age-related decline in systemic immunologic capacity may be specifically related to better tolerance of cardiac allografts seems to be a possibility. It may be necessary to have somewhat different immunosuppressive protocols for younger and older patients.—J.J. Collins, Jr., M.D.

Development of Coronary Artery Disease in Cardiac Transplant Patients Receiving Immunosuppressive Therapy With Cyclosporine and Prednisone

Barry F. Uretsky, Srinivas Murali, P. Sudhakar Reddy, Bruce Rabin, Ann Lee, Bartley P. Griffith, Robert L. Hardesty, Alfredo Trento, and Henry T. Bahnson
(Presbyterian Univ. Hosp., Pittsburgh, and Univ. of Pittsburgh)
Circulation 76:827–834, October 1987 5–41

Cyclosporine may provide good protection against chronic allograft rejection, but it is associated with moderate to severe hypertension, which itself may be a risk factor for coronary disease in heart transplant recipients. Annual coronary arteriography was done prospectively in transplant recipients, who numbered 57 in the first year, 30 in the second, and 14 in the third. All patients were adults given orthotopic cardiac transplants and long-term cyclosporine and prednisone for immunosuppression.

Coronary artery disease was diagnosed in 18% of the patients 1 year after cardiac transplantation, in 27% at 2 years, and in 44% at 3 years. Coronary disease was associated with the occurrence of at least two major rejection episodes. Autopsy of two patients dying of coronary disease showed subintimal inflammatory cellular infiltration in coronary artery lesions.

Coronary artery disease developing after cardiac transplantation probably represents chronic tissue rejection and the tissue response to rejection. If circulating immunoglobulins are involved, other approaches (e.g., use of platelet-inhibiting drugs) may be worth exploring. It is not clear whether coronary deaths will increase in number within 1–3 years after operation.

▶ The evidence for an immunologic component in the development of atherosclerosis in cardiac transplant recipients seems unassailable. Is it possible that atherosclerosis in the general population may also be an expression determined by immunologic phenomena? Is it through the immune system that hereditary influences are expressed? Much needs to be done.—J.J. Collins, Jr., M.D.

Biopsy Assessment of Fifty Hearts During Transplantation

S. Darracott-Čulanković, D. Wheeldon, R. Cory-Pearce, J. Wallwork, and T.A.H. English (Papworth Hosp., Cambridge, and St. Thomas' Hosp., London)

J. Thorac. Cardiovasc. Surg. 93:95–102, January 1987 5–42

The success of cardiac transplantation depends largely on the quality of the donor heart and on effective myocardial protection during storage. The biopsy findings in 50 donor hearts were reviewed. Full-thickness biopsy specimens were taken from the left ventricular apex using a Tru-Cut needle.

Fifteen of the 50 hearts had poor birefringence before excision and transport, and values were unchanged after implantation. The hearts were stored at 4 C in crystalloid cardioplegic solution. Two thirds of the hearts with poor birefringence required inotropic support after implantation. Twenty-two other hearts deteriorated during transplantation; half received inotropic support. None of the 13 hearts that were unchanged required inotropic support.

Improved protection of donor hearts during transportation is needed. Quantitative estimates of birefringence in myocardial biopsies provide a rapid and reliable indicator of the viability of donor hearts before they are excised, and of their functional status during transplantation.

Autoperfusion of the Heart and Lungs for Preservation During Distant Procurement

Robert L. Hardesty and Bartley P. Griffith (Univ. of Pittsburgh)

J. Thorac. Cardiovasc. Surg. 93:11–18, January 1987 5–43

Combined transplantation of the heart and lungs provides long-term survival for patients with end-stage cardiopulmonary disease; however, donor procurement is a problem. Autoperfusion of the heart and lungs preserves the organs and permits distant procurement. The authors describe their experiences with 20 heart and lung grafts that were obtained distantly.

A modified Starling preparation is used to maintain coronary and pulmonary arterial blood flow (Fig 5–25). The heart pumps fresh, heparinized, normothermic donor whole blood, augmented with glucose and regular insulin, into a reservoir suspended at 100 cm to maintain pressure within a closed segment of aorta, which in turn perfuses the coronary arteries. The lungs are ventilated by hand. The preparation is encased in a sterile plastic bag and floated in a normothermic electrolyte solution inside a special container (Fig 5–26). The internal diameter (ID) and length

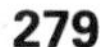

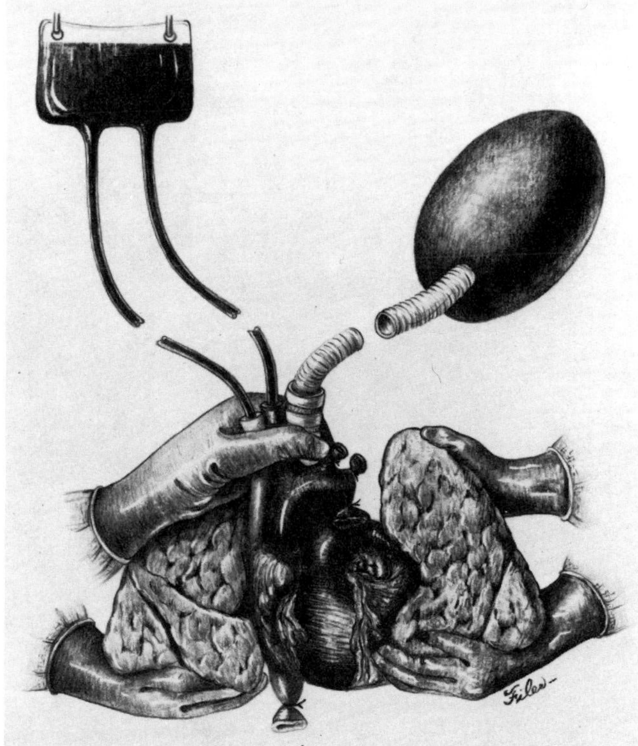

Fig 5–25.—The autoperfusing modified Starling preparation provides pulmonary arterial and coronary arterial flow to preserve the heart and lungs. (Courtesy of Hardesty, R.L., and Griffith, B.P.: J. Thorac. Cardiovasc. Surg. 93:11–18, January 1987.)

of the cannula within the innominate artery, 3/8 in. ID by 4 in., and the internal diameters of the arterial tubing, 1/2 in. ID, and venous tubing, 1/4 in. ID, are critical to avoid excessive preloading and afterloading.

Of 20 autoperfusing heart and lung grafts successfully transported and subsequently implanted, 14 grafts were considered well preserved. In 4 recipients, it was not possible to determine the adequacy of preservation; in 1, preservation was unsatisfactory; and in 1, donor selection was responsible for poor cardiac function. There were four deaths among patients who received well-preserved organs, but deaths were not caused by poor preservation.

Ten patients, who would otherwise have died, are alive as a result of the autoperfusion technique allowing for distant procurement.

▶ As the number of acceptable candidates for cardiac or cardiopulmonary transplantation continues to increase farther and farther beyond the available supply of donor organs, important considerations are necessary to ensure a fair and equitable distribution of organs (1). As important as the administrative

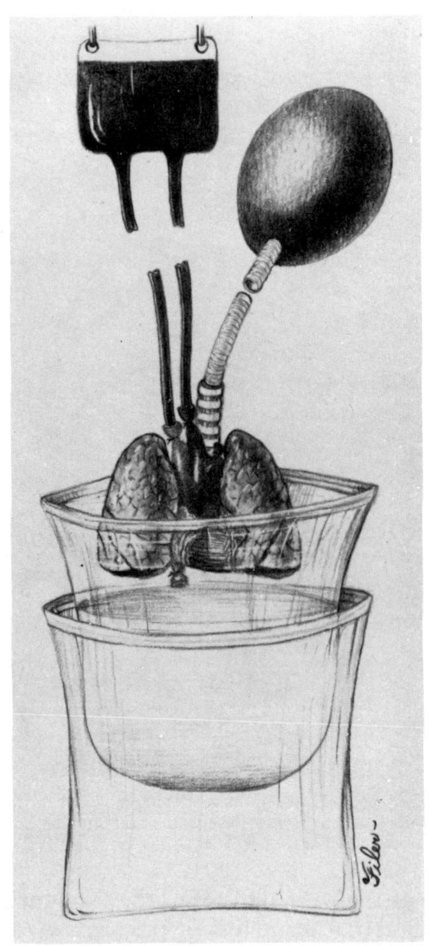

Fig 5–26.—The autoperfusing heart and lungs are contained within a sterile plastic bag. (Courtesy of Hardesty, R.L., and Griffith, B.P.: J. Thorac. Cardiovasc. Surg. 93:11–18, January 1987.)

problems are, the scientific ones are pertinent to selection of the best matches, the greatest number of usable organs, and the best possible management of donor organs at harvesting, during transportation, and after implantation (2,3).

The reports by Hardesty and Griffith and by Darracott-C̄ulanković and associates (Abstracts 5–42 and 5–43) emphasize efforts to improve safe transport and evaluation of organs. Birefringence is a quick technique for evaluation of the metabolic state of cardiac muscle that may have promise as a clinical tool for initial evaluation of donor hearts as well as for monitoring techniques of preservation and reperfusion. The autoperfusion technique suggested by Hardesty and Griffith may allow more consistent success with heart-lung transplants when it is not feasible to have donor and recipient in close proximity.—J.J. Collins, Jr., M.D.

References

1. Robertson, J.A.: Transplantation of the heart: Supply and distribution of hearts for transplantation: Legal, ethical, and policy issues. *Circulation* 75:77–87, 1987.
2. Beeman, S.K., Shuman, T.A., Perna, A.M., et al.: Intermittent reperfusion extends myocardial preservation for transplantation. *Ann. Thorac. Surg.* 43:484–489, 1987.
3. Swanson, D.K., Myerowitz, D., Watson, K.M., et al.: A comparison of blood and crystalloid cardioplegia during heart transplantation after 5 hours of cold storage. *J. Thorac. Cardiovasc. Surg.* 93:687–694, 1987.

Myocardial Protection

Free Radicals and Cardioplegia: Allopurinol and Oxypurinol Reduce Myocardial Injury Following Ischemic Arrest

D.J. Chambers, M.V. Braimbridge, and D.J. Hearse (St. Thomas' Hosp., London)

Ann. Thorac. Surg. 44:291–297, September 1987 5–44

Reactive oxygen intermediates may account for some reoxygenation-induced injury after open heart surgery. The occurrence of such injury might be reduced by adding free radical scavengers to the cardioplegic solution. Alternatively, the production of free radicals can be inhibited. The isolated working rat heart model of cardiopulmonary bypass was used to evaluate the specific xanthine oxidase inhibitors, allopurinol and oxypurinol.

Both allopurinol and oxypurinol, its primary active metabolite, significantly improved postischemic functional recovery when added chronically or acutely to the cardioplegic or reperfusion solution during normothermic ischemic arrest. Under hypothermic conditions, however, allopurinol conferred added protection when used as pretreatment or during reperfusion. It was effective when added to the cardioplegic solution.

Allopurinol and oxypurinol enhance the protective effect of cardioplegic solution in the isolated working rat heart model of cardiopulmonary bypass, presumably by inhibiting xanthine oxidase activity and preventing the formation of oxygen-derived free radicals. Pretreatment of cardiac surgery patients with allopurinol reportedly prevents metabolic changes and cell damage during and after cardiopulmonary bypass.

Reperfusion With ATP-$MgCl_2$ Following Prolonged Ischemia Improves Myocardial Performance

Gary S. Kopf, Irshad Chaudry, Spyros Condos, and Arthur E. Baue (Yale Univ.)

J. Surg. Res. 43:114–117, August 1987 5–45

The conditions of reperfusion are important in determining reversibility after a prolonged period of hypothermic global ischemia. A canine model of cardiopulmonary bypass with systemic hypothermia of 28 C and 2.5 hours of aortic cross-clamping was used to determine whether infusion of adenosine triphosphate (ATP)-magnesium chloride ($MgCl_2$) during reperfusion would enhance functional recovery. Crystalloid cardioplegia was infused every 20 minutes during ischemia, and reperfusion lasted for 20 minutes before bypass was withdrawn. The study animals received ATP, 1 mg/kg per minute, and $MgCl_2$, 0.33 mg/kg per minute, during reperfusion.

Recording of Starling curves 15 minutes and 45 minutes after bypass showed complete functional recovery in the experimentally treated dogs, whereas control animals had markedly reduced hemodynamic performance and myocardial compliance. The myocardial water content was higher in control animals (81% vs. 66%).

Reperfusion with ATP-$MgCl_2$ solution after 2.5 hours of hypothermic ischemia in the dog leads to improved postischemic hemodynamics and better recovery of myocardial compliance. It is not clear whether ATP-$MgCl_2$ molecules pass the plasma membrane, but this treatment may be a useful adjunct during reperfusion after a prolonged hypothermic ischemic insult.

▶ These two reports (Abstracts 5–44 and 5–45) on progress in the general area of myocardial protection represent welcome departures from the usual investigations of various combination of ingredients solutions for cardioplegia. Since many patients undergoing cardiac surgery are already taking allopurinol, it might be of considerable interest to obtain metabolic measurements on those patients for comparison with otherwise similar patients not taking allopurinol. Perhaps something may be learned.

In the report of Kopf and associates (Abstract 5–45) the inclusion of ATP-$MgCl_2$ probably requires more experimental investigation prior to clinical application. The general concept of addition of high-energy phosphates seems reasonable on the surface. However, the difficulty in transporting ATP across the intact cell membrane has precluded serious investigation as to the utility of including ATP in perfusates. If ATP can be supplied to the intracellular milieu, it may be possible to achieve better myocardial protection. Further studies to confirm, refute, or explain the observations reported by these authors are awaited with interest.—J.J. Collins, Jr., M.D.

Arrhythmia Surgery

Cryoablative Techniques in the Treatment of Cardiac Tachyarrhythmias

David A. Ott, Arthur Garson, Jr., Denton A. Cooley, Richard T. Smith, and Jeffrey Moak (Texas Heart Inst., Texas Children's Hosp., and St. Luke's Episcopal Hosp., Houston)

Ann. Thorac. Surg. 43:138–143, February 1987 5–46

For drug-resistant, incessant, or life-threatening cardiac tachyarrhythmias, surgery is recommended in selected patients. Recently, cryoablative techniques have been demonstrated to be effective in eliminating foci or pathways causing tachycardia when used alone or in conjunction with surgery.

Of 175 patients treated surgically for cardiac tachyarrhythmias, 53 underwent confirmatory operative mapping and definitive operation using cryoablative procedures. Sixteen patients had supraventricular tachycardia caused by Kent bundle in the right anterior or posterior paraseptal location, 6 patients had permanent junctional reciprocating tachycardia, and 19 had atrial ectopic tachycardia. Of 19 infants with critical ventricular tachycardia, 13 were treated with cryoablation at the site of the ectopic focus, either alone or combined with excision of the area.

In patients with Kent bundle, cryoablation was successful in eliminating tachycardia in 15 of 16 patients; cryoablation was successful in all patients with permanent junctional reciprocating tachycardia and in all infants with critical ventricular tachycardia. The success rate was 83.3% in patients having atrial ectopic tachycardia, but was 100% successful in patients having a single focus.

Cryoablative techniques have a high rate of cure when used either alone or in combination with other treatments in selected cases of tachyarrhythmias.

Technical Considerations in the Surgical Approach to Multiple Accessory Pathways in the Wolff-Parkinson-White Syndrome

Jay G. Selle, Will C. Sealy, John J. Gallagher, John M. Fedor, Robert H. Svenson, and Samuel H. Zimmern (Sanger Clinic, the Heineman Found., and Charlotte Mem. Hosp., Charlotte, N.C.)

Ann. Thorac. Surg. 43:579–584, June 1987 5–47

Because nearly 20% of patients with Wolff-Parkinson-White (WPW) syndrome have multiple atrioventricular accessory pathways, standard operative procedures must be modified in order to divide these pathways.

Of 90 patients operated on for WPW syndrome, 18 had multiple accessory pathways. In 10 patients with a right free wall and a posterior septal accessory pathway, approach was by a right atriotomy with the posterior septal dissection extended onto the right free wall area. In 3 patients with a left free wall and a posterior septal accessory pathway, approach began with a right atriotomy for the posterior septal space dissection. This was followed by an atrial septotomy to expose the left free wall area (table).

In 39 attempts, 38 pathways were successfully divided. Two months postoperatively, one posterior septal accessory pathway reappeared and was removed by catheter.

There are potential difficulties in patients with a left free wall accessory pathway and an accessory pathway in any other of the three anatomical areas. Three methods of exposure are possible: right atriotomy and left atriotomy, right atriotomy with atrial septotomy, and right atriotomy with posterior septal extension. In this study, the third technique was preferred.

Patients with multiple accessory pathways should have as successful

APPROACHES TO ACCESSORY PATHWAYS FOR SUCCESSFUL DIVISION*

Method of Approach	Combination of Pathways: No.	Combination of Pathways: Anatomical Location
Left atriotomy	Single or multiple	LFW
Right atriotomy	Single or multiple	RFW, PS, AS
	Multiple combined	RFW + PS, RFW + AS, PS + AS
Right atriotomy + Left atriotomy + Atrial septotomy	Multiple combined LFW +	PS, RFW, AS
With posterior septal extension	Posterior LFW +	PS

*LFW = left free wall; RFW = right free wall; PS = posterior septal; AS = anterior septal.

(Courtesy of Selle, J.G., et al.: Ann. Thorac. Surg. 43:579–584, June 1987.)

surgical outcomes as patients with single pathways if the surgeon has an organized knowledge of the various methods of approach.

▶ Continued advances in the surgical management of disabling or threatening tachyarrhythmias holds great promise for the future as well as providing patients currently with relief from many types of tachyarrhythmia. These two publications (Abstracts 5–46 and 5–47) provide an up-to-date review of available surgical techniques. While the utilization of surgery for interruption of conducting pathways in the heart is an exciting area of cardiac surgery, it is also an area in which changes will be occurring rapidly in the future and in which substantial experience is necessary to achieve predictable favorable results. Under these circumstances, it does not seem reasonable to have an ever-increasing number of institutions performing an ever-diminishing number of cases each year. It is one area in which regionalization is not only reasonable but, in my opinion, essential.—J.J. Collins, Jr., M.D.

Miscellaneous Topics

Mixed Venous Oxygen Saturation as a Predictor of Cardiac Output in the Postoperative Cardiac Surgical Patient

Donald J. Magilligan, Jr., Robert Teasdall, Roy Eisinminger, and Edward Peterson (Henry Ford Hosp., Detroit)

Ann. Thorac. Surg. 44:260–262, September 1987 5–48

The mixed venous oxygen saturation (Sv_{O_2}) is reported to be helpful in managing critically ill patients. The value of monitoring cardiac output using Sv_{O_2} was studied in 25 unselected patients in the first 24 hours after cardiac surgery. Measurements of Sv_{O_2} obtained with a fiberoptic pulmonary artery catheter were compared with values determined by the thermodilution cardiac index. Most of the patients underwent coronary bypass surgery.

All patients survived operation, and none required prolonged pharmacologic support. The mean correlation between Sv_{O_2} and the cardiac index was 0.05, not significantly different from zero. The mean correlation between changes in these parameters was significant, but the correlation coefficient was only 0.19. Correlation did not improve after adjustment for multiple clinical variables. The Sv_{O_2} did not predict a cardiac index of less than 2 L/minute/sq m.

The mixed venous oxygen saturation is not predictive of cardiac index in cardiac surgery patients to an extent that would be clinically helpful.

▶ Despite previous studies casting doubt on the usefulness of mixed venous oxygen saturation as an indicator of cardiac output in postoperative cardiac surgical patients, reliance on this measurement continues to be used widely. Potentially hazardous interventions should not be undertaken based principally on this measurement.—J.J. Collins, Jr., M.D.

The Etiologic Spectrum of Constrictive Pericarditis

James Cameron, Stephen N. Oesterle, John C. Baldwin, and E. William Hancock (Stanford Univ.)

Am. Heart J. 113:354–360, February 1987 5–49

It is important to diagnose constrictive pericarditis as a cause of congestive heart failure because it is potentially curable. Constrictive pericarditis has been reported after open heart surgery; since this procedure is relatively common, it is important to examine the etiologic spectrum of constrictive pericarditis.

Ninety-five patients who underwent pericardiectomy for constrictive pericarditis from 1970 to 1985 were studied. Parietal and visceral pericardiectomy was undergone by 80 patients; 15 patients had parietal pericardiectomy alone. Cardiopulmonary bypass was required by 46 patients to facilitate dissection; 7 patients had associated procedures requiring the heart-lung machine. Patients were classified according to etiology during the entire time frame (Table 1) and then separated into pre- and post-1980 cases (Table 2).

Overall, 42% of cases were idiopathic, 31% were postradiotherapy; and 11% were postsurgical. The remainder were divided among a variety of causes. However, when pre- and post-1980 etiology were considered separately, the picture changed. Post-1980, causes were evenly divided among idiopathic, postradiotherapy, and postsurgical, with 29% each;

TABLE 1.—CAUSE IN 95 CASES OF CONSTRICTIVE PERICARDITIS

Cause	*No. (%)*
Idiopathic	40 (42%)
Postradiotherapy	29 (31%)
Postsurgical	10 (11%)
Postinfective	6 (6%)
Connective tissue disorder	4 (4%)
Neoplastic	3 (3%)
Dialysis	2 (2%)
Sarcoidosis	1 (1%)

(Courtesy of Cameron, J., et al.: Am. Heart J. 113:354–360, February 1987.)

TABLE 2.—ETIOLOGIC SPECTRUM BEFORE AND AFTER 1980

	Before 1980 (n = 61)	*After 1980 (n = 34)*
Idiopathic	30 (49%)	10 (29%)
Postradiotherapy	19 (31%)	10 (29%)
Postsurgical	0 (0%)	10 (29%)
Miscellaneous	12 (20%)	4 (12%)

(Courtesy of Cameron, J., et al.: Am. Heart J. 113:354–360, February 1987.)

12% had miscellaneous causes (see Table 2). Ten patients had constrictive pericarditis following open heart surgery.

Postradiotherapy continues to be an important cause of constrictive pericarditis, but postsurgical constriction has recently contributed significantly to the total number of cases. Idiopathic cases are also found in substantial numbers. Cases secondary to malignancy, bacterial and fungal infection, uremia, and connective tissue disorders were relatively few. In the postradiotherapy cases, the period from initial treatment until presentation was significantly longer after 1980 than prior to 1980.

▶ In the course of time, the etiology for many mechanical aberrations of cardiac function tends to change. This is certainly true of constrictive pericarditis. The authors have presented the experience from one academic center that has had an active radiotherapy unit for some years. While this change in the etiology of pericarditis may not be precisely what is observed in other institutions throughout the country, it does serve to emphasize that the old order is not static.—J.J. Collins, Jr., M.D.

Primary Repair of Traumatic Aortic Disruption

Lawrence R. McBride, Stephen Tidik, Joseph C. Stothert, Hendrick B. Barner,

George C. Kaiser, Vallee L. Willman, and D. Glenn Pennington (St. Louis Univ.)
Ann. Thorac. Surg. 43:65–67, January 1987 5–50

Prompt surgical repair is indicated in traumatic disruption of the thoracic aorta. Most repairs are made by prosthetic graft; only 4% of recent cases were repaired by primary anastomosis. A retrospective study was undertaken to evaluate 22 patients who underwent repair of acute traumatic rupture of the aorta by prosthetic graft or by primary anastomosis.

The patients had all suffered deceleration injuries as a result of motor vehicle accidents. The operative procedure was determined by the surgeon; in 64% of patients, a modified Gott shunt was used. Primary anastomosis was performed in 68% of patients. Wherever possible, intercostal arteries were preserved. Ligation of no more than one pair of intercostal arteries was usually required for sufficient mobilization, although additional branches were sometimes temporarily occluded. Sufficient mobilization permitted transected end to be approximated with gentle traction.

There was an overall survival rate of 82%; in the shunt group, technical problems related to the shunt contributed to the deaths of 3 patients. One patient died intraoperatively; postoperative morbidity usually stemmed from associated injuries. Aortic cross-clamp time averaged 37 minutes for primary anastomosis and 58 minutes for insertion of a prosthetic graft.

Primary repair of aortic tears has several advantages, including shorter aortic cross-clamp time, reduced risk of infection, and reduced risk of pseudoaneurysm formation from suture dehiscence. Although primary anastomosis is more technically demanding, successful application of this technique is feasible in most patients if adequate mobilization of the proximal and distal aorta can be obtained. Preservation of the intercostal arteries is important for the success of this procedure.

▶ This series of patients in whom traumatic aortic disruption was treated by primary anastomosis is, as the authors point out, contrary to customary practice among most cardiothoracic surgeons today. However, the authors also argue that elimination of prosthetic material is a useful concept. Furthermore, they demonstrate that in their experience primary anastomosis actually required a shorter clamp time than the utilization of a prosthetic interposition graft. If, as they demonstrate, these two desirable outcomes can be achieved, it would seem reasonable that more patients should be treated by primary anastomosis and fewer by prosthetic interposition.—J.J. Collins, Jr., M.D.

6 Hypertension

Introduction

Along with a number of significant advances in our understanding of mechanisms that raise blood pressure and of therapies that may lower it, two simple truths emerged during 1987 that will markedly change the management of hypertension. First, we are overtreating many patients because of our reliance on too few office blood pressure measurements both to make the diagnosis and to evaluate therapy. Second, our therapy has not provided the expected protection against coronary disease, the most serious consequence of an elevated blood pressure.

The recognition of these two truths will certainly change our practices. First, the majority of patients, those whose pressures on initial examination are only mildly elevated and who are in no immediate danger, will be more carefully evaluated by multiple readings taken both in the office and, increasingly, out of the office by either self-recordings or ambulatory automatic recordings. Second, treatment will increasingly involve various nondrug and drug therapies that will be monitored more assiduously and aimed more carefully toward the greatest possible reduction in our patients' cardiovascular risk.

To elucidate these points and the other major advances made during 1987, the synopses that follow of the 50 articles published since the last YEAR BOOK that I have selected are arranged in this sequence:

- A restatement of the risks of hypertension.
- New insights into the mechanisms that may cause hypertension.
- The overall status of current management, with emphasis on the probable reasons that it has failed to protect against coronary disease.
- An update on the use of various nondrug and drug therapies of hypertension, with emphasis upon newer agents and the therapy of complicated patients, including the elderly and those with secondary causes.

Norman M. Kaplan, M.D.

Risks of Hypertension

▶ ↓ Hypertension has long been recognized as one of the major risk factors for premature cardiovascular disease. As we shall see, the recognition of both its major role as a risk factor and its frequency has lead to a massive campaign to identify and treat the 40 to 60 million Americans who have an elevated blood pressure. However, unlike the comment attributed to Mae West that "Too much of a good thing is wonderful," I believe we have gone too far in both diagnosing and treating hypertension and that too much of what may be considered "a good thing" has turned out not to be "wonderful."

Before looking at the evidence that our current practices may need to be revised, let's remind ourselves of the risks of hypertension with evidence from the grand-daddy of cardiovascular epidemiology—the Framingham Study.—N.M. Kaplan, M.D.

The Relative Importance of Selected Risk Factors for Various Manifestations of Cardiovascular Disease Among Men and Women From 35 to 64 Years Old: 30 Years of Follow-up in the Framingham Study

Joseph Stokes III, William B. Kannel, Philip A. Wolf, L. Adrienne Cupples, and Ralph B. D'Agostino (Boston Univ.)

Circulation 75(Suppl. V):V-65–V-73, June 1987 6–1

The risk profiles for various manifestations of cardiovascular disease differ substantially from one another. The authors examined the differences in risk profiles for the 5,070 men and women in the original Framingham cohort.

The Framingham Study was a long-term prospective study of cardiovascular disease begun in 1948. The subjects were initially free of cardiovascular disease and subsequently had some manifestation of cardiovascular disease between the ages of 35 and 64 years in a 30-year follow-up period. A standard cardiovascular examination was performed on participating subjects every 2 years. The risk factors examined in this study were recorded at each of the first 15 examinations. Systolic blood pressure contributed more consistently and more significantly to the risk of coronary heart disease, stroke and transient ischemic attacks (TIAs), intermittent claudication, and congestive heart failure than did any of the other standard risk factors.

The serum total cholesterol level made a significant contribution to the risk of cardiovascular disease, particularly to coronary heart disease; it was not a significant predictor of stroke or TIAs. The blood glucose concentration was strongly and significantly correlated with intermittent claudication and congestive heart failure; it also contributed to the risk of coronary and cerebral vascular disease in women. The contribution of obesity was most consistent for coronary heart disease and also contributed to the risk of congestive heart failure in women. An inverse relationship was found between obesity and the risk of intermittent claudication in men. The contribution to risk of cigarette smoking was strong and consistent for various manifestations of cardiovascular disease, except for stroke, TIA, and congestive heart failure in women. Hematocrit made a significant contribution to the risk of stroke and TIA and to intermittent claudication in men. Although limited VC was a risk factor for both sexes, it was more useful for estimating risk for women than for men.

This study demonstrated that hypertension contributed most consistently to short-term risk of all manifestations of cardiovascular disease. Differences were found between sexes and among age groups. These patterns have biologic, clinical, and statistical significance.

▶ Systolic blood pressure is equal to serum cholesterol and cigarette smoking as a risk factor for coronary heart disease in men and greater than the other two in women. It is quantitatively more of a risk for stroke but is a significant risk for all cardiovascular diseases in both men and women. Systolic pressures have been used because they have turned out to be a more reliable measure than diastolic pressures, but both readings give virtually identical prognostic information.

Confirmation of the importance of hypertension comes from necropsy data, as summarized by William C. Roberts (*Am. J. Cardiol.* 60:1E–8E, 1986). Hypertension is present in more than 50% of patients with coronary events, in more than 75% of patients with cerebrovascular events, and in more than 90% of patients with aortic dissection.

The applicability of the Framingham Study data to the larger population has been validated by a 10-year follow-up of 14,407 adults aged 25–74 years who were selected from 100 locations as a representative sample of the American population in the National Health and Nutrition Examination Survey from 1971 to 1975 (NHANES I) (Leaverton et al.: *J. Chronic Dis.* 40:775–784, 1987).

Another epidemiologic survey of newly diagnosed hypertensives aged 40–69 years makes a point not examined in the Framingham cohort: the 5-year risk for cardiovascular complications, compared with normotensive subjects of similar age, is inversely related to the age of onset (Buck et al.: *Hypertension* 9:204–208, 1987). The highest rate of complications occurred in those whose age of onset was 40–49 years, the lowest rate in the group whose age of onset was 60–69 years.

One of the components of the Framingham risk data base is left ventricular hypertrophy (LVH) as seen by ECG. Some of the Framingham cohort have now been subjected to echocardiography (echo) and, not surprisingly, LVH echo turns out to be a risk factor and much more common than LVH by ECG.—N.M. Kaplan, M.D.

The Spectrum of Left Ventricular Hypertrophy in a General Population Sample: The Framingham Study

Daniel D. Savage, Robert J. Garrison, William B. Kannel, Daniel Levy, Sandra J. Anderson, Joseph Stokes III, Manning Feinleib, and William P. Castelli (Natl. Heart, Lung, and Blood Inst., Bethesda, Md., and Boston Univ.)

Circulation 75(Suppl. I):I-26–I-33, January 1987 6–2

Until recently, limited information has been available on the prevalence and features, including severity, of various forms of left ventricular hypertrophy (LVH) in the general population. The Framingham Study subjects were assessed by echocardiography, which allows more precise evaluation on the severity and types of LVH than does electrocardiography.

The authors examined 510 men and 855 women, aged 59–90 years, from the original Framingham cohort by M-mode echocardiography. Offspring and spouses (1,718 men and 1,892 women, aged 17–75 years) were also examined. The severity of echo LVH, as determined by left ventricular mass indexed to body surface area, ranged from 101 gm/sq m in women and 132 gm/sq m in men to more than 400 gm/sq m. The prevalence of electrocardiographically assessed LVH increased proportionately with increased echocardiographic left ventricular mass. Women with left ventricular mass indexes greater than 200 gm/sq m were three to four times more likely to have electrocardiographic LVH than men with similar increases of echocardiographic left ventricular mass index.

Echo LVH prevalence ranged from 6.6% in the younger women in the offspring study to 33% in the older women in the cohort study; the range for men was 8.6% to 23.7%, respectively. A spectrum of forms was found: eccentric-dilated, eccentric-nondilated, concentric, and disproportionate septal thickness. The forms varied in prevalence in the various age-sex groups. Each form of echo LVH was associated with higher systolic blood pressures at the time of echocardiographic examination and over the previous 30 years compared with blood pressures of Framingham subjects without echo LVH.

These results demonstrate the wide spectrum of hypertrophy found in a general population sample. The differences noted support the value of using a continuous variable to describe echo LVH so that degree of hypertrophy is emphasized, instead of a somewhat arbitrary cutpoint. Preliminary follow-up data have already suggested prognostic significance of echo LVH in patients with hypertension.

▶ These data confirm the association of LVH by echo with increasing blood pressure. But the value of echocardiography is likely greater for the early detection of left ventricular dysfunction, which is usually an abnormal diastolic filling pattern (Phillips et al.: *J. Am. Coll. Cardiol.* 9:317–322, 1987). This study and others (Smith et al.: *J. Am. Coll. Cardiol.* 8:1449–1454, 1986; Agati et al.: *Int. J. Cardiol.* 17:177–186, 1987) have shown that reversal of myocardial hypertrophy and improved diastolic function can be seen by echo when the blood pressure is lowered by most any medication save direct vasodilators (e.g., hydralazine) or, in some studies, diuretics.

The recognition of LVH and dysfunction by echo may eventually turn out to be a clinically useful part of the evaluation and follow-up of hypertensive patients. However, at present, it costs too much and it likely doesn't add much to simpler and less expensive indices of cardiac involvement.

Nonetheless, even children with minimally elevated blood pressure have been found to have LVH by echo. This brings us to consider the problem of hypertension in children, since the disease likely begins early in life and, if prevention will ever be possible, it will have to begin long before most patients are identified as hypertensive.—N.M. Kaplan, M.D.

Tracking and Prediction of Blood Pressure in Children

Virginia V. Michels, Erik J. Bergstralh, Verna R. Hoverman, W. Michael O'Fallon, and William H. Weidman (Mayo Clinic and Found.)

Mayo Clin. Proc. 62:875–881, October 1987 6–3

Several longitudinal studies of blood pressure (BP) among school-age children have failed to identify any factors that could be strongly linked to the development of hypertension in adulthood. However, a significant, although weak, correlation between an initial and a subsequent BP measurement in the same patient has been reported. The authors conducted a 9-year BP tracking study in a sample of schoolchildren to determine whether such measurements were of any clinical value in predicting an individual child's future BP level.

From a BP screening program comprising 3,666 schoolchildren in Rochester, Minn., 69 boys and 73 girls, aged 5.9–9.5 years at the time of the original BP screening, underwent a second BP measurement 9 years later. Weight and height were also recorded at both the original screening and at follow-up. All examinations were performed in a schoolroom.

There was a direct correlation between body size at the original screening and body size at follow-up. A significant correlation was observed between initial and subsequent raw systolic BPs. Correlations of systolic BP based on percentiles for age, height, and weight were smaller, but still statistically significant. However, correlations of raw diastolic BP were significant only for boys. Correlations of diastolic BP did not improve when percentiles for age, height, and weight were included.

The degree of BP correlation observed in this study was not sufficient to permit accurate prediction of subsequent BP levels on the basis of a single casual BP measurement in an individual child.

▶ Despite the relatively weak predictive value of a single or even repeated blood pressure measurement in children, all children should have measurements taken, and those above the 90th percentile for age should be carefully followed and evaluated, using guidelines published by a National Heart, Lung, and Blood Task Force (Horan, M.J., Simaiko, A.R.: *Hypertension* 10:115–121, 1987).

What is clear is that large weight gain is often associated with a large increase in blood pressure (Visser et al.: *J. Hypertens.* 5:367–370, 1987). The one preventive measure that can safely be applied is maintenance of near normal weight. Fat babies often turn into fat and hypertensive adults.

The hypertensive process likely starts very early in life. The next section examines recent articles on the pathophysiology of the disease, again with the hope that an understanding of its mechanisms will lead to the ability to prevent it or abort it before it becomes permanent.—N.M. Kaplan, M.D.

Pathophysiology of Hypertension

▶ ↓ In 1987, no major breakthroughs occurred in our understanding of what causes hypertension. But some intriguing clues were uncovered that suggest that, at least for a significant portion of those with "essential" hypertension—which I believe is better called "primary"—hyperinsulinemia may play a key role by inducing hypertrophy of the arterial vessel wall. The high plasma insulin levels seen in many with hypertension, particularly if they have upper body obesity, connects three common conditions: hypertension, obesity, and glucose intolerance or diabetes.

Before noting the evidence linking this triad, we will review some of 1987's more mundane but useful basic discoveries about the abnormal hemodynamics seen in hypertension.—N.M. Kaplan, M.D.

Arterial Hemodynamics in Human Hypertension

C.T. Ting, Kenneth P. Brin, S.J. Lin, S.P. Wang, M.S. Chang, Benjamin N. Chiang, and Frank C.P. Yin (Veterans Gen. Hosp., Taichung, Taiwan, and Johns Hopkins Univ.)

J. Clin. Invest. 78:1462–1471, December 1986 6–4

Few studies have examined the hemodynamics accompanying hypertension in detail. Differences in aortic impedance between normotensive and hypertensive individuals were studied in age-matched normotensive and hypertensive Chinese patients, all of whom were likely to be free of atherosclerosis.

Impedance was measured in 8 normotensive subjects, with a mean blood pressure of 96.7 mm Hg, and in 11 hypertensive subjects, with a mean blood pressure of 122.2 mm Hg, undergoing cardiac catheterization at rest, during nitroprusside, and handgrip exercises before and after β blockade with propranolol. Hypertensives had higher resistance than normotensive subjects (2,295 vs. 1,713 dyn-s/cm^5). Characteristic impedance in hypertensive subjects was 145.7 dyn-s/cm^5 compared with 93.9 dyn-s/cm^5 in normotensives. Total external power in hypertensives was 1,579 vs. 1174 mW in normotensives. In hypertensive patients, peripheral reflections (ratio of backward to forward wave components) was 0.54 vs. 0.44 in normotensive subjects. The first zero crossing of impedance phase angles was 4.15 Hz in hypertensives vs. 2.97 Hz in normotensives. These abnormalities were eliminated with vasodilation, and differences between groups were not exacerbated when pressure was increased during handgrip exercises. Resistance and reflections were further increased by β blockade.

These results demonstrate distinct differences in the arterial hemodynamics of hypertensive patients compared with normotensive individuals. In addition to the well-documented higher arterial resistance, aortic impedance at rest is characterized by a larger modulus of the first harmonic, higher characteristic impedance, a right shift of the entire spectrum, and greater wave reflections, abnormalities that are all eliminated with nitroprusside. Further increases in resistance, first modulus of impedance, and wave reflections occur during generalized β blockade. These vascular abnormalities could not all be attributed to higher blood pressure; some of the changed hemodynamics can be attributed to an increased smooth muscle tone that is further unmasked during β blockade.

▶ This study is the more valuable because it was done in new-onset hypertensives who were likely free of atherosclerosis. Therefore, the increased resistance, impedance, and wave reflections probably represent the basic hemodynamic mechanisms for high arterial pressure, all likely related to increased vascular tone.

Others have demonstrated reduced arterial and venous compliance, reflecting intrinsic alterations of the vascular wall (Safer, M.E., London, G.M.: *Hypertension* 10:133–139, 1987). When small subcutaneous resistance vessels from matched normotensives and hypertensive subjects were examined, those from hypertensives had increased thickness of the media but essentially unchanged smooth muscle function, suggesting that the heightened tone and pressor responsiveness seen in hypertension is mainly explained by the altered vascular structure (Aalkjaer et al.: *Circ. Res.* 61:181–186, 1987).

This leads us to consider the way in which smooth muscle hypertrophy develops. Here we enter some new and exciting territory.—N.M. Kaplan, M.D.

Slow Pressor Mechanisms in Hypertension: A Role for Hypertrophy of Resistance Vessels?

Anthony F. Lever (Western Infirmary, Glasgow, Scotland)

J. Hypertension 4:515–524, 1986 6–5

Disagreement exists on the cause of essential hypertension and on the mechanism by which arterial pressure is raised in secondary hypertension. Most of the suggested mechanisms are quick-acting and only slightly abnormal; the rise in blood pressure, however, is too large to have resulted from one abnormality acting alone. Thus, it is postulated that two processes are at work in hypertension—an initiating abnormality and a slow amplifier, such as whole-body autoregulation, a change of pressure-natriuresis in the kidney, or a feedback mechanism involving vascular hypertrophy and arterial pressure.

Primary hyperaldosteronism, Cushing's syndrome, pheochromocytoma, and renin-secreting tumors are conditions in which the cause of hypertension is known but the rise in pressure is slower and more pronounced than would be expected from the properties of the causative agent. Folkow proposed that overactivity of a pressor mechanism causes a small increase in pressure, and the resulting hypertrophy amplifies the pressor signal by positive feedback, producing further hypertension and hypertrophy (Fig 6–1). The initiating cause may be small and quick-acting and is specific for a particular form of hypertension, whereas the amplification is slowly progressive, ultimately large, and probably nonspecific.

Another potential stimulus to feedback is from a trophin or mitogen of vascular smooth muscle; the mechanism of hypertension would be increased trophin activity. Vascular hypertrophy would result, followed by a rise in blood pressure and the beginning of amplification. Sympathetic nerves, catecholamines, angiotensin II, growth hormone, insulin, and insulin-like growth factor I (ILGF-I) are trophins or mitogens that may act in this way. Acromegaly, early type II diabetes, obesity, and essential

(a) First hypothesis

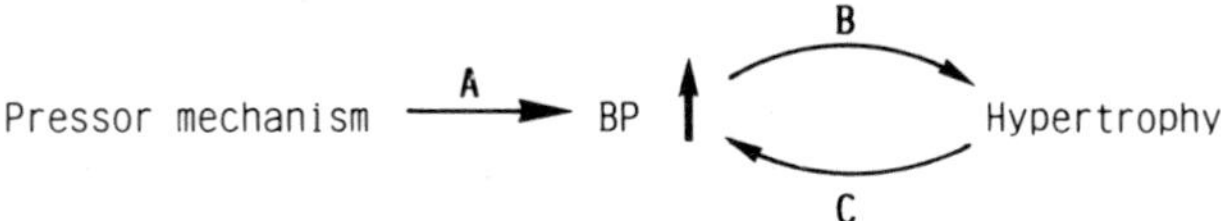

(b) Second and third hypotheses

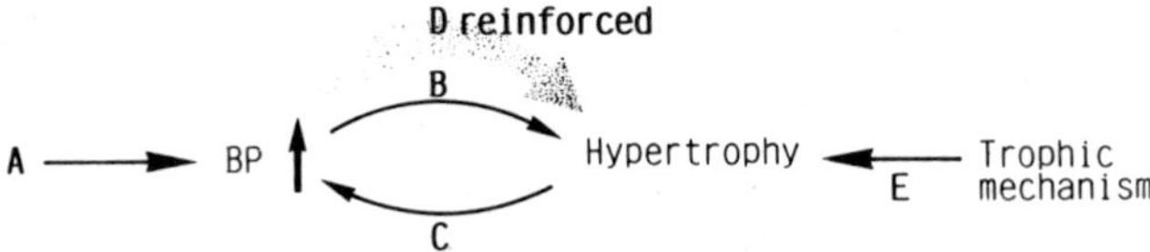

Fig 6–1.—Folkow's proposals. **a,** first hypothesis states that minor overactivity of a pressor mechanism (A) raises blood pressure slightly, initiating positive feedback (BCB) and a progressive rise in blood pressure. **b,** second and third hypotheses are similar to the first, with the addition of an abnormal or "reinforced" hypertrophic response to pressure (D) and increase of an agent causing hypertrophy directly (E). (Courtesy of Lever, A.F.: J. Hypertension 4:515–524, 1986.)

hypertension are characterized by hypertension and vascular disease. Levels of vascular growth factors are increased in each of those conditions; GH and ILGF-I are increased in acromegaly; and either ILGF-I or insulin is increased in essential hypertension, early type II diabetes, and obesity.

If hypertension does develop by a double process, it is likely that the primary cause will be most apparent in early stages; in the later stages, the cause will be concealed by the increasing contribution from hypertrophy. Also, a particular form of hypertension may be wrongly judged to have no cause if each mechanism is considered insufficiently abnormal alone to have produced the hypertension.

▶ As we have seen, the primary hemodynamic fault responsible for the persistence of higher blood pressure is an increased vascular tone and resistance. The mechanisms likely involve a constantly changing interaction between two sets of opposing forces, one contracting, the other relaxing the resistance vessels. Each of these, in turn, involves numerous hormonal and neural inputs that are transmitted into a smaller number of intracellular messages with free intracellular calcium as the final mediator.

The specific changes in both contraction and relaxation that may be involved in human hypertension remain unknown. However, considerable knowledge has been gained concerning the way by which interactions between certain agonists and their membrane receptors (the first messenger) lead to the generation of second messengers, which in turn may regulate the mobilization of intracellular calcium, the third and final messenger for smooth muscle contraction.

Along with contraction, biochemical effects of various stimulants of vascular cells may be responsible for conversion of quick-acting but transient and rather small pressor effects into long-lasting and larger rises in blood pressure by the induction of vascular wall hypertrophy. As summarized in this lovely review by Lever, the hypothesis is an extension of the proposal made by Folkow in the 1950s that rises in pressure induce hypertrophy which, in turn, feedbacks to raise pressure further (Fig 6–1). Since hypertrophy of resistance vessels seems to come not after but either before or in parallel with the rise in blood pressure (Mulvany, J.: *Hypertension* 5:129–136, 1987), Lever proposes that various trophic mechanisms may cause hypertrophy directly. These trophins are thought to activate the metabolism of phosphoinosotide within the membrane of vascular smooth muscle cells leading through a series of steps to an increased cell alkalinity, which has been proposed as the signal of hyperplasia and hypertrophy via stimulation of DNA synthesis (Griendling et al.: *Hypertension* 9(suppl. III):181–185, 1987).

As noted by Lever, there are various specific trophins that could be responsible for the vascular hypertrophy that sustains the elevated blood pressure in certain known forms of secondary hypertension: growth hormone in acromegaly; angiotensin II in renovascular hypertension; catecholamines in pheochromocytoma; aldosterone in primary aldosteronism. Although these may also be involved in primary (essential) hypertension, another potential candidate is supported by increasingly strong evidence, namely insulin. Insulin receptors are found on blood vessels; insulin causes proliferation of vascular smooth muscle in culture; infusion of insulin into one femoral artery of the diabetic dog causes vascular hypertrophy on that side only. As will be noted in the next abstract, patients with primary (essential) hypertension have increased levels of plasma insulin and such increased levels may explain the commonality of diabetes, obesity, and hypertension.

Such conjecture is of more than academic interest. Vascular and cardiac hypertrophy are responsible not only for the rise in blood pressure but also for many of the complications of hypertension. Although hypertrophy may come and go independently of blood pressure, they usually are in close approximation and the prevention or reversal of hypertrophy may increasingly be the primary goal for the control of hypertension.

The other forces that modulate blood pressure are those involved in vascular relaxation, another new arena that is receiving attention (Kaiser and Sparks: *Arch. Intern. Med.* 147:569–573, 1987). Vasodilation induced by some endogenous neurotransmitters such as acetylcholine and 5-hydroxytryptamine involves the local release of an endothelium-derived relaxing factor (EDRF) which appears to be nitric oxide; EDRF and other vasodilators, including exogenous nitrovasodilators and atrial natriuretic factor, have been linked to elevations of cyclic guanosine 3′,5′-monophosphate (cGMP). The manner by which cGMP induces vascular relaxation remains uncertain with data to support inhibition of the flux or sensitivity of calcium, the hydrolysis of phosphatidylinositol, and the phosphorylation of contractile proteins.

The rapidly advancing knowledge of basic mechanisms controlling both contraction and relaxation of vascular smooth muscle promises to explain a great deal of the pathophysiology of hypertension and offers the prospect of more effect targeted therapy.

In particular, the possible role of insulin is looming very large indeed.—N.M. Kaplan, M.D.

Insulin Resistance in Essential Hypertension

Eleuterio Ferrannini, Giuseppe Buzzigoli, Riccardo Bonadonna, Maria Antonietta Giorico, Marco Oleggini, Linda Graziadei, Roberto Pedrinelli, Luigi Brandi, and Stefano Bevilacqua (Univ. of Pisa, Italy)
N. Engl. J. Med. 317:350–357, Aug. 6, 1987 6–6

High blood pressure is prevalent in obese patients and in patients with diabetes, both conditions with insulin resistance. A study was done to determine whether hypertension is associated with insulin resistance independently of obesity and glucose intolerance.

Thirteen patients, aged 38 ± 2 years, with untreated essential hypertension, normal body weight, and normal glucose tolerance were studied. Insulin sensitivity was measured using the euglycemic insulin-clamp technique, glucose turnover was measured using [^{3}H] glucose isotope dilution, and whole-body glucose oxidation was measured using indirect calorimetry. All measures of glucose metabolism were normal in the postabsorptive state. During steady-state euglycemic hyperinsulinemia, hepatic glucose production and lipolysis were found to be effectively suppressed, and glucose oxidation and potassium disposal were stimulated normally. However, total insulin-induced glucose uptake was significantly impaired: 3.8 ± 0.32 vs. 6.31 ± 0.42 mg per minute per kilogram of body weight in 11 age- and weight-matched control subjects. Thus, nonoxidative glucose disposal—glycogen synthesis and glycolysis—accounted for the defect in overall glucose uptake. Total glucose uptake was found to be inversely related to systolic or mean blood pressure.

This study gives preliminary evidence that essential hypertension is an insulin-resistant state. It is concluded that resistance involves glucose but not lipid or potassium metabolism, is located in peripheral tissues but not the liver, is restricted to nonoxidative pathways of intracellular glucose disposal, and is directly correlated with the severity of hypertension.

▶ This study is the first to document peripheral insulin resistance in *nonobese* patients with primary hypertension. Many previous articles, going back to 1966, have shown that peripheral blood insulin levels are increased in many hypertensive persons, whether obese or not.

Lever's review (Abstract 6–5) pointed out the possible role of insulin as a trophic factor for vascular hypertrophy. High insulin levels could raise the blood pressure in at least two other ways: by stimulation of the sympathetic nervous system and by renal retention of sodium (Reaven and Hoffman: *Lancet* 1:435–436, 1987).

High insulin levels are present in obese subjects, who also have peripheral insulin resistance. The connection between hyperinsulinemia, obesity, and hypertension is seen even among adolescents (Rocchini et al.: *Hypertension* 10:267–273, 1987). To fit it all together, when these kids lost weight (by diet and exercise), their blood pressures fell in relation to a fall in plasma insulin.

Look out for insulin: it may prove to be a major player in the pathophysiology of much hypertension, particularly that seen in obesity and diabetes.

Obviously, there's more to hypertension, including abnormal handling of sodium, stress, and other hormones. Before examining some of these elements, let's take a detour to look at an interesting comparison between men and women with hypertension that may, in fact, add further support to the connection between upper body obesity, hyperinsulinemia, and hypertension.—N.M. Kaplan, M.D.

Disparate Cardiovascular Findings in Men and Women With Essential Hypertension

Franz H. Messerli, Guillermo E. Garavaglia, Roland E. Schmieder, Kirsten Sundgaard-Riise, Boris D. Nunez, and Celso Amodeo (Ochsner Clinic and Alton Ochsner Medical Found., New Orleans)

Ann. Intern. Med. 107:158–161, August 1987 6–7

Based on data from the Framingham cohort, it has been shown that women have a 66% lower risk of stroke, a 50% lower risk of developing coronary artery disease or congestive heart failure, and a 33% lower risk of dying suddenly than men with the same level of arterial pressure. The reason for these differences in morbidity and mortality is not clearly understood. Therefore, a study was done to assess the cardiovascular findings in 100 women with mild hypertension who were carefully matched to 100 men on the basis of arterial pressure, age, race, and body surface area.

Systemic hemodynamic, volume, and endocrine findings were measured. The female subjects had a slightly but significantly lower diastolic pressure than the male patients, even though a close match of arterial pressure between the two groups was attempted. Women with essential hypertension were found to have a higher cardiac index, left ventricular ejection time, and pulse pressure. Women also had a slightly faster heart rate and a lower total peripheral resistance than men with the same arterial pressure. The women's blood volume was slightly more contracted than that of the men, as were total blood volume and erythrocyte mass. Mean arterial pressure correlated directly with total peripheral resistance in both men and women. However, a shift to the left of the regression line noted in men meant that for every given level of blood pressure, total peripheral resistance, and therefore the risk of systemic hypertensive vascular disease, was higher in men than in women with essential hypertension.

This study demonstrated that total peripheral resistance was lower and systemic blood flow higher in premenopausal women than in men for any given level of arterial blood pressure. Women were found to be hemodynamically younger than men of the same chronologic age. Women's vascular resistance is lower and their arterial pressure surges with less isometric stress. Thus, a pathophysiologic mechanism was identified for the epidemiologic observation that essential hypertension is associated with less cardiovascular disease in women than in men.

▶ This nicely done comparison may provide a logical explanation for what has been long noted: women tolerate hypertension better than men. There's likely a hormonal reason behind it all: testosterone increases the deposition of fat in the upper body and this, in turn, is associated with higher plasma insulin levels (Peiris et al.: *J. Clin. Endocrinol. Metab.* 64:162–169, 1987). It has been known, at least since 1940, that those with upper body obesity have more hypertension (Robinson and Brucer: *Arch. Intern. Med.* 66:393–417, 1940), so once again we have the deadly triangle: upper body obesity, hypertension, and hyperinsulinemia.

We will now look at some 1987 publications on other possible factors involved in the pathogenesis of primary hypertension. The first set of these relate to possible defects in the transport of sodium into cells. For some time, there has been strong evidence that hypertensive persons have increased sodium within their cells that may directly cause a rise in free intracellular calcium levels, which in turn are responsible for cell contraction.

Sodium is normally kept low within cells compared to extracellular fluids by a number of mechanisms (Fig 6–2). Defects in one or more of these may be found in blood cells of hypertensive patients, which are easily obtained for study and which hopefully provide a mirror to what is going on within vascular tissue as well. The major control mechanism for sodium transport is the Na^+-K^+ ATPase pump, usually measured by ouabain-sensitive Na^+ efflux. In addition, Na^+, K^+ cotransport and Na^+, Li^+ countertransport have been found to be altered in some hypertensive persons. The Na^+-Li^+ exchange may be an indicator of the activity of another important regulator of cell function, the Na^+-H^+ exchanger.—N.M. Kaplan, M.D.

Kinetic Study of Na^+-K^+ Pump in Erythrocytes From Essential Hypertensive Patients

Javier Diez, Patrick Hannaert, and Ricardo P. Garay (Inst. of Health and Med. Res., Paris)

Am. J. Physiol. 252:H1–H6, January 1987 6–8

Different investigators have found Na^+-K^+ pump activity in essential hypertension to be low, normal, or high. The authors investigated this transport system in a study of the interaction of the Na^+-K^+ pump with internal Na^+ in erythrocytes from 38 normotensive control subjects and 49 subjects with essential hypertension.

The hypertensive subjects were 24 women and 25 men, aged 26–60 years; controls were 13 women and 25 men, aged 19–60 years. Venous blood was collected, and erythrocytes were prepared. Ouabain-sensitive Na^+ efflux was taken as a measure of pump activity. In 6 of the hypertensive patients, the Na^+-K^+ pump showed an apparent dissociation constant for internal Na^+ above an upper normal limit of 7 mmole/L at cells. Four of these 6 subjects showed an increase in the maximal rate of ouabain-sensitive Na^+ efflux above an upper normal limit of 11 mmole/L

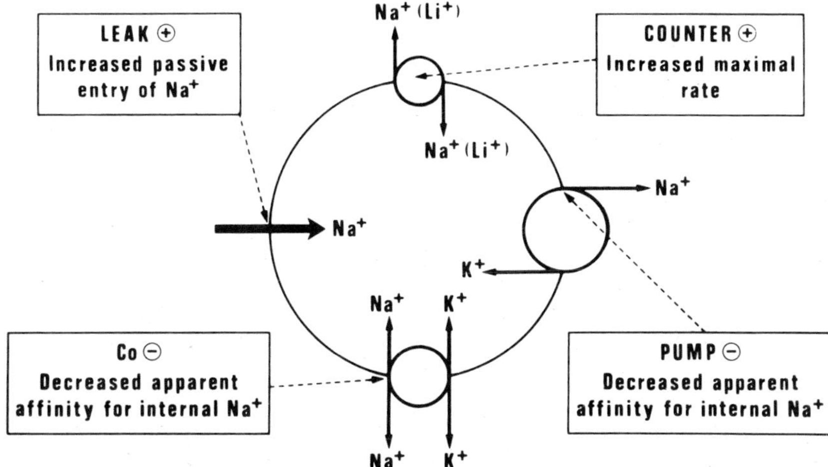

Fig 6–2.—Stable Na^+ transport abnormalities in erythrocytes from patients with essential hypertension: LEAK ⊕, increased passive entry of Na^+; Co ⊖, decreased apparent affinity of the Na^+-K^+ cotransport system for internal Na^+; COUNTER ⊕, increased maximal rate of Na^+-Li^+ countertransport; PUMP ⊖, decreased apparent affinity of the Na^+-K^+ pump for internal Na^+. (Courtesy of Diez, J., et al.: Am. J. Physiol. 252:H1–H6, January 1987.)

of cells/hour. In repeated determinations during a period of 1–3 years, these abnormalities proved stable (Fig 6–2). A kinetic study of other erythrocyte Na^+ transport pathways revealed that 16 hypertensive subjects had a low apparent affinity of the Na^+-K^+ cotransport system for internal Na^+, 10 had increased Na^+-Li^+ countertransport fluxes, and 11 had increased Na^+ leak. None of these abnormalities was seen in the 6 hypertensive subjects with abnormal pump fluxes. Four of these 6 subjects showed an increased maximal rate of outward Na^+-K^+ cotransport. Basal erythrocyte Na^+ content of these 6 hypertensive subjects was within the normal range.

▶ Diez et al. find various combinations of sodium transport defects in red cells from hypertensive subjects which obviously do not fit a single pattern. Why the differences are seen in subjects who all have apparently uncomplicated primary hypertension, who are not taking any medications, and who have no other known confounding feature, remains a major mystery.

The explanation may be that these defects are epiphenomena, unrelated to the basic defect responsible for hypertension, or that they are simply markers for the basic defect. Nonetheless, they may be correlated to both the high blood pressure and the increased vascular resistance.—N.M. Kaplan, M.D.

Red Blood Cell Li^+- Na^+ Countertransport, Na^+-K^+ Cotransport, and the Hemodynamics of Hypertension

Alan B. Weder, M. Andrew Fitzpatrick, Barbara A. Torretti, Alan L. Hinderliter, Brent M. Egan, and Stevo Julius (Univ. of Michigan)

Hypertension 9:459–466, May 1987 6–9

Essential hypertension is characterized by increased systemic vascular resistance. Earlier observations relating quantitative disturbances of red blood cell (RBC) Li^+-Na^+ countertransport and Na^+-K^+ cotransport to essential hypertension fueled speculation that similar abnormalities may affect vascular smooth muscle cells. The authors examined Li^+-Na^+ countertransport and Na^+-K^+ cotransport activities in 65 white men.

Self-determined blood pressure (BP), invasive systemic hemodynamic pattern, limb venous compliance, and RBC Li^+-Na^+ countertransport and Na^+-K^+ cotransport activities were measured in 23 normotensive men, 22 men with borderline hypertension, and 20 men with mild essential hypertension. The Li^+-Na^+ countertransport activity was found to be positively and significantly correlated with self-determined systolic BP and systolic and diastolic BP measured directly in the hemodynamic laboratory. These correlations were independent of potentially confounding variables. Analysis of the hemodynamic determinants of BP also revealed a significant positive correlation of countertransport with vascular resistance, but not with cardiac output or CI. High RBC Na^+-K^+ cotransport activity was not independently associated with hypertension or with a characteristic hemodynamic pattern; however, it was related to decreased venous compliance.

These observations confirm and extend previous findings of a positive correlation of casual clinic BP determinations and countertransport in white patients. It appears that Na^+-K^+ cotransport may be altered secondarily by factors related to hypertension and may be a valid marker for abnormalities of the venous system in hypertension. The authors believe that Li^+-Na^+ countertransport deserves further study as a marker for the genetic substrate of essential hypertension.

▶ Of more pathophysiologic consequence than these alterations in cotransport and countertransport may be higher rates of Na^+-H^+ exchange.—N.M. Kaplan, M.D.

Increased Platelet Na^+-H^+ Exchange Rates in Essential Hypertension: Application of a Novel Test

A. Livine, R. Veitch, S. Grinstein, J.W. Balfe, A. Marquez-Julio, A. Rothstein
(The Hosp. for Sick Children and Toronto Western Hosp., Toronto)
Lancet 1:533–536, March 7, 1987 6–10

The plasma membrane Na^+-H^+ exchanger, a ubiquitous system, is believed to play a physiologic role in intracellular pH regulation; in the control of cell growth and proliferation; in stimulus-response coupling in white cells and platelets; in the metabolic response to hormones and the regulation of cell volume; and in the transepithelial transport of Na^+, H^+, HCO_3^-, $C1^-$, and organic ions. Enhanced sodium-proton exchange may have a role in the pathogenesis of hypertension. Researchers have suggested that the enhanced Na^+-Li^+ exchange in erythrocytes may indicate the presence of changed Na^+-H^+ exchange activity. Na^+-H^+ exchange was measured in platelets obtained from normotensive subjects and patients with essential hypertension using an assay based on electronic cell sizing.

Study subjects included 20 normotensive persons, 8 normotensive persons with a family history of hypertension, 15 hypertensive patients receiving medication, and 7 hypertensive patients not receiving any antihypertensive medication. Na^+-H^+ exchange was measured indirectly in platelets as the rate of amiloride-sensitive and sodium-dependent volume gain of cells suspended in sodium-proportionate. The cytoplasmic acidification induced by the permeant propionic acid activated the exchanger; volume changes coupled to Na^+ uptake were measured by cell sizing with a Coulter counter and Channelyzer. The exchanges rate constants were 13.1 in the first normotensive group; 15.5 in the normotensive group with family history of hypertension; 18.4 in the hypertensive patients receiving medication; and 25.6 in the unmedicated, hypertensive patients.

These results substantiate earlier suggestions that the Na^+-H^+ antiport is altered in hypertension and indicate a higher exchange activity in platelets of patients with essential hypertension than in normotensive individuals. This is the first report of Na^+-H^+ exchange activity changes associated with essential hypertension in humans. Enhanced Na^+-H^+ activity has previously been reported in lymphocytes, neutrophils, and platelets of spontaneously hypertensive rats. Measurement of Na^+-H^+ exchange in platelets may be useful in diagnosing essential hypertension. Currently, no single index of cation transport distinguishes clearly between normotensive and hypertensive persons. Simultaneous assessment of multiple sodium transport systems may be of more diagnostic value than single measurements.

▶ Not only is this assay simple and rapid, but it requires only a small amount of plasma. Beyond serving as a possible diagnostic test for primary hypertension, it may also reflect a basic abnormality that leads to hypertension in various possible ways. In the kidney, proximal tubular sodium reabsorption is largely via Na^+-H^+ exchange; an increase in Na^+-H^+ exchange might increase sodium reabsorption. In vascular smooth muscle, increased Na^+-H^+ exchange would increase intracellular sodium concentration. Moreover, cell growth and proliferation is affected by intracellular pH and this is, in turn, influenced by Na^+-H^+ exchange. Increased exchange in smooth muscle cells could stimulate vascular hypertrophy.

The previous three abstracts (6–8, 6–9, and 6–10) refer to possible defects in sodium transport which may secondarily increase intracellular calcium and, thereby, lead to increased vascular contraction, tone and resistance. Past work has suggested that a circulating Na^+-K^+ pump inhibitor, possibly of hypothalamic origin, may be increased as a response to initial volume expansion in hypertension (Haber and Haupert: *Hypertension* 9:315–321, 1987). This putative circulating pump inhibitor would lead to an increase in renal sodium excretion but at the same time increase intracellular sodium. A circulating factor has been found in plasma from patients with primary hypertension that increases intracellular free calcium in normal platelets. Whether this works by inhibiting the Na^+-K^+ pump remains to be seen.—N.M. Kaplan, M.D.

Effects of a Circulating Factor in Patients With Essential Hypertension on Intracellular Free Calcium in Normal Platelets

Armando Lindner, Margaret Kenny, and Alice J. Meacham (VA Med. Ctr. and Univ. of Washington, Seattle)

N. Engl. J. Med. 316:509–513, Feb. 26, 1987 6–11

The role of calcium in essential hypertension is the subject of considerable controversy. Some researchers have reported that intracellular free, or cytosolic, calcium is increased in the platelets of patients with essential hypertension. To investigate the possibility that the high cytosolic calcium concentration may be caused by a circulating plasma factor, platelets from normotensive subjects were incubated with plasma infiltrates from patients with essential hypertension.

Twenty normotensive volunteers, aged 25–53 years and 31 patients with essential hypertension, aged 28–72 years, were studied. The patients received no previous medication or treatment for at least 2 weeks before the study. All had diastolic blood-pressure readings above 95 mm Hg after sitting for 5 minutes. The cytosolic calcium concentration in platelet was measured and found to be significantly increased in the platelets of hypertensive patients compared with control subjects. After incubation with plasma from the untreated hypertensive patients, the cytosolic calcium concentration in normal platelets increased by 80 ± 15%. After incubation with plasma from patients in whom hypertension was well controlled by calcium-influx blockers, normal platelet cytosolic calcium concentration increased 129 ± 33%. By contrast, the cytosolic calcium concentration was unchanged after incubation with plasma from normotensive subjects. After platelets from the patients were incubated with plasma from the normotensive controls, cytosolic calcium concentration decreased by more than 30%, into the normal range.

These findings suggest that plasma from patients with essential hypertension contains a substance that increases the cytosolic calcium concentration in platelets. Cytosolic calcium acts as a trigger for vascular smooth-muscle cell concentration; if the plasma factor acts on these cells as it acts on platelets, it may be responsible for the increased peripheral vascular resistance associated with hypertension.

▶ The preceding four abstracts (6–8 to 6–11) are only a small sample of a voluminous literature on possible defects in sodium transport across cells and intracellular calcium in the pathogenesis of hypertension. For those wanting more, an entire supplement of the journal *Hypertension* covered the subject of cation transport and natriuretic factors (Tosteson: *Hypertension* 10[suppl I] 1987).

While the search for a possible natriuretic factor of hypothalamic origin has gone for over 30 years, the atrial natriuretic hormone (or factor) has been completely identified and synthesized and extensively studied since De Bold first found it in 1981.—N.M. Kaplan, M.D.

Cardionatrin: A Cardiac Hormone

A. Fournier and A. De Bold (Centre Hospitalier Universitaire, Amiens, France, and Ottawa Civic Hosp., Ottowa, Canada)

Presse Med. 16:349–352, Feb. 28, 1987 6–12

Until the late 1970s, the heart was considered to be only a pump that ensures the circulation of blood. In 1981, De Bold conducted experiments in rats that demonstrated that atrial extracts contain a protein that produces transient natriuresis and a fall in arterial pressure. Within 5 years these findings led not only to the identification, but also to the biosynthesis, of a new hormone, atrial natriuretic factor (ANF), or cardionatrin.

Secretion of ANF is stimulated by distention of the right and left atria, which explains why it plays an essential role in cardiovascular homeostasis. Atrial natriuretic acts mainly as an antagonist of two systems, the renin-angiotensin-aldosterone system, and the adrenergic system. The vasodilative effect of ANF has been demonstrated in vitro by its antagonistic activity on vasoconstriction induced by angiotensin II, noradrenaline, and vasopressin. This effect can be demonstrated in the absence of endothelium.

While the diuretic and natriuretic effects of ANF are now well understood, its effect on renal function has not yet been well explained. It was initially thought that the effect of ANF on renal function was due to increased glomerular filtration secondary to vasodilatation of the afferent artery, and to increased renal blood flow. However, later studies have shown that ANF can increase natriuresis without increasing glomerular filtration or renal blood flow. More recent studies have shown that renal blood flow actually decreases with constant ANF infusion.

▶ The *physiologic* role of ANF seems fairly certain: a rapid mediator of sodium excretion whenever the central circulation is expanded. However, the *pathophysiologic* role of ANF in hypertension, heart failure, and any other disease remains uncertain. Specifically, levels are not increased in patients with primary hypertension (Zachariah et al.: *Mayo Clin. Proc.* 62:782–786, 1987). However, the exaggerated excretion of sodium (natriuresis) seen after volume loads in low-renin hypertensives may be caused by enhanced secretion of ANF (Matsubara et al.: *Am. J. Cardiol.* 60:708–714, 1987).

In addition to the article by Fournier and De Bold—chosen because the second author is the discoverer of the peptide, but inaccessible to many because it is in French—excellent reviews of ANF are available, including that of Lang et al. (*J. Hypertens.* 5:255–271, 1987).

Meanwhile, that old devil sodium remains a likely culprit, at least in the half or so of the hypertensive population who are "sodium sensitive," i.e., who have a rise in blood pressure when given sodium and a fall in blood pressure when deprived of sodium. There's been no easy way to determine sodium sensitivity, but Weinberger and coworkers in Indianapolis have noted a significant correlation with haptoglobin phenotypes, which could turn out to be clinically usable (*Hypertension* 10:443–446, 1987). Meanwhile, Hollenberg, Williams, and coworkers at the Brigham in Boston continue to characterize those sodium-sensitive subjects as being "nonmodulators" of various mechanisms that normally regulate sodium homeostasis (Rabinowe et al.: *Hypertension* 10:404–408, 1987).

Just when most have accepted an important role for sodium, at least in the sodium-sensitive half, Kurtz et al. (*N. Engl. J. Med.* 317:1043–1048, 1987) have shown that the anionic component of the sodium salt "can influence the ability of that salt to increase blood pressure." Specifically, they found that variations in sodium chloride intake did change blood pressure but that equimolar amounts of sodium citrate did not. Although both induced comparable weight gain and sodium retention, only NaCl increased plasma volume, which may be the reason it raised blood pressure.

Regardless, sodium chloride is what most of us consume in excessive amounts and I continue to believe a modest reduction to around 75–100 mmoles per day (4.3–5.8 gm of sodium chloride per day or 1.7–2.3 gm of sodium per day) or roughly half of current average consumption makes good sense—as we shall cover later under the section on nondrug therapy.

Meanwhile, excess sodium intake and abnormal sodium transport do not exhaust the list of probable factors involved in the pathogenesis of hypertension. Guyton continues to emphasize the necessity for a defect in renal function (*Hypertension* 10:1–6, 1987). Behavioral scientists continue to emphasize hyperreactivity to stress (Melamed: *Psychsom. Med.* 49:217–225, 1987), possibly connected to a greater inhibition of anger (Boutelle et al.: *Psychiatry* 50:206–217, 1987).

On the other hand, poor blacks who have a strong personality predisposition to cope actively with psychosocial environmental stressors (referred to as John Henryism) have been found to have more hypertension (James et al.: *Am. J. Epidemiol.* 126:664–673, 1987). Regardless, the higher mortality in poor and uneducated people with hypertension likely reflects their lesser access to adequate health care. In the Hypertension Detection and Follow-up Program, those with less than a high school education who were given routine care in the community had a 5-year death rate twice as high as those with more than a high school education, whereas both groups given more intensive care in special clinics had equally lower death rates (HDFP Cooperation Group: *Hypertension* 9:641–646, 1987).

Lastly, sympathetic nervous hyperactivity with or without more stress may be involved. A decrease in central dopaminergic activity may be responsible (Os et al.: *J. Hypertens.* 5:191–197, 1987). This fits with a blood pressure lowering effect from dopamine$_1$-receptor agonists, such as fenoldopam (Glück et al.: *Hypertension* 10:43–54, 1987).—N.M. Kaplan, M.D.

Benefits and Costs of Therapy

▶ ↓ The foregoing review of last year's advances in understanding what causes hypertension leaves an unsettled feeling: a few more pieces of the mosaic puzzle may be in place, but the overall picture still cannot be made out. Therefore, lacking the knowledge needed to prevent the disease, we must continue to do what is necessary to treat it.

The treatment of hypertension is now the leading indication for visits to physicians and for the use of prescription drugs in the United States. But in 1987 a number of publications provided evidence that our rush to treat all hypertension may be partly misguided and inappropriate. At the least, they suggest that elevated blood pressure be better documented before the diagnosis is made or therapy begun and that greater caution be taken not to lower the blood pressure too much.—N.M. Kaplan, M.D.

Progress in the Battle Against Hypertension: Changes in Blood Pressure Levels in the United States From 1960 to 1980

Andrew L. Dannenberg, Terence Drizd, Michael J. Horan, Suzanne G. Haynes, and Paul E. Leaverton (Natl. Heart, Lung, and Blood Inst., Bethesda, Md., Natl. Ctr. for Health Statistics, Hyattsville, Md., and Univ. of South Florida, Tampa)

Hypertension 10:226–233, August 1987 6–13

Intensive efforts to identify and treat people with hypertension have been under way for many years. Changes in blood pressure levels in the United States were evaluated based on nationally representative health examination surveys conducted by the National Center for Health Statistics in 1960–1962, 1971–1974, and 1976–1980.

These surveys were designed to assess certain aspects of health of the U.S. noninstitutionalized population, based on clinical histories and physical examinations of representative individuals selected by complex probability sampling techniques. The first survey reached 7,710 people; the second, 19,572; the third, 18,209. The findings are national estimates based on weighted observations. The first blood pressure determination in each survey was the most comparable among the surveys and thus was used in the analysis.

Analysis of age-adjusted data for persons, aged 18–74 years, including those taking antihypertensive medication, indicated that mean systolic blood pressure declined 5 and 10 mm Hg for whites and blacks, respectively, between the first and third surveys. The proportion of people with systolic blood pressure of 140 mm Hg or higher fell 18% and 31% in whites and blacks, respectively. The proportion with undiagnosed hypertension decreased by 17% among whites and 59% among blacks. The proportion of those taking antihypertensive medications increased by 71% and 31% in whites and blacks, respectively.

Differences noted between the first and third surveys were statistically significant. Changes in diastolic blood pressure levels were not significant among race-sex groups. The proportion of people with definitive hypertension—systolic blood pressure equal to or greater than 160 mm Hg and/or diastolic pressure equal to or greater than 95 mm Hg and/or taking antihypertensive medication—declined among blacks and rose slightly among whites.

The changes in blood pressure levels and prevalence of hypertension noted in these surveys were those anticipated and were consistent with other reports. Overall, there were decreases in mean and median systolic blood pressure and in the proportion of people with systolic blood pressures of 140 mm Hg or higher. No consistent changes in diastolic blood pressure measurements were seen, for reasons not fully understood. The improvements noted were most marked among black adults, who were at the greatest risk at the beginning of the study period.

▶ This review of the excellent data from large national surveys performed from 1960 to 1980 documents the improvements made over this time in the control of hypertension, but also calls attention to the need for additional attention to a large segment of the population who remain at risk. It is particularly upsetting to see that the proportion of persons with definitive hypertension (> 160/95 mm Hg) rose slightly among whites, despite the greater proportion of diagnosed and treated persons.

Nonetheless, the more widespread treatment of hypertension has clearly been shown to reduce mortality and morbidity from strokes.—N.M. Kaplan, M.D.

The Changing Pattern of Hypertension and the Declining Incidence of Stroke

W. Michael Garraway and Jack P. Whisnant (Mayo Clinic and Found.)
JAMA 258:214–217, July 10, 1987 6–14

Mortality due to stroke has been declining in the United States for more than 50 years. Population-based studies in Rochester, Minn., have reflected this decline in stroke mortality. In Rochester, the major contributing factor to this phenomenon has been a decrease in the incidence of stroke. It is not known whether the declining incidence of stroke in this community has been accompanied by changes in risk factors, especially hypertension. The authors examined changes in recognition and control of hypertension in this community from 1950 to 1979.

Between 1950–1959 and 1970–1979, the prevalence of diastolic blood pressure (BP) greater than or equal to 105 mm Hg decreased 26% in men and 70% in women. The prevalence of BPs of at least 95 mm Hg declined by 5% in men and 58% in women. Increasing control of hypertension was found to have an almost inverse linear relationship with the decreasing incidence of stroke in women, but the incidence of stroke in men did not decline until 10 years after improvement in the control of BP began. The percentage of hypertensive patients whose condition was not under control in treatment or who were without treatment decreased from 66% in 1950–1959 to 21% in 1970–1979.

Improvements in the detection and control of mildly and moderately increased BP in Rochester were found to occur in the same period in which there was a major decline in the incidence of stroke.

Improved awareness, as manifested by the recording of BP in the medical records, and better control of BP through treatment probably contributed to this change.

▶ In the original article Figure 2 shows a very dramatic crossing of two lines: a raising control of hypertension and a falling incidence of stroke.

It is important to realize that these data show a falling *incidence* of stroke (and not better management of people who have had a stroke). This is what the treatment of hypertension is supposed to do: prevent the cardiovascular complications that accompany high blood pressure.

As good as these data should make us all feel, the picture is not so clear or promising for prevention of the number one cardiovascular complication of hypertension—coronary heart disease (CHD). We've made little or no progress in reducing the role of hypertension in what remains the number one cause of mortality in our population.

The following series of articles examines two probable reasons why the treatment of hypertension has not been found to protect against CHD: the metabolic side effects of the drugs used, and the inadvertent lowering of blood pressure too much in those with borderline coronary perfusion.—N.M. Kaplan, M.D.

Failure to Reduce Cholesterol as Explanation for the Limited Efficacy of Antihypertensive Treatment in the Reduction of CHD: Examination of the Evidence From Six Hypertension Intervention Trials

S. Heyden, K.A. Schneider, and G.J. Fodor (Duke Univ. Med. Ctr., Durham, N.C. and St. John's Hosp., Newfoundland)

Klin. Wochenschr. 65:828–832, September 1987 6–15

Several studies of hypertension intervention have shown a marked reduction in mortality from cerebrovascular disease, but no comparable effect on coronary heart disease (CHD). Concomitant hypercholesterolemia is a possible explanation. The authors reviewed the results of six long-term randomized trials which were reported in 1980–1985: the Oslo Study, the Multiple Risk Factor Intervention Trial (MRFIT), the Australian National Blood Pressure Study, the International Prospective Primary Prevention Study in Hypertension (IPPPSH), the Medical Research Council (MRC) Trial, and the European Working Party on High Blood Pressure.

Both the Oslo and British MRC studies reported very high average levels of cholesterol and failed to show protection against CHD with intensive treatment. In the Australian and American MRFIT studies, coronary mortality was reduced in hypertensives who had lower levels of cholesterol. In the European Working Party study patients with markedly lowered blood pressure and levels of cholesterol had lower cardiac mortality than placebo recipients. In the IPPPSH study higher levels of cholesterol in hypertensives who were given a β-blocker or diuretic therapy were associated with an increased risk of myocardial infarction.

Cholesterol appears not to be a risk factor in cerebrovascular disease.

Failure to lower the level of cholesterol by antihypertensive treatment will, however, explain a lack of effect on CHD. It is suggested that dietary treatment be used if the level of cholesterol is 200–260 mg/dl. Lipid-lowering drugs are recommended for patients with levels of cholesterol that exceed 260 mg/dl.

▶ As this review and that of MacMahon et al. (*Prog. Cardiovasc. Dis.* 29(suppl. 1):99–118, 1986) document, the failure to protect against CHD by treatment of hypertension may reflect the failure to lower serum cholesterol and even to raise it further by the lipid-raising effects of diuretics and non-ISA β-blockers, the primary drugs used in all of the major trials.

Another reason for the failure to reduce CHD mortality in those trials that used fairly high doses of diuretic and that did not require correction of diuretic-induced hypokalemia is the induction of ventricular ectopic activity. The issue as to whether diuretic-induced hypokalemia does induce cardiac arrhythmias remains unresolved: some find a definite connection (Cohen et al.: *Am. J. Cardiol.* 60:548–554, 1987); others do not (Bause et al.: *Am. J. Cardiol.* 59:874–877, 1987). As reviewed by Poole-Wilson (*J. Hypertens.* 5:(suppl. 3):S51–S55, 1987), the issue may be unresolved, but the prudent course is to prevent or treat diuretic-induced hypokalemia.—N.M. Kaplan, M.D.

Cardiovascular Morbidity in Relation to Change in Blood Pressure and Serum Cholesterol Levels in Treated Hypertension: Results From the Primary Prevention Trial in Göteborg, Sweden

Ola Samuelsson, Lars Wilhelmsen, Ove K. Andersson, Kjell Pennert, and Göran Berglund (Sahlgrenska Hosp. and Osstra Hosp., Univ. of Göteberg, Sweden)
JAMA 258:1768–1776, Oct. 2, 1987 6–16

Despite a favorable effect of antihypertensive treatment on overall cardiovascular disease (CVD) morbidity, the total mortality and morbidity from CVD are still higher in treated hypertensive patients than in normotensive subjects or the total population. This study was done to determine the relationship between control of blood pressure (BP) and control of serum cholesterol levels with regard to prognosis for CVD and coronary heart disease (CHD) during long-term antihypertensive treatment.

The study population included 686 hypertensive men, aged 47–54 years, who were followed for up to 12 years. Either a β-blocker or a thiazide diuretic were given as first-line treatment, but drug regimens were adapted as needed to attain a BP of below 160/95 mm Hg. After 5 years of treatment, 73% of the patients were taking β-blockers, including 14% who were taking β-blockers as single-drug therapy, and 48% were taking a thiazide diuretic, including 16% who were taking thiazides as single-drug therapy.

Statistical analysis of the data showed that a combined reduction of BP and serum cholesterol levels was essential in order to reduce the incidence of CVD. The beneficial effect of BP reduction was small if serum cholesterol levels reduction in both BP and cholesterol levels resulted in a sub-

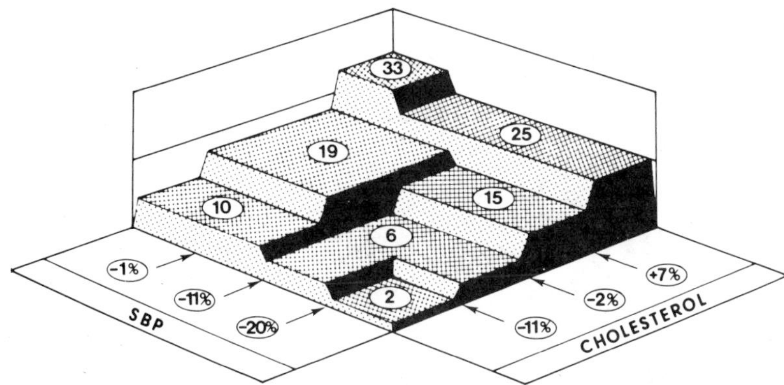

Fig 6–3.—All coronary heart disease morbidity during the 4th to 12th year of antihypertensive treatment in relationship to relative change during initial 3 years of follow-up) on both systolic blood pressure (SBP) and serum cholesterol levels (quartiles). Rates adjusted for risk at entry. (Courtesy of Samuelsson, O., et al.: JAMA 258:1768–1776, Oct. 2, 1987.)

stantial reduction in CVD and CHD mortality (Fig 6–3). An unexpected finding was that for mean in-study systolic and diastolic BP, there seemed to be a level below which further reduction of BP had no additional benefit from treatment.

In addition to reducing the BP in middle-aged hypertensive men, serum cholesterol levels need also to be reduced in order to improve the prognosis. However, it may be unfavorable to reduce the BP below a certain level in these patients.

▶ This study was not a randomized controlled one, as were the six reviewed in the preceding abstract. But it makes two important points, the first portrayed in Figure 6–3. As shown, the high rate of CHD was minimally reduced by even significant reduction in blood pressure if the serum cholesterol level was not lowered simultaneously. No attempt was made in this trial to alter cholesterol levels, so presumably the changes in the patients' serum cholesterol levels reflected either beneficial dietary changes or harmful antihypertensive drug effects. The message is clear: both blood pressure and cholesterol must be lowered to protect against CHD.

The second major point is that CHD morbidity fell as blood pressure was reduced to a systolic level of 143 or a diastolic level of 86, but that it rose again when blood pressure was reduced to below those levels.

The next article makes the same point with exactly the same critical level of diastolic blood pressure, 85 mm Hg.—N.M. Kaplan, M.D.

Benefits and Potential Harm of Lowering High Blood Pressure

John M. Cruickshank, Jeffrey M. Thorp, and F. James Zacharias (Imperial Chemical Industries PLC, Macclesfield, England, Wythenshawe Hosp., Manchester, England, and Clatterbridge Hosp., Merseyside, England)

Lancet 1:581–584, March 14, 1987 6–17

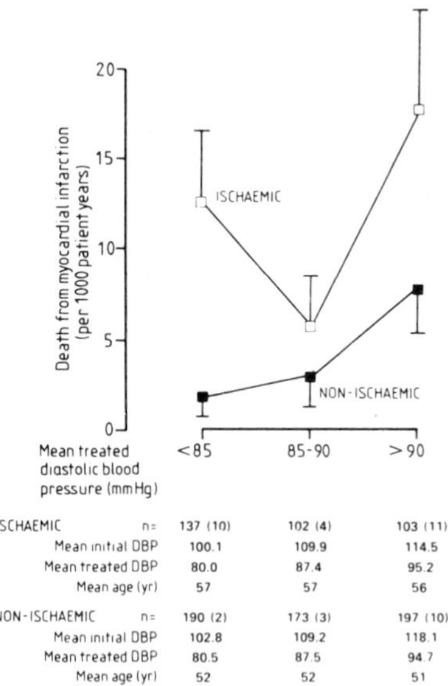

		<85	85-90	>90
ISCHAEMIC	n=	137 (10)	102 (4)	103 (11)
	Mean initial DBP	100.1	109.9	114.5
	Mean treated DBP	80.0	87.4	95.2
	Mean age (yr)	57	57	56
NON-ISCHAEMIC	n=	190 (2)	173 (3)	197 (10)
	Mean initial DBP	102.8	109.2	118.1
	Mean treated DBP	80.5	87.5	94.7
	Mean age (yr)	52	52	51

Fig 6–4.—Relation between mortality (SEM shown) from myocardial infarction in ischemic and nonischemic patients and treated diastolic blood pressure (age-adjusted). Number of deaths is given in parentheses. (Courtesy of Cruickshank, J.M., et al.: Lancet 1:581–584, March 14, 1987.)

Many studies have shown that lowering high blood pressure (BP) prevents strokes; however, it confers no obvious benefit in preventing coronary heart disease events and deaths. Lowering a raised diastolic BP (DBP) to below about 90 mm Hg may be associated with an increase in coronary events. A study was done to investigate whether lowering BP resulted in a better prognosis for patients with moderate to severe hypertension.

The original study subjects were 939 hypertensive patients, aged 17–77 years, who were followed up for as long as 10 years (mean, 6.1 years); 37 were lost to follow-up. Patients received a median dose of 100 mg of atenolol daily; 79% received 50–100 mg per day. Of the initial 939 patients, 72 received atenolol alone, 345 also took a diuretic, 244 also took a diuretic and a vasodilator, and 278 also took a diuretic and other medications. There were 91 deaths: 40 from myocardial infarction, 21 from stroke, 12 from cancer, and 18 from other causes. Initial BP was a poor predictor of mortality from myocardial infarction, but treated systolic blood pressure was a strong predictor. The relationship was J-shaped, confined to those with evidence of ischemic heart disease, between frequency of death due to myocardial infarction and treated DBP (Fig 6–4). The frequency was lowest at a treated DBP of 85–90 mm Hg and rose with treated DBP on either side of this range.

These findings strongly support those of others that indicate that lowering DBP (phase V) to below about 85 mm Hg in both younger and older patients is likely to increase the incidence of death from myocardial infarction. However, it appears that not all patients are at risk: only those with evidence of ischemic heart disease displayed the J-curve relation between death from myocardial infarction and treated DBP.

▶ In this study, a β-blocker was the primary drug but most also took a diuretic. The increase in CHD mortality when the diastolic blood pressure was brought down to below 85 mm Hg was limited to the 40% of the patients who had evidence for preexisting ischemic heart disease on entry into the trial, exactly as noted in the preceding abstract.

The lesson is clear: those with borderline myocardial perfusion because of underlying coronary artery disease may be harmed by a lowering of blood pressure to a level most of us have accepted as the appropriate goal of therapy. This likely reflects the limited ability of the coronary circulation to dilate and thereby increase blood flow as blood pressure is reduced, the process of autoregulation (Strandgaard and Haunsø: *Lancet* 2:658–660, 1987).

Since so many hypertensive persons have coronary disease, and since it may not be recognized or be recognizable before institution of therapy, the lesson must be remembered whenever antihypertensive therapy is begun.

There is another fact to this important issue: what we record in the office may turn out to be a much higher blood pressure than what the patient has out of the office. Therefore, we may be lowering blood pressure too much in many patients and thereby putting them, inadvertently, at greater risk.—N.M. Kaplan, M.D.

Are Some Hypertensive Patients Overtreated? A Prospective Study of Ambulatory Blood Pressure Recording

Bernard Waeber, Urs Scherrer, Antonio Petrillo, Jacques Bidiville, Jürg Nussberger, Gérard Waeber Jean-René Hofstetter, and Hans R. Brunner (Univ. of Vaudois and Polyclinique Médicale, Lausanne, Switzerland)

Lancet 2:732–734, Sept. 26, 1987 6–18

Blood pressure measurements that are taken in the office are not always a reliable predictor of future cardiovascular events, and it remains uncertain whether lowering blood pressure reduces the incidence of coronary heart disease. There is some indication that too great a reduction in diastolic pressure may have an adverse effect.

Thirty-four subjects with uncontrolled diastolic blood pressure despite antihypertensive therapy were studied. Sitting pressures were 95 mm Hg or higher at the outset. Measurements of ambulatory pressure were made with the Remler M2000, a patient-activated noninvasive device. Attempts were made to reduce office pressures to 90 mm Hg within a 3-month period.

Half the patients initially had ambulatory diastolic blood pressures of 90 mm Hg or below. Systolic pressures followed the same pattern. Target office diastolic pressure of 90 mm Hg or below was achieved in 11 of these 17 patients and in 7 of the 17 who initially had higher ambulatory pressure. Ambulatory pressure also decreased in the latter group.

Monitoring of ambulatory blood pressure can identify those hypertensive patients whose pressure only seems uncontrolled when measured in the office of a physician. Subjects with normal ambulatory pressures do not appear to benefit from further adjustments in drug therapy. The risks of overtreatment require further study.

▶ It is obvious that office readings may be higher than those recorded out of the office. These patients were evaluated with automatic ambulatory monitors, equipment that is expensive and cumbersome. The same careful monitoring that I believe should be obtained on all patients, both to document the presence of hypertension and to monitor its response to therapy, can be obtained by less expensive, easier to use home blood pressure measurements.—N.M. Kaplan, M.D.

Changing Relation Between Home and Clinic Blood-Pressure Measurements: Do Home Measurements Predict Clinic Hypertension?

P.L. Padfield, B.A. Lindsay, J.A. McLaren, A. Pirie, and M. Rademaker (Western General Hosp., Stockbridge Health Ctr., Edinburgh)

Lancet 2:323–324, Aug. 8, 1987 6–19

Increasing evidence suggests that blood pressure measurements taken in a clinic by a physician or nurse may be less accurate predictors of ultimate risk than measurements taken at home. Thus, self-measurement has become more common. Ambulatory or self-monitored blood pressure is believed to be lower at home than that recorded in a clinic, but it is not clear whether this difference persists in patients who regularly attend blood pressure clinics. A study was done to test the hypothesis that repeated measurement in the clinic might be replaced by a simple assessment of blood pressure by the patient at home.

Fifty-three men and 61 women were identified in a family health center as having diastolic pressures of 95 mm Hg or greater after three readings were taken at the clinic with the patients seated. The patients were instructed in the use of the Copal UA 231/251 electronic sphygmomanometer and took a series of readings at home over a 3-day period. Repeated blood pressure measurements were then taken at the clinic at 2 and 4 weeks. Blood pressure measurements were found to decrease on successive clinic visits. At the final visit, only 31 men and 28 women had diastolic pressures of 95 mm Hg or greater.

Average daytime home measurements were 155 (2)/94 (2) mm Hg, significantly lower than the average screening blood pressure measurements, but not significantly lower than measurements taken at the third clinic visit. In 79% of patients, home blood pressure measurements were successful in predicting outcome at the third clinic visit. Home-monitored pressures suggested normotension when the third clinic visit diastolic blood pressure reading was still above 95 mm Hg in 16 patients, 14% of the total group.

Home monitoring was found to be a practicable and acceptable alternative to repeated clinic measurements in the initial assessment of patients with hypertension. It is highly likely that electronic sphygmomanometers will play a greater role in the management of hypertensive patients.

▶ The instrument used was an electronic semiautomatic sphygmomanometer, of the sort that is readily available for $50 to $75 and that can be used by anyone capable of inflating the balloon. A microphone picks up the Korotkoff sounds, and an electronic printer displays the systolic and diastolic levels so that the patient doesn't need to use a stethoscope or be able to read the gauge.

The use of such equipment should become routine in the management of all patients with hypertension (Kaplan: *Am. J. Cardiol.* 60:1383–1386, 1987). We can thereby avoid the problem of "white-coat" hypertension so graphically shown in the next abstract.—N.M. Kaplan, M.D.

Alerting Reaction and Rise in Blood Pressure During Measurement by Physician and Nurse

Giuseppe Mancia, Gianfranco Parati, Guido Pomidossi, Guido Grassi, Roberto Casadei, and Alberto Zanchetti (Univ. of Milan)

Hypertension 9:209–215, February 1987 6–20

Previous studies have shown that blood pressure (BP) measurements made by a physician may trigger an altering reaction that increases BP for several minutes. The BP was monitored by continuous intra-arterial recording in 46 subjects to determine whether the alarm reaction and BP and heart rate increases attenuate when the physician's visit is repeated several times or when a nurse measures the BP.

Subjects were either normotensive or had mild or moderate essential hypertension with no sign of severe target organ damage. None received antihypertensive treatment during the period from 2 weeks before admission until the end of the study. Sixteen patients received repeated physician visits throughout a 2-day period of intra-arterial BP monitoring. In the early part of the physician's first visit, the peak mean BP and heart rate increased 22.6 ± 1.8 mm Hg and 17.7 ± 1.7 beats per minute, respectively; these increases were also seen in the physician's three subsequent visits. Less pronounced pressor and tachycardic responses observed initially also were virtually identical in the four visits. By contrast, in the remaining 30 subjects, the BP and heart rate rises that occurred during the nurse's visit were 46.7% and 42.1% less than those that occurred during the physician's visit (Fig 6–5). The late and less pronounced pressor and tachycardic responses were also significantly reduced during the nurse's visit.

It appears that the error of overestimation of BP inherent in cuff BP measurement by a physician cannot be avoided by repeated visits by the physician during a short span of time. However, it can be reduced if BP measurements are obtained by a nurse. It has been debated whether BP values obtained in the absence of an emotional pressor response provide a better index for clinical evaluation of hypertension. Although more ev-

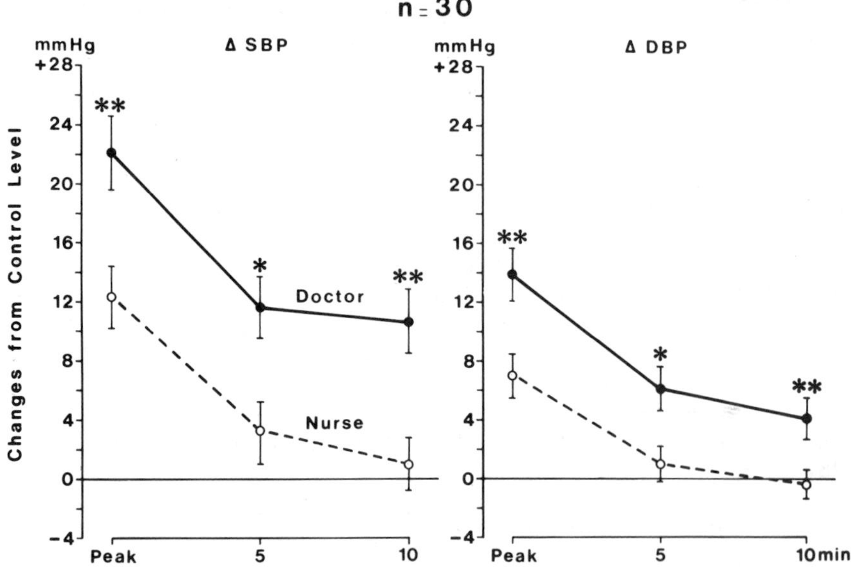

Fig 6–5.—Comparison of maximal rises in systolic blood pressure (SBP) and diastolic blood pressure (DBP) in 30 subjects at the fifth and tenth minutes of visits by a physician and a nurse. Data are expressed as mean (± SEM) change from a control value obtained 4 minutes before each visit (* indicates $P < .05$; **, $P < .005$). (Courtesy of Mancia, G., et al.: Hypertension 9:209–215, February 1987.)

idence is needed, the results of several studies suggest that reduction or avoidance of the BP overestimation inherent in traditional procedures may be of clinical value.

▶ The dramatic rise in blood pressure when it was taken by the doctor was lessened when it was taken by the nurse. Good reason to let your nurse take all the blood pressures.

These were all hospitalized patients, and what they experienced may be more than what your office patients would experience. Nonetheless, the real point of this study is that the blood pressure usually rises when it is taken by a health professional. Two messages: first, take at least three readings on each visit, and have at least three separate office visits to overcome the alerting reaction (Watson et al.: *J. Hypertens.* 5:207–211, 1987); second, have patients take their own blood pressures at home.

I strongly believe in the value of home blood pressure measurement. What is lacking, however, is certain evidence that the long-term home blood pressure levels are more predictive of the development of the complications that accompany hypertension than are the office readings. Such evidence is mounting (Parati et al.: *J. Hypertens.* 5:93–98, 1987), but we need more.—N.M. Kaplan, M.D.

Non–Drug Therapy

▶ ↓ As more and more people with minimally elevated blood pressure are being identified, there is an obvious need for greater care in ensuring that they have enough persistent hypertension to benefit from antihypertensive drug therapy, with its various costs. At the same time, there is an even greater potential value for the adroit use of various nondrug therapies that may lower the blood pressure and at the same time reduce other cardiovascular risk factors, while costing the patient little in the way of side effects or bothersome interference with the quality of life.

The next ten abstracts provide evidence that various (but not all) nondrug therapies may be helpful. The first relates to weight reduction for those who are obese, in view of evidence that obese hypertensives may not have as much increased risk from cardiovascular disease as do thin hypertensives (Barrett-Connor, E., Khaw, K.T.: *Circulation* 72:53–60, 1985).—N.M. Kaplan, M.D.

Does Obesity Protect Hypertensives Against Cardiovascular Disease?

Ellen Bloom, Dwayne Reed, Katsuhiko Yano, and Charles MacLean (Honolulu Heart Program and the Natl. Heart, Lung, and Blood Inst.)

JAMA 256:2972–2975, Dec. 5, 1986 6–21

Two recent studies have reported that obesity may protect hypertensive patients against cardiovascular disease (CVD). This possibility was investigated by the Honolulu Heart Program, a prospective epidemiologic study of CVD in a cohort of Japanese-American men, aged 45–65 years, who have been followed up for 12 years.

A total of 7,554 men free of CVD and cancer at baseline were studied. The combined effect of body mass index (BMI), as a measure of obesity, and blood pressure on coronary heart disease and CVD incidence was determined. In both normotensive and hypertensive men, rates of coronary heart disease and CVD were higher in the most obese than in the nonobese men. Blood pressure-BMI interaction was not significant for any CVD end point. Hypertension was associated with higher rates of coronary heart disease and CVD at all levels of BMI.

These findings support the conclusion that hypertension is associated with an increased risk of CVD in both obese and nonobese men. The relationship of blood pressure and CVD did not vary with BMI level. Thus, no evidence was found to support the hypothesis that obesity confers a protective effect on the relationship of hypertension to CVD incidence. These results were not altered when the variation by BMI level in smoking habit, alcohol intake, cholesterol and glucose levels, and the use of antihypertensive medication were controlled for.

▶ This survey finds that obesity does not protect the hypertensive from cardiovascular disease although those who are lean may be at greater risk (Goldbourt et al.: *Hypertension* 10:22–28, 1987). Since weight reduction will usually lower the blood pressure (Jarrett et al.: *J. Epidemiol. Community Health* 41:145–151, 1987), all who are overweight should be encouraged to lose weight, preferably before antihypertensive drug therapy is started.

As noted earlier, those whose obesity is predominantly deposited in the upper body (abdominal or apple-shaped) rather than in the lower body (gluteal or pear-shaped) suffer a greater likelihood of having hypertension and abnormal blood lipids, placing them at greater risk (Baumgartner et al.: *Am. J. Epidemiol.* 126:614–628, 1987).

Next to weight reduction for the obese, moderate sodium restriction probably has the most to offer for the overall hypertensive population, either by itself or in combination with antihypertensive drugs. Sodium restriction tends to raise renin-angiotensin levels, thereby limiting the lowering of blood pressure that can be achieved. The concomitant use of drugs that inhibit the renin-angiotensin system should be particularly effective.—N.M. Kaplan, M.D.

Moderate Sodium Restriction With Angiotensin Converting Enzyme Inhibitor in Essential Hypertension: A Double Blind Study

Graham A. MacGregor, Nirmala D. Markandu, Donald R.J. Singer, Francesco P. Cappuccio, Angela C. Shore, and Giuseppe A. Sagnella (Charing Cross and Westminster Med. School, London)

Br. Med. J. 294:531–534, Feb. 28, 1987 6–22

Theoretically, the combination of moderate sodium restriction and an angiotensin-converting enzyme inhibitor should overcome the disadvantages of both treatments given alone. A study of moderate sodium restriction was done in 15 patients who had mild to moderate essential hypertension and who were already taking captopril.

The average supine blood pressure (BP) of the patients when they were not receiving treatment and when sodium was unrestricted was 162/107 mm Hg. Patients received 50 mg of captopril twice a day. After 1 month, the average supine BP had decreased to 149/94 mm Hg. Patients were then instructed to reduce their sodium intake to about 80 mmoles per day. Two weeks later, they were entered into a double-blind, randomized crossover study to compare the effect of ten slow Sodium tablets (100 mmoles of sodium chloride) with matching placebo tablets while captopril therapy and dietary sodium restriction continued. After the patients had taken placebo for 1 month, the mean supine BP was 137/88 mm Hg, and the mean urinary sodium excretion was 83 mmole/24 hour. After the patients had taken Slow Sodium tablets for 1 month, the mean supine BP was 150/97 mm Hg, and the mean sodium excretion was 183 mmole/24 hour, the mean supine BP during moderate sodium restriction therefore decreased by 9% and correlated significantly with the reduction in urinary sodium excretion.

These findings suggest that moderate reduction in sodium intake combined with use of an angiotensin-converting enzyme inhibitor is effective in decreasing the BP in patients with essential hypertension. This approach overcomes some of the objections to salt restriction alone and to converting enzyme inhibitors alone.

▶ It's nice to see that what is theoretically logical works in practice. There are also theoretical reasons why potassium supplements may lower blood pressure, and this too seems to be true in clinical practice (Svetkey et al.: *Hypertension* 9:444–450, 1987, Siani et al.: *Br. Med. J.* 294:1453–1456, 1987). However, I'm not sure that it is worthwhile unless potassium depletion is present.

However, even a little extra potassium as provided in one or two extra servings of fresh fruits and vegetables a day may have benefits beyond any antihypertensive effect.—N.M. Kaplan, M.D.

Dietary Potassium and Stroke-Associated Mortality: A 12-Year Prospective Population Study

Kay-Tee Khaw and Elizabeth Barrett-Connor (Univ. of California, San Diego, and Univ. of Cambridge, England)

N. Engl. J. Med. 316:235–240, Jan. 29, 1987 6–23

The most important known risk factor for stroke is hypertension. Research suggests that a high dietary intake of potassium is associated with lower blood pressure. A high potassium intake has been reported to protect against stroke in hypertensive rats, although blood pressure (BP) was not affected. The relation between the 24-hour dietary potassium intake at baseline and subsequent stroke-associated mortality was studied in a population-based cohort of 859 men and women, aged 50–79 years.

From 1972 to 1974, 82% of all adult residents of a white upper-middle-class community participated in a heart disease risk factor survey. A 15% random sample plus all subjects identified as having hyperlipidemia at the first visit participated in a second evaluation. The subjects were followed up for 12 years. The 356 men and 503 women in the current analysis had no personal history of heart attack, heart failure, or stroke at baseline examination. The baseline distribution of the reported 24-hour intake of nutrients and of cardiovascular risk factors, according

Age-Adjusted 12-Year Stroke-Associated Mortality Rates According to Tertile of Potassium Intake at Base Line in Men and Women Aged 59 to 79 Years

	Men			Women		
	Potassium intake	No.	Rate/100	Potassium intake	No.	Rate/100
	mmol			*mmol*		
	<59	118	3.4	<49	167	5.3
	≥59–76	119	2.4	≥49–66	168	2.1
	≥76	119	0.0	≥67	168	0.0
Relative risk for lowest tertile vs. top two tertiles			2.6			4.8
P value			0.16			0.01

(Courtesy of Khaw, K.-T., and Barrett-Connor, E.: N. Engl. J. Med. 316:235–240, Jan. 29, 1987.)

to 12-year stroke-mortality status, were examined, adjusting for age with use of analysis of variance.

In general, higher mean blood pressures, higher fasting plasma glucose levels, and a higher proportion of smokers were noted among those who subsequently had a stroke; however, the differences in this small cohort were significant only for systolic blood pressure in women and fasting plasma glucose level in men. Only mean age and calorie-adjusted potassium intake were significantly lower in both men and women who later had a stroke-associated death compared with all other subjects. The mean 24-hour potassium intake was 64 mmoles; the range was 17 to 154 mmoles. The stroke rates, according to the tertile of potassium intake (table), suggest a dose response, with no stroke-associated deaths in the highest tertile. For those with potassium intake in the lowest tertile, the relative risks for stroke compared with those in the top two tertiles combined were 2.6 in men and 4.8 in women.

Potassium intake tended to be inversely and independently related to a reduction in stroke in men and women. The effect appeared independent of age, systolic BP, serum cholesterol level, fasting plasma glucose level, obesity, and cigarette smoking. Despite the large imprecision in estimating dietary intake and the relatively small number of stroke-associated deaths in this study, the association observed was strong.

▶ The protection against stroke that was noted with the higher dietary potassium intake is almost too good to be true. But there are animal data of protection against cerebral and renal damage, so an extra banana or two a day shouldn't hurt and may be much better than chicken soup.

Which brings us to milk and cheese, the major dietary sources of calcium. David McCarron and coworkers at the University of Oregon have popularized the concept that hypertensives consume less calcium and that calcium supplements will lower blood pressure. I disagree with both the theory and the practice, but I do believe a small proportion of hypertensives may lower their blood pressure when given extra calciums.—N.M. Kaplan, M.D.

The Calcium Deficiency Hypothesis of Hypertension: A Critique

Norman M. Kaplan and Roderick B. Meese (Univ. of Texas, Dallas)
Ann. Intern. Med. 105:947–955, December 1986 6–24

Recent reports have linked essential hypertension to calcium deficiency, rather than excess. The authors reviewed the evidence used to support this hypothesis and the theoretical construct used to explain it.

Several studies have shown that hypertensive subjects have a lower dietary calcium intake than normotensive subjects. However, these studies suffer from methodologic shortcomings, and the relationship between dietary calcium and blood pressure remains uncertain. Some researchers have reported a lower serum concentration of ionized calcium in hypertensive subjects than in normotensive subjects. Many studies, however, show small differences, which may reflect nonspecific alterations. Current

EFFECT OF CALCIUM SUPPLEMENTS ON BLOOD PRESSURE

Author (Reference)	Subjects	Study Design	Calcium Supplement		Blood Pressure Response
			Dose	Duration	
	n		*g*		
Normotensive persons					
Belizan et al.	30	Parallel with placebo	1	22 wks	↓ diastolic 6%-9%
McCarron and Morris	32	Crossover with placebo	1	8 wks	No change
Sunderrajan and Bauer	7	Crossover with placebo	1	6 wks	↑ 5/2 mm Hg
Hypertensive persons					
McCarron and Morris	48	Crossover with placebo	1	8 wks	↓ 4/2 mm Hg (supine)
Resnick et al.	15	Open, no placebo	2	5 mos	↓ diastolic 4 mm Hg
Grobbee and Hofman	90	Double-blind parallel with placebo	1	12 wks	↓ diastolic 2.3 mm Hg
Strazzullo et al.	15	Crossover with placebo	1	15 wks	↓ mean blood pressure 0.6 mm Hg
Singer et al.	18	Crossover with placebo	1.6	4 wks	No change
Meese et al.	26	Double-blind crossover with placebo	0.8	8 wks	↓ 0.4 mm Hg sitting mean blood pressure

(Courtesy of Kaplan, N.M., and Meese, R.B.: Ann. Intern. Med. 105:947–955, December 1986.)

data on this subject are inconsistent: some researchers find higher levels in platelets from hypertensive patients, but some do not.

It has been reported that patients with essential hypertension excrete more calcium in their urine. A likely explanation for this finding is increased intake and excretion of sodium. The hypothesis further holds that the putative vasoconstricting effect of calcium depletion is somehow revealed in a compensatory increase in parathyroid hormone. However, research findings do not necessarily support this, and may in fact weaken this hypothesis. There are few published studies on the effects of dietary calcium supplementation in humans (table). In these studies, the response to calcium has been variable.

It appears that there is little support for the basic premise of the calcium deficiency hypothesis—that the limited changes in extracellular calcium concentration seen in patients with essential hypertension could have the proposed paradoxical effects on vascular contraction and relaxation. The authors believe that the calcium deficiency hypothesis cannot now be accepted, but that it deserves further investigation.

▶ I cannot comment further on our own writing except to say that subsequent experience has supported my belief that hypertension is not related to calcium deficiency and that calcium supplements likely will not lower blood pressure in most people.

However, I may be wrong.—N.M. Kaplan, M.D.

Blood Pressure and Metabolic Effects of Calcium Supplementation in Normotensive White and Black Men

Roseann M. Lyle, Christopher L. Melby, Gerald C. Hyner, James W. Edmondson, Judy Z. Miller, and Myron H. Weinberger (Purdue Univ., West Lafayette, Ind., and Indiana Univ., Indianapolis)

JAMA 257:1772–1776, April 3, 1987 6–25

A possible relationship between dietary calcium and blood pressure has been noted in observational and experimental research. The authors carried out a randomized, double-blind, placebo-controlled study to examine the effect of calcium supplementation on blood pressure in 21 normotensive black men and 54 normotensive white men.

After a 4-week baseline period, in which blood pressure was measured weekly, volunteer subjects, aged 19–52 years, were randomized within racial groups to either a treatment or placebo group for 12 weeks. The treatment group received 1,500 mg of calcium per day. Multiple blood pressure measurements were taken every 2 weeks in the seated and supine positions, using a random baseline sphygmomanometer. The treatment group ended with lower seated and supine systolic and diastolic blood pressure than the placebo group. No differences were seen between racial groups. Seated and supine mean arterial blood pressure values were also lower in the calcium group compared with the placebo group. The overall blood pressure-lowering effect was not correlated with the response of total and ionized serum calcium levels, total inorganic phosphorus, parathyroid hormone, or overnight urinary electrolyte values.

Supplementation with 1,500 mg per day of calcium, in a divided dose of 500 mg three times a day, produced modest but significantly lower systolic and diastolic blood pressure in seated and supine positions in white and black men compared with a placebo group. Differences in mean arterial pressure were small (2–3 mm Hg), but consistent. No difference in response was seen between the races.

▶ This study was done in normotensives. Calcium supplements have also been found to lower blood pressure by 4–5 mm Hg in a group of healthy pregnant women during the last trimester (Villar et al.: *Obstet. Gynecol.* 70:317–322, 1987).

However, we (Meese et al.: *Am. J. Med. Sci.* 294:219–224, 1987) and others (Zoccali et al.: *J. Hypertens.* 4(suppl. 6):S676–S678, 1986) continue to find little overall effect. On the other hand, hypertensives may have hypercalciuria (likely induced by excessive sodium intake), which will lower ionized calcium levels and cause a slight degree of secondary hyperparathyroidism, as shown in animals with volume-expanded forms of hypertension (Kageyama, Y., Bravo, E.L.: *Hypertension* 9(suppl. III):166–170, 1987). The increased PTH levels may raise the blood pressure. If extra calcium is given and ionized calcium raised, the PTH levels will be normalized, so that the blood pressure could fall—but at the cost of even more hypercalciuria.

In view of the evidence noted earlier that hypertension is associated (? caused) by increased intracellular calcium (Lechi et al.: *Hypertension* 9:230–235, 1987), I believe the best course is to encourage normal dietary calcium intake but not to give extra calcium in hopes of lowering blood pressure.

We'll find out, sooner or later, who's right. In the meantime, let's watch out for the saturated fat in many dairy products while increasing unsaturated fat intake.—N.M. Kaplan, M.D.

Associations of Dietary Fat, Regional Adiposity, and Blood Pressure in Men

Paul T. Williams, Stephen P. Fortmann, Richard B. Terry, Susan C. Garay, Karen M. Vranizan, Nancy Ellsworth, and Peter D. Wood (Stanford Univ.)

JAMA 257:3251–3256, June 19, 1987 6–26

The low incidence of cardiovascular disease and hypertension among Mediterranean populations may be partly due to dietary factors, particularly a relatively high intake of monounsaturated fat as olive oil. A cross-sectional survey of 76 middle-aged American men was done to investigate the relationship between monounsaturated fat intake and blood pressure (BP).

The subjects were sedentary men, aged 30–55 years, with resting BPs below 160/100 mm Hg. Nutritional components, as grams per 4,200 kJ, from 3-day food records were examined in association with resting BP. Systolic and diastolic BPs were found to correlate significantly and inversely with consumption of monounsaturated fat. Polyunsaturated fat intake also correlated inversely with diastolic BP; however, this relationship became nonsignificant after adjustments were made for an index of regional adiposity that characterizes male-type obesity patterns. The correlations with monounsaturated fat intake were found to be specific to oleic acid; the correlation with polyunsaturated fat intake was specific to linoleic acid. Multiple regression analysis was done, and 18.2% of the variance in systolic BP and 23.2% of the variance in diastolic BP were found to be related to monounsaturated and polyunsaturated fat consumption and regional adiposity.

These correlations reveal a significant, unexplained association between increasing levels of monounsaturated fat intake and decreasing levels of systolic and diastolic BP. Polyunsaturated fat consumption was also found to correlate inversely with diastolic BP. Causality remains to be determined.

▶ The Mediterranean diet, rich in olive oil, garlic, and wine, may be protective against cardiovascular disease in general and hypertension in particular. Too few controlled intervention trials have been done to settle the blood pressure issue, but pasta with lots of olive oil and garlic, some seafood, and Chianti cannot possibly be bad.

However, too much Chianti may undo all the advantages.—N.M. Kaplan, M.D.

Alcohol Consumption and Hypertension

Stephen MacMahon (Natl. Heart, Lung, and Blood Inst., Bethesda, Md.)

Hypertension 9:111–121, February 1987 6–27

For many years, it has been recognized that persons with high alcohol consumption have an increased prevalence of hypertension. Recent studies have suggested that an independent association exists between alcohol intake and blood pressure (BP) levels in samples from general populations. The authors reviewed 30 cross-sectional population studies on this subject.

Most researchers reported small but significant elevations in BP in persons who drank three or more alcoholic beverages a day when compared with nondrinkers. In 25% of the studies reviewed, increases in BP were also reported at lower levels of alcohol consumption. In about 40% of the studies, the BP of nondrinkers was found to be greater than that of persons who had consumed one to two drinks a day. In one study from the United States and one from Australia, the maximum contribution to the prevalence of hypertension of alcohol consumption of more than two drinks a day was estimated to be 5% to 7%; it was greater in men than in women because of greater alcohol consumption.

In five studies, a prospective association of alcohol intake with changes in BP was found. In a small number of experimental studies, short-term decreases in BP accompanied alcohol restriction in normotensive and hypertensive subjects. Uncontrolled observations of heavy drinkers suggest that the effect on BP of alcohol withdrawal may be lasting.

The available evidence clearly indicates that BP, the prevalence of hypertension, and the rate of increase in BP over time are significantly elevated in heavy drinkers. Alcohol withdrawal may result in a decrease in BP in such patients, and BP may even drop to normotensive levels after a period of abstinence. However, definite conclusions about the long-term effects of alcohol restriction on moderate drinkers require more research.

▶ My reading of the extensive literature so nicely summarized in this review is that an ounce of ethanol per day, as contained in two portions of beer, wine, or whiskey, will not raise blood pressure but will protect against coronary heart disease. On the other hand, the evidence that 2 ounces or more of ethanol per day will raise blood pressure continues to mount (Lang et al.: *J. Chronic Dis.* 7:713–720, 1987). Excess alcohol intake is likely the most common cause of reversible hypertension among men.

Those who are under high levels of stress may drink more, and the combination may be particularly bad for blood pressure (De Frank et al.: *Psychosom. Med.* 49:236–249, 1987).—N.M. Kaplan, M.D.

Stressful Work Conditions and Diastolic Blood Pressure Among Blue Collar Factory Workers

Karen A. Matthews, Eric M. Cottington, Evelyn Talbott, Lewis H. Kuller, and Judith M. Siegel (Univ. of Pittsburgh and Univ. of California, Los Angeles)

Am. J. Epidemiol. 126:280–291, August 1987 6–28

The relation of stressful work conditions to blood pressure is of considerable interest. The authors studied the relation between stressful work conditions that were due to the nature of the work, organizational structure, or interactions with coworkers, and diastolic blood pressure in 288 male blue collar workers aged 40–63 years. The men had worked for 10 years or longer at one of two plants in Pittsburgh. Forty-seven men who had been treated for previously diagnosed hypertension were excluded.

Several work conditions were significant predictors of diastolic blood pressure when age, body mass, alcohol and cigarette use, and family history of hypertension were controlled for. Overall job dissatisfaction was a predictive factor. Men with higher diastolic pressure had relatively little opportunity for promotion, had participated little in work decisions, and had an uncertain job future. These subjects reported a lack of support by coworkers and foremen, as well as difficulty in communicating with others. Overall job satisfaction was related to lower diastolic pressure in men who were rated as having good overall working conditions.

These findings support a role for stressful work conditions in higher diastolic blood pressure, independently of major risk factors for hypertension. Satisfaction with work and working in a relatively good environment appear to protect against elevated diastolic blood pressure.

▶ Relief of stress by whatever manner, including improved working conditions, may lower blood pressure. Relaxation training at the worksite, however, doesn't seem to help reduce blood pressure much more than simply monitoring the blood pressure among either unmedicated mild hypertensives (Chesney et al.: *Psychosom. Med.* 49:250–263, 1987) or poorly controlled, treated patients (Agras et al.: *Psychosom. Med.* 49:264–273, 1987).

Another form of relaxation—for many but not, I'm sorry to say, for me—is exercise, and it more likely provides an antihypertensive effect.—N.M. Kaplan, M.D.

Antihypertensive and Volume-Depleting Effects of Mild Exercise on Essential Hypertension

Hidenori Urata, Yoichi Tanabe, Akira Kiyonaga, Masaharu Ikeda, Hiroaki Tanaka, Munehiro Shindo, and Kikuo Arakawa (Fukuoka Univ., Japan)
Hypertension 9:245–252, March 1987 6–29

Despite widespread interest in nonpharmacologic therapy for hypertension, physical exercise had not been accepted as an effective antihypertensive therapy. There have been no well-controlled studies of such factors as age, sex, and race, and the related mechanisms of the antihypertensive effects of exercise remain unclear. A study was done to confirm the depressor effects of exercise and to analyze changes in hemodynamics.

Twenty Japanese subjects with essential hypertension were clinically observed for 4 weeks and then randomly divided into two groups. The first group, consisting of four men and six women, aged 51.4 ± 2.8 years, agreed to physical training using bicycle ergometer exercise with the intensity at blood lactate threshold for 1 hour three times a week for 10 weeks. The second group, also four men and six women aged 51 ± 2.9 years, did no particular physical training and were examined once a week. Changes in blood pressure and hemodynamic and humoral factors of the exercise group were compared with those of the control group.

Blood pressure and whole blood and plasma volume indices were significantly reduced in the exercise group compared with controls. The change in ratio of serum sodium to potassium was found to correlate positively with the change in systolic blood pressure. Plasma norepinephrine concentrations at rest and at the work load of blood lactate threshold during graded exercise tests were also significantly reduced in the exercise group after 10 weeks of exercising. The change in the resting level of plasma norepinephrine correlated positively with the change in mean blood pressure. These changes were not seen in the control group. Body weight and urinary sodium excretion showed no significant change in either group.

In this controlled study in well-matched subjects, the antihypertensive effect of mild exercise training was confirmed. Reduction in blood volume and reduction in plasma norepinephrine concentration were apparently associated.

▶ This is another well-controlled study that confirms an antihypertensive effect of regular isotonic exercise, likely mediated by a dampening of sympathetic nervous activity.

No one has put all of these various nondrug therapies together. The result could be a phenomenal antihypertensive interaction, but it's more likely that only so much can be obtained by any or all of them. Which leads us to consider what will work with more certainty but with more potential side effects—the rapidly expanding group of antihypertensive drugs.—N.M. Kaplan, M.D.

Antihypertensive Drugs

▶ ↓ The list keeps growing although no new classes of drugs were added in 1987. What we now have is essentially seven classes of drugs: (1) diuretics; (2) central α-agonists; (3) α-blockers; (4) β-blockers; (5) direct vasodilators; (6) converting enzyme inhibitors; and (7) calcium entry blockers.

For a number of reasons, our use of the available drugs is rapidly changing, as noted in the next two abstracts.—N.M. Kaplan, M.D.

Rational Therapies for Hypertension: Is Step 1 of Stepped Care Archaic?
Harriet P. Dustan (Univ. of Alabama, Birmingham)
Circulation 75:96–100, January 1987 6–30

Because of the bewildering array of antihypertensive drugs with many different mechanisms of action, the Joint National Committees on the Detection Evaluation, and Treatment of Hypertension (JNC) provided physicians with "stepped care" guidelines, indicating first-treatment drugs and alternative therapies as needed. New information suggests that step 1 of stepped care is archaic, that different types of hypertension should be treated more specifically, and that racial factors are more important in therapy response than was previously thought, rendering therapies appropriate for white patients ineffective for black patients.

Much of the hypertension that physicians treat is mild. The 1984 JNC report recommends stepped care for patients with diastolic pressures of 95 mm Hg or above, the first step being half a dose of a diuretic or a β blocker, with increase if needed. However, accumulating evidence suggests that rational therapy for mild hypertension is not stepped care, but the use of a drug that reduces sympathetic vasomotor outflow or blocks adrenergic receptors, both α and β types. Ample evidence shows that mild hypertension has a neurogenic component. Hemodynamic and humoral characteristics of borderline hypertension have been defined, and some patients with mild hypertension have been found to have increased plasma renin activity and plasma norepinephrine concentrations. Plasma norepinephrine levels appear to be higher in younger hypertensive patients.

Research on hypertension in black patients clearly establishes diuretic therapy as the first-line treatment of choice for all but the most severe forms of hypertension. For patients with severe essential hypertension, the approach should not be step 1 of stepped care, but a direct attack on arteriolar vasoconstriction through the use of a potent vasodilator; initial therapy with sublingual nifedipine followed by oral nifedipine or minoxidil has proved effective.

The next few years will see development of more specific therapies and recommendations on how best to use different types of drugs in treating hypertension. The usefulness of angiotensin-converting enzyme inhibitors and calcium-channel blockers will be determined. Hypertension in the elderly is another topic that should be clarified in the near future.

Evolution of the Clinical Management of Hypertension: Emerging Role of "Specific" Vasodilators as Initial Therapy

Victor J. Dzau (Harvard Univ.)

Am. J. Med. 82(Suppl. IA):36–43, Jan. 5, 1987 6–31

Essential hypertension is characterized by elevated systemic vascular resistance that may reflect increased sympathetic tone, activation of the renin-angiotensin system, or structural and cellular abnormalities (e.g., those involving calcium) of the blood vessel wall. The goal of therapy should be to reduce vascular tone through the use of a specific blocker of neurohormonal mechanisms or a nonspecific vasodilator. The use of vasodilators as initial therapy in patients with hypertension is reviewed, with emphasis on metabolic side effects, effects on left ventricular hypertrophy, hemodynamic effects, and mechanism of action.

Vasodilators are not equally effective in all patients. Important considerations are pathophysiology, patient characteristics, mechanism of drug action, long-term efficacy, and metabolic effects. Studies have suggested that there is a better response to angiotensin converting enzyme inhibitors in young and middle-aged patients, while the elderly may have more of a response to calcium channel blockers. Alpha$_1$-adrenergic blockers seem to be effective for all age groups. In black patients, calcium channel blockers and α_1-adrenergic blockers are generally more effective than angiotensin converting enzyme inhibitors; neither of these drugs adversely affects serum potassium, glucose, or plasma lipid levels. In fact, studies suggest that α_1-adrenergic blockers may decrease low-density lipoprotein cholesterol and triglyceride levels and increase high-density lipoprotein cholesterol levels. Calcium channel blockers may have a negative inotropic effect and improve cardiac diastolic relaxation, unlike α-adrenergic blockers and angiotensin-converting enzyme inhibitors.

Commonly used antihypertensive regimens have not reduced the incidence of myocardial infarction or sudden death. This has prompted the evaluation of alternative antihypertensive drugs. Ideally, an antihypertensive agent should be efficacious, with little or no development of patient tolerance in long-term therapy, have few bothersome side effects, and have no adverse effects on other cardiovascular risk factors.

▶ These two experts (Abstracts 6–30 and 6–31) both agree that we must go beyond "diuretic-first, step-care" to incorporate new and proved antihypertensive agents that offer the likelihood of better long-term protection against coronary disease and less interference with the quality of life. Dr. Dustan (Abstract 6–30) likes diuretics for most hypertensive blacks, adrenergic inhibitors for most younger patients, and vasodilators for those with more severe degrees of hypertension. Dr. Dzau (Abstract 6–31) prefers one or another vasodilator, including α-blockers, ACE inhibitors, and calcium entry blockers. My view leans toward Dr. Dzau's.

What we all have to realize is that there is no one right answer. We are blessed with a variety of effective drugs. As the Fourth Joint National Committee report (published in the *Archives of Internal Medicine* in May 1988) indicates, the best course is to pick and choose from various classes, the choice based largely on the type of patient. Whatever the first choice, if it doesn't work or causes side effects the wise course is to stop it and substitute another drug from another class.

The next nine abstracts review recent experience with the major classes of drugs now available.—N.M. Kaplan, M.D.

Beta-Blockers Versus Diuretics in Hypertensive Men: Main Results From the HAPPHY Trial

Lars Wilhelmsen, Göran Berglund, Dag Elmfeldt, Timothy Fitzsimons, Heinz Holzgreve, James Hosie, Per-Erik Hörnkvist, Kjell Pennert, Jaakko Tuomilehto, and Hans Wedel (Univ. of Göteborg, Östra Hosp., Göteborg, Sweden, and other institutions on behalf of the Heart Attack Primary Prevention in Hypertension Trial Research Group)

J. Hypertension 5:561–574, October 1987 6–32

When the Heart Attack Primary Prevention in Hypertension (HAPPHY) Trial was first designed in 1975–1976, thiazide diuretics and β-blockers were as first-line drugs in the treatment of hypertension. Because some results indicated that β-blockers are effective in the treatment of myocardial infarction, it was hypothesized that they might also reduce the incidence of myocardial infarction and sudden coronary death in hypertensive patients who had no evidence of coronary heart disease (CHD). The purpose of the HAPPHY Trial was to compare the effectiveness of β-blockers in the prevention of primary CHD with that of thiazide diuretics.

The study population included 6,569 men, aged 40–64 years, with mild to moderate hypertension, defined as a diastolic blood pressure of 100–130 mm Hg, who were randomized to undergo treatment with a thiazide diuretic (n = 3,272), either bendroflumethiazide or hydrochlorothiazide, or treatment with a β-blocker (n = 3,297), either atenolol or metoprolol. Men with previous CHD, stroke, or other serious diseases were excluded. Patients were assessed at 6-monthly intervals.

There was no difference in the incidence of CHD between the two groups, and the total mortality in both groups was similar. The BP-reducing effect was also similar for both study groups. The incidence of fatal stroke tended to be lower in the β-blocker-treated group than in the thiazide-treated group. Although the percentage of patients withdrawn because of side effects was similar for both study groups, β-blocker-treated patients reported a higher incidence of side effects.

The most important finding of the HAPPHY Trial was that neither thiazide diuretics nor β-blockers reduced the incidence of CHD morbidity and mortality among the participants in this study.

▶ This was not a controlled trial of therapy versus nontherapy, since all patients were treated. However, it provides further evidence that β-blockers, which have been shown to provide secondary prevention of CHD to those who have already had an MI, are no better than diuretics in providing primary protection against CHD.

Since all were treated, we do not know if treatment reduced the overall rate of cardiovascular disease. However, we know that both diuretics and non-ISA β-blockers, the drugs used in the HAPPHY trial, will often cause lipid derangements that may reduce their ability to reduce CHD. Therefore, there is a growing attraction toward other types of drugs that are equally effective as antihypertensives but that do not alter lipids.—N.M. Kaplan, M.D.

Alpha-$_1$-Adrenergic Blockade and Lipoprotein Metabolism in Essential Hypertension

Claudia Ferrier, Carlo Beretta-Piccoli, Peter Weidmann, and Rubino Mordasini (Univ. of Bern, Switzerland)

Clin. Pharmacol. Ther. 40:525–530, November 1986 6–33

Terazosin, a new quinazoline compound with sympatholytic activity mediated by postsynaptic α_1-adrenergic blockade, has been shown effective in lowering blood pressure. Its half-life is about 12 hours, longer than that of prazosin, which explains its long-lasting antihypertensive action. To determine the effect of this new compound on lipid metabolism, serum lipoproteins, and certain important blood pressure-modulating factors, 4 women and 11 men, aged 31–61 years, with mild to moderate essential hypertension were studied. Five subjects had type II hyperlipoproteinemia of mild degree and 1 had mild type IV hyperlipoproteinemia.

Terazosin was given in one daily dose for 8 weeks at weekly increasing doses of 2, 5, 10, and 20 mg. Terasozin reduced arterial pressure after 8 weeks from 153/103 to 143/96 mm Hg, but did not modify body weight, heart rate, blood volume, plasma renin activity, aldosterone and catecholamine levels, or serum cholesterol, triglycerides, and their lipoprotein fractions. Blood pressure control was not achieved in 9 patients with terazosin alone, and the diuretic methyclothiazide, 2.5 mg, was added. Eight weeks after the initiation of combined therapy, blood pressure decreased further, and serum lipids and lipoprotein fractions did not change compared with placebo or terazosin alone.

In this study, the treatment of 15 patients with mild to moderate essential hypertension with the selective postsynaptic α_1-adrenergic antagonist terazosin for 8 weeks did not produce significant changes in cholesterol or triglyceride metabolism. Results suggest that terazosin does not unfavorably affect lipid metabolism. The addition of the diuretic methyclothiazide in 9 patients was not associated with variations in serum total or low-density lipoprotein cholesterol levels; thus, α_1-blockade may prevent the thiazide-related alterations in cholesterol metabolism.

▶ These data show that the new once-a-day α_1-blocker, terazosin, will lower blood pressure modestly, without adversely changing lipids. Similar or even better results have been shown for prazosin and yet another α_1-blocker, doxazosin (Hjortdahl et al.: *Acta Med. Scand.* 221:427–434, 1987). Therefore, the α-blockers as a class provide an antihypertensive effect that may be limited by a tendency toward fluid retention if they are used alone (Izzo et al.: *Am. J. Cardiol.* 60:303–308, 1987), but which is usually accompanied by a lowering of total cholesterol.

The other advantage of this class of drugs is the ability to increase cardiac output during physical activity, unlike the impairment seen with β-blocker which may reduce the ability of patients to exercise. Beta-blockers may also cause some other undesirable effects, including some within the CNS.—N.M. Kaplan, M.D.

Central Nervous System Effects of β-Adrenergic–Blocking Drugs: The Role of Ancillary Properties

John B. Kostis and Raymond C. Rosen (Rutgers Med. School, New Brunswick, N.J.)

Circulation 75:204–212, January 1987 6–34

β-Adrenergic–blocking drugs, widely used to treat hypertension, angina, arrhythmias, and other noncardiovascular conditions, may have adverse effects on the CNS. The effects of four β-blockers with different ancillary properties were compared on objective and subjective measures of CNS function in 30 healthy men.

Atenolol, metoprolol, propranolol, and pindolol were tested. The subjects, aged 23–40 years, were randomly assigned to take drug or placebo for five 1-week periods separated by 2-week washout periods. At the end of each treatment period, evaluations were performed, including multistage exercise stress testing; questionnaire assessment of mood state, sexual function, and sleep habits; tests of psychomotor function; and overnight polysomnographic sleep measures. Each of the drugs had significant effects on sleep continuity: the mean number of awakenings was 6.4 ± 5 for pindolol, 6.3 ± 3.8 for propranolol, 7.2 ± 4.7 for metoprolol, and 3.6 ± 2.9 for atenolol. The mean number of awakenings for those taking placebo was 3.9 ± 2.7.

Time of wakefulness was 20.6 ± 27 minutes for pindolol, 15.5 ± 23 minutes for propranolol, 19.5 ± 24.3 minutes for metoprolol, 10.2 ± 11.6 minutes for atenolol, and 9.2 ± 74.5 minutes for placebo. Rapid eye movement sleep time was significantly affected only by pindolol; it was 74.5 ± 19.0 minutes for those receiving placebo and 54.5 ± 21.9 minutes for those taking pindolol. Rapid eye movement latency was 175 ± 60.7 minutes with pindolol and 95.4 ± 43.8 minutes with placebo. Subjects also reported increased wakefulness and greater restlessness with the lipophilic β-blockers on subjective measures. Higher depression scores were found to be associated with pindolol and propranolol, but other measures of psychomotor and sexual function did not show a consistent pattern of results. During exercise, all β-blockers depressed heart rate.

These findings provide strong evidence that the CNS effects of β-blockers are modulated by the ancillary properties of the drugs, such as lipophilicity and intrinsic sympathomimetic activity.

▶ Although this carefully performed study confirms that various β-blockers may have diverse adverse effects on sleep and other CNS functions, the bad rap that propranolol received from a survey of antidepressant medication use (Avorn et al.: *JAMA* 225:357–360, 1986) may not be warranted. At least, no more depressive symptoms were noted in a group of patients taking a β-blocker than in a group receiving other medications (Carney et al.: *Am. J. Med.* 83:223–226, 1987).

Nonetheless, the various side effects noted with both diuretics and β-blockers have made the two newly approved classes of antihypertensives—calcium blockers and ACE inhibitors—even more attractive.—N.M. Kaplan, M.D.

Calcium-Channel Blockers in Systemic Hypertension

William H. Frishman, Jack A. Stroh, Steven M. Greenberg, Theresa Suarez, Adam Karp, and Harry B. Peled (Albert Einstein College of Medicine, New York)

Curr. Probl. Cardiol. 12:285–346, May 1987 6–35

Calcium-channel blockers interfere with the normal transmembrane flux of extracellular calcium ions, on which vascular tissue depends for contraction or impulse generation. These agents decrease the contractile activity of the heart and promote coronary and systemic vasodilatation. These effects constitute the clinical rationale for using calcium-channel blockers in the treatment of ischemic heart disease, hypertrophic cardiomyopathy, and certain arrhythmias. Because systemic vasodilatation is expected to reduce elevated blood pressure, clinicians have become interested in using calcium antagonists in the management of systemic hypertension.

The calcium antagonists have been used alone and in combination with other antihypertensive drugs. Their use has also been investigated in hypertensive crisis and in patients with angina pectoris. The calcium-channel blockers have been shown to be remarkably safe in the treatment of hypertension. Side effects include headache, dizziness, gastrointestinal effects, flushing, paresthesia, decreased sinoatrial or atrioventricular node conduction, congestive heart failure, hypotension, pedal edema, and worsening of angina. The overall frequencies of these effects from diltiazem, verapamil, and nifedipine range from 5% to 20%. There appear to be no adverse effects on concentrations of glucoregulatory hormones, parathyroid hormone, plasma lipids and lipoproteins, uric acid, and serum electrolytes when therapeutic doses are used. Calcium-channel blockers are contraindicated for patients with serious cardiac conduction abnormalities and patients with overt congestive heart failure.

Scientific rationale and clinical investigation have suggested that calcium-channel blockers may have an important role in the treatment of systemic hypertension. Further clinical research and use will ultimately define their place in the stepped-care approach to hypertension.

▶ The advantage of calcium-channel blockers in the treatment of systemic hypertension, as listed in the article, are (1) no deleterious effects on lipid profile and glucoregulatory hormones; (2) no kaluretic actions; (3) safety of use in patients with bronchospasm, peripheral vascular disease, and renal dysfunction; (4) little incidence of depression and sexual dysfunction; (5) effectiveness in treating coexisting angina pectoris and/or arrhythmias; and (6) effectiveness in treating black as well as white patients, old and young patients. The disadvantages are that calcium–channel blockers can exacerbate congestive heart failure and can adversely affect atrioventricular and sinus node function.

The advantages far outweigh the disadvantages. Moreover, these agents do not impair responses to physical or mental stress.—N.M. Kaplan, M.D.

Disparate Hemodynamic Responses to Mental Challenge After Antihypertensive Therapy With Beta Blockers and Calcium Entry Blockers

Roland E. Schmieder, Heinz Rueddel, Herman Neus, Franz H. Messerli, and August W. Von Eiff (Univ. of Bonn, West Germany, and Ochsner Clinic and Alton Ochsner Med. Found., New Orleans)

Am. J. Med. 82:11–16, January 1987 6–36

Because pressure readings at patients' work sites are of greater prognostic value for coronary artery disease fatality and correlate better with the degree of left ventricular hypertrophy than casual pressure readings, the impact of any antihypertensive agent on cardiovascular reactivity during stress is most important. The hemodynamic response to mental challenge was investigated in 40 men with mild essential hypertension.

Twenty patients were treated with the β adrenoreceptor blocker, oxprenolol, and 20 received the calcium entry blocker, nitrendipine. Cardiovascular reactivity was assessed during two mental arithmetic tasks before and 6 months after treatment by continuously measuring systolic and diastolic pressure with the ultrasonic Doppler device, heart rate by electrocardiography, and stroke volume by impedance cardiography. Patients in both treatment groups had equal arterial pressure decreases and the same pressures at rest. In patients taking nitrendipine, mental challenge provoked an increase in stroke volume and a decrease in total peripheral resistance similar to that in the pretreatment phase. In contrast, oxprenolol reversed the hemodynamic response pattern to a distinct decrease in stroke volume and an increase in total peripheral resistance. Attenuated heart rate responses and larger increases in diastolic pressure were found in the β-blocker group compared with the calcium entry blocker group.

These results demonstrated that although β-blockers and calcium blockers produce equal decreases in arterial pressure, β-blockers evoke an abnormal hemodynamic response to mental challenge, whereas calcium entry blockers preserve the physiologic reactivity pattern of the untreated state.

▶ This study shows that the response to mental stress is well preserved during therapy with calcium entry blockers. Similarly, the response to physical stress is well maintained (Mooy et al.: *Clin. Pharmacol. Ther.* 41:490–495, 1987).

Another potential advantage of this group of drugs is their ability to preserve or to increase renal blood flow (Sunderrajan et al.: *Am. Heart J.* 114:383–388, 1987). This may eventuate in a slight natriuresis and a greater likelihood that their antihypertensive effect will not be blunted by volume retention so that diuretics will be less needed with them.

There is some evidence that the effectiveness of calcium entry blockers may, in fact, be blunted by concomitant use of a diuretic or a lower sodium intake.—N.M. Kaplan, M.D.

The Effects of Bendroflumethiazide Added to Nifedipine in Patients With Hypertension

A.V. Zezulka, J.S. Gill, and D.G. Beevers (Dudley Road Hosp., Birmingham, England)

J. Clin. Pharmacol. 27:41–45, January 1987 6–37

Calcium-channel blocker therapy does not normalize blood pressure in all hypertensive patients, and additional drugs are sometimes necessary. It has been suggested that combining a calcium-channel blocker with a diuretic may not produce additional hypertensive effect and may aggravate biochemical side effects. The authors studied the blood pressure changes and metabolic consequences of adding the thiazide diuretic, bendroflumethiazide, to the calcium-channel blocker, nifedipine, in 17 patients with essential hypertension.

Patients had persistent mild to moderate hypertension that was uncontrolled by treatment with nifedipine slow-release tablets, 20 mg twice daily. Eight patients received bendroflumethiazide, 5 mg, before, and 9 received the same dose of the drug after taking placebo in a double-blind, randomized cross-over trial. Supine systolic and diastolic blood pressure were significantly reduced in both groups after therapy with bendroflumethiazide: 170/108 to 156/98 mm Hg and 166/105 to 150/96 mm Hg, respectively. In patients taking the drug before placebo, the treatment effect was sustained into the placebo period without significant difference between placebo and the end of the drug therapy phase, which was attributed to a carry-over effect of active treatment. A reduction in serum potassium level and a rise in serum uric acid concentration were seen.

A further reduction of blood pressure can be obtained by adding bendroflumethiazide to the treatment of patients whose hypertension is uncontrolled with nifedipine alone. The adverse metabolic changes seen were those that would be expected from this combination.

▶ Similar enhancement of the effectiveness of diltiazem by the addition of hydrochlorothiazide has been reported (Massie et al.: *Ann. Intern. Med.* 107:150–157, 1987). Nonetheless, calcium entry blockers seems equally effective with a high sodium intake as with a low sodium intake (Nicholson et al.: *Ann. Intern. Med.* 107:329–334, 1987), and these drugs may be particularly effective in hypertensives who are presumably volume-expanded, as reflected by low levels of plasma renin activity (Resnick et al.: *Hypertension* 19:254–258, 1987). Thus, calcium entry blockers may be particularly efficacious in low-renin hypertension, a general characteristic of elderly and black patients.

On the other hand, drugs that directly inhibit the renin-angiotensin system might be expected to be less effective in patients with low renin activity. The most direct inhibitors of this system are the angiotensin-converting enzyme (ACE) inhibitors, three of which are now available. In practice, they appear to be slightly less effective, overall, in blacks and elderly hypertensives. But these drugs seem to offer some special advantages for patients with renal insufficiency.—N.M. Kaplan, M.D.

Renal Protective Effect of Strict Blood Pressure Control With Enalapril Therapy

John H. Bauer, Garry P. Reams, and Sunder M. Lal (Univ. of Missouri)
Arch. Intern. Med. 147:1397–1400, August 1987 6–38

The effect of strict blood pressure control on progression of renal disease in patients with essential hypertension has not been well defined. Twenty-three patients, aged 33–68 years, with essential hypertension were evaluated prospectively for 3 years to assess their renal function response to either enalapril or enalapril-hydrochlorothiazide therapy. The mean dose of enalapril was 15 mg per day when used alone, and 20.7 mg per day when used in combination with hydrochlorothiazide (mean dose, 51.5 mg per day). A 4.5- 5-gm sodium diet was advised.

Blood pressure was well controlled with either enalapril or enalapril-hydrochlorothiazide therapy. Glomerular filtration rate, as assessed by serum creatinine level, creatinine clearance, or inulin clearance, was maintained, while effective renal plasma flow showed a sustained 17% increase throughout the observation period. Twelve patients initially exhibiting moderately impaired renal function (initial inulin clearance $\leq$ 13 ml per second) demonstrated a 50% increase in inulin clearance and 39% increase in para-aminohippurate clearance in the first year, and 33% and 47% increases in the third year, respectively. Filtration fraction and urinary protein excretion were unchanged. Patients initially exhibiting normal renal function showed no changes in renal function indices.

Long-term blood pressure control with the angiotensin-converting enzyme inhibitor enalapril or enalapril-hydrochlorothiazide is associated with preservation or improvement in renal function. The renal protective effects of enalapril in patients with moderately impaired renal function can be due to mitigation of the effects of angiotensin II and/or to concurrent reduction of glomerular capillary hydraulic pressure.

▶ As we shall see in Abstract 6–47, there is a particular interest in preservation of renal function in patients with diabetic nephropathy, and ACE inhibitors are currently under careful scrutiny for this purpose.

In the meantime, ACE inhibitors are being used increasingly and proving effective as monotherapy (Sassano et al.: *Am. J. Med.* 83:227–235, 1987) or in combination with a diuretic (Webster et al.: *J. Hypertens.* 5:457–460, 1987) or with a calcium entry blocker for those with more severe hypertension (Singer et al.: *Hypertension* 9:629–633, 1987).

A large part of the growing enthusiasm for this class of drugs is the widely held belief that they cause fewer side effects than other agents, as noted in reports of large-scale post-marketing surveillance (Cooper et al.: *J. Royal Coll. Gen. Pract.* 37:346–349, 1987; Chalmers et al.: *Br. J. Clin. Pharmacol.* 24:343–349, 1987).

However, a side effect that was claimed to be quite rare—cough—turns out to be quite common, with reports of a frequency as high as 10% of patients (Fuller and Choudry: *Br. Med. J.* 295:1025–1026, 1987). The cough may reflect increased levels of bradykinin. Another, more serious but much less common problem is the inability to sustain fluid volume and blood pressure in the face of gastrointestinal fluid loss from acute diarrheal diseases (Murray and Matthews: *Postgrad. Med. J.* 63:385–387, 1987).

All in all, ACE inhibitors are another effective group of antihypertensive drugs, neither the magic bullet nor the totally benign agents that some (mainly their manufacturers) claim. They are particularly useful as vasodilatory drugs, as in hypertensive patients with peripheral vascular disease who may be made worse by β-blockers (Roberts et al.: *Lancet* 2:650–653, 1987).

A proper comparison of drugs from all seven classes for the two main characteristics that are needed from an antihypertensive drug—long-term protection from all cardiovascular complications and little interference with the quality of life—has not been done and likely will never be done. However, short-term comparisons have been made as to their efficacy, and they all come out pretty much the same.—N.M. Kaplan, M.D.

Comparison of Nifedipine, Prazosin and Hydralazine Added to Treatment of Hypertensive Patients Uncontrolled by Thiazide Diuretic Plus Beta-Blocker

L.E. Ramsay, L. Parnell, and P.C. Waller (Royal Hallamshire Hosp., Sheffield, England)

Postgrad. Med. J. 63:99–103, February 1987 6–39

In the 10% to 30% of patients who fail to respond adequately to two drugs, a third will be needed to control the blood pressure. Some third-line drugs have been shown to be ineffective or to produce unacceptable adverse effects. Nifedipine, prazosin, and hydralazine were compared as third-line drugs in 93 patients with hypertension uncontrolled by bendrofluazide, 5 mg, plus atenolol, 100 mg, administered daily in a 6-month open random parallel group trial.

Patients had supine blood pressure greater than 140 mm Hg systolic or 95 mm Hg diastolic at each of three visits during a 4-week run-in period. Thirty-one patients received nifedipine, up to 60 mg per day, 31 received prazosin up to 20 mg per day, and 31 received hydralazine, up to 200 mg per day. Treatment was stopped because of side effects in 29% of patients: 8 from nifedipine, 7 from prazosin, and 12 from hydralazine. Changes in supine blood pressure did not differ significantly among the three drugs. Target blood pressure was attained at 6 months by 52% of the patients receiving nifedipine, 45% receiving prazosin, and 33% receiving hydralazine. The effect on serum biochemical variables did not significantly differ among the three drugs. Headache, flushing, and edema were common with nifedipine, tiredness and drowsiness with prazosin, and headache with hydralazine.

Antihypertensive effect, withdrawal rate, total number of side effects, and effect on serum biochemical variables were similar for nifedipine, prazosin, and hydralazine. The pattern of adverse effects differed. It is concluded that nifedipine is an acceptable third-line antihypertensive drug that may have some advantage over hydralazine and prazosin.

▶ Most trials simply comparing two drugs of different classes turn out to show them as equally effective. This study compared three different vasodilatory drugs as the third drug in patients not adequately controlled by a diuretic and a β-blocker. Other trials have shown that calcium entry blocker (e.g., nifedipine) and ACE inhibitors (e.g., captopril) are equally effective as third drugs (Potter and Beevers: *J. Clin. Pharmacol.* 27:410–414, 1987).

In patients who are in serious trouble with very high blood pressure, one or another rapidly acting drug is needed. Oral nifedipine has become quite popular and, as might be expected, cases of tissue hypoperfusion have appeared (O'Mailia et al.: *Ann. Intern. Med.* 107:185–186, 1987). Other choices include sublingual isosorbide and intravenous labetalol.—N.M. Kaplan, M.D.

The Use of Isosorbide in the Treatment of Severe, Uncontrolled Hypertension

Héctor Fontanet, Juan C. García, Juan Del Río, Manuel Martínez-Maldonado (Univ. of Puerto Rico and the VA Hosp., San Juan)

Arch. Intern. Med. 147:426–428, March 1987 6–40

In this double-blind, randomized study the safety and effectiveness of sublingual isosorbide dinitrate was compared to that of placebo and to conventional antihypertensive therapy. Twenty-five severe arterial hypertension patients with diastolic blood pressure (DBP) above 120 mm Hg were enrolled.

Of 11 who received isosorbide dinitrate, 10 mg, blood pressure (BP) dropped from 205/131 to 166/106 mm Hg at 120 minutes. Mean BP drop in the 8 receiving placebo was 203/130 to 193/122 mm Hg at 120 minutes; the BP dropped to 161/105 mm Hg 120 minutes after this group received sublingual isosorbide. Two hours after the single dose of isosorbide, the patients were given standard antihypertensive drug therapy. Of these 19 patients, 9 had achieved steady BP control at 24 hours, whereas 5 of the 6 control patients who received only conventional therapy were under good control at 24 hours. It appears that sublingual isosorbide safely and effectively lowers systolic BP and DBP in patients with severe uncontrolled arterial hypertension without obvious complications. Nevertheless, use of the isosorbide does not appear to offer any clear-cut advantages over standard oral treatment.

Intravenous Labetalol for Treatment of Postoperative Hypertension

John B. Leslie, Robert W. Kalayjian, Mark A. Sirgo, John R. Plachetka, and W. David Watkins (Duke Univ. and Glaxo Inc., Research Triangle Park, N.C.)

Anesthesiology 67:413–416, September 1987 6–41

Postoperative hypertension may be related to increased levels of circulating catecholamines, and it requires urgent treatment. The use of labetalol, an α- and β-receptor blocker, in controlling acute postoperative hypertension was evaluated in 15 patients who were hypertensive after receiving general anesthesia. Labetalol was given intravenously if the systolic pressure was 170 mm Hg or higher or if the diastolic pressure was 100 mm Hg for longer than 10 minutes, without apparent inciting factors. The initial dose was 0.25 mg/kg in 2 minutes and the maximum dose was 1.5 mg/kg over 40 minutes.

One patient required only the initial dose of labetalol and 8 required more than two doses. The average dose was 1.4 mg/kg. Pressures remained under control 4 hours after treatment with labetalol. No untoward effects of the treatment were observed.

When labetalol is given in a step-wise manner, it is a safe and effective means of controlling acute postoperative hypertension. None of the present patients had adverse side effects, such as may occur after the use of α- or β-adrenergic blocking agents.

▶ I doubt that isosorbide offers much, (Abstract 6–40) but IV labetalol seems to be an excellent choice for those needing quick reduction in blood pressure but not needing IV nitroprusside, with the attendant requirement that blood pressure be constantly monitored.

Hypertension after coronary artery bypass surgery is common, likely caused by a massive catecholamine surge. The short-acting IV β-blocker esmolol may be a particularly good way to treat this type of hypertension (Gray et al.: *Am. J. Cardiol.* 59:887–891, 1987).

Hypertension after carotid endarterectomy is also common and may be severe. It likely reflects preexisting interference with cerebral autoregulation and should also be treated aggressively (Skydell et al.: *Arch. Surg.* 122:1153–1155,

1987). Caution is advised against the use of hydralazine and other drugs that may reflexly increase cardiac output and thereby cerebral perfusion (Abstract 6–39).—N.M. Kaplan, M.D.

Treatment of the Elderly

▶ ↓ As more and more people live longer, the number of elderly hypertensive persons will continue to expand since about half of people older than 65 have either combined systolic and diastolic hypertension or isolated systolic hypertension (ISH). All of these people are at increased risk for cardiovascular catastrophes, particularly stroke. However, at least for those with ISH, much of that risk may reflect underlying atherosclerosis, hypertension being more of an innocent bystander rather than an active participant.

Not only are we unsure of the dangers posed by ISH in the elderly, we are also uncertain about the ability of antihypertensive therapy to reduce those dangers. A proper placebo-controlled trial, the Systolic Hypertension in the Elderly Program (SHEP), is under way using a low dose of the diuretic, chlorthalidone, as first therapy. Preliminary results from a pilot study of 551 patients are encouraging: after an average of 34 months, more than 80% are still enrolled, side effects have been relatively infrequent, compliance has been excellent, and those receiving therapy have shown a greater fall in blood pressure than those taking placebo–but there has been no difference in complication rates (Perry et al.: *J. Hypertens.* 4(suppl.6):S21–S23, 1986).

Obviously, we must await the completion of the full study to reach any conclusions. In the next 5 years or so, until the results are in, there will likely be a slow but steady increase in the active therapy of elderly hypertensives with drugs. On the basis of fairly good evidence, such therapy can be justified for the elderly with diastolic hypertension (Davidson and Caranasos: *Arch. Intern. Med.* 147:1933–1937, 1987). Although the evidence for benefit is not available for the elderly with ISH, I believe any person with a systolic blood pressure above 170 who has a reasonable life expectancy at any age deserves to be gently and gradually treated to bring the systolic blood pressure below 160.

The next two abstracts provide some general guidelines and specific evidence about such therapy.—N.M. Kaplan, M.D.

An Approach to Limiting the Adverse Effects of Therapy for Hypertension in the Elderly

Martin J. Bass (Univ. of Western Ontario)
Can. Fam. Physician 33:213–216, January 1987 6–42

Elevated blood pressure (BP) and medication side effects are common in patients older than 65 years. The benefits and side effects of drug treatment for high BP in the elderly must be considered carefully.

To determine whether an elderly patient really has high BP, a cuff appropriate to the arm size must be used, more than one reading should be taken as the basis for diagnosis, and the possibility of the presence of stiff brachial arteries, which would falsely elevate BP readings, should be considered. It is crucial to know which elderly patients will benefit from hypotensive therapy. Treatment is recommended for patients 65–74 years old if the diastolic BP is 100 mm Hg or above, and treatment may be of value if the systolic BP is greater than 200 mm Hg. If associated problems exist, treatment is recommended or may be of value for that age group if the diastolic BP is 90 mm Hg or above and the systolic BP is 180 mm Hg or above. For persons older than 75 years, treatment is recommended only if the diastolic BP is greater than 120 mm Hg. For those with target-organ involvement, treatment of BPs above 180/100 mm Hg may be beneficial.

Thiazide is generally considered the optimal drug to begin therapy; the dose should be no more than half that used for middle-aged patients. The optimal starting dose of hydrochlorothiazide is 12.5 mg once a day. Many researchers believe that dosages above 25 mg a day produce many more side effects and confer little extra hypotensive effect.

Careful monitoring of elderly hypertensive patients is essential, also important is the patient's role in selecting therapy; decisions should be made jointly by a knowledgeable physician and an informed patient.

▶ Dr. Bass and the Canadian Consensus Conference on Hypertension in the Elderly (*Can. Med. Assoc. J.* 135:741–745, 1986) are more conservative than I would be, certainly in regard to limiting treatment to those older than 75 years to those with diastolic blood pressure above 120 mm Hg. The longer I live, the more bothered I am with the arbitrary placement of age limits for anything. If a patient is 95 years old but in reasonably good overall condition so that there is a good chance she'll (it's much more likely that the patient will be a woman) be around at 100, I would unquestionably offer antihypertensive therapy if the diastolic BP is above 105 mm Hg and maybe even 100.—N.M. Kaplan, M.D.

Systemic Systolic Hypertension in the Elderly: Correlation of Hemodynamics, Plasma Volume, Renin, Aldosterone, Urinary Metanephrines and Response to Thiazide Therapy

Suman Vardan, Milton H. Dunsky, Norma E. Hill, Saktipada Mookherjee, Harold Smulyan, and Robert A. Warner (State Univ. of New York, Syracuse)
Am. J. Cardiol. 58:1030–1034, November 1986 6–43

Systolic hypertension in the elderly is associated with increased mortality and morbidity. Its pathogenesis remains unclear. A study was done to clarify the relation of the hemodynamics of systolic hypertension to plasma volume, plasma renin, and aldosterone levels, and 24-hour urinary metanephrine excretion and to investigate the effect of thiazide diuretic therapy on these variables.

Twenty-four men (mean age, 63 ± 1.7 years) with systemic systolic hypertension were assessed before and after 1 month of therapy with oral hydrochlorothiazide, 50 mg/day. Before therapy, the mean plasma volume was 2,664 ± 96 ml, the CI was 3.9 ± 0.2 L/minute/sq m, the stroke volume index was 52 ± 2 ml/beat/sq m, the systemic vascular resistance was 1,351 ± 80 dynes s cm^{-5}, the plasma aldosterone concentration was 8.6 ± 1 ng/dl, and the 24-hour urinary excretion of metanephrines was 0.371 ± 0.044 mg. After renin-sodium profiling of 23 subjects, 12 were classified as normal, and 11 as having low renin values. None had high renin values. Multiple regression analysis showed that systolic blood pressure correlated most closely to the 24-hour urinary excretion of total metanephrines, explaining 28% of the variability in systolic blood pressure (BP). Systolic and diastolic BPs decreased after 1 month of hydrochlorothiazide therapy (50 mg per day), with concomitant reduction in systemic vascular resistance. Patients with either normal or low renin values had normal plasma volume and responded similarly to thiazide diuretic therapy without symptomatic side effects.

This study confirms previous hemodynamic observations in patients with systolic hypertension. Average direct intra-arterial diastolic BP was normal, whereas the mean values of cardiac output and stroke volume were elevated. In most patients, the systemic vascular resistance was higher in relation to cardiac output. After therapy, 90% had a decrease in systolic BP of more than 10 mm Hg. No adverse effects were seen in the 1-month follow-up period.

▶ This article and a follow-up after a year of therapy (Vardan et al.: *Am. J. Cardiol.* 60:388–390, 1987) provide excellent data on the baseline hemodynamics and hormonal levels of elderly patients with ISH and the effects of diuretic therapy on these measurements.

The relatively large dose of hydrochlorothiazide (HCT) provided excellent antihypertensive effect with appropriate hemodynamic changes and few side effects. After a full year, the effects were well maintained, still with no difference between the low or normal renin subgroups.

Diuretics in low doses, i.e., 12.5–25 mg of HCT, are widely believed to be the easiest drugs to use in the elderly. I believe they should be given with a potassium-sparer, since hypokalemia can be a problem in the elderly as in the younger. Myers (*Arch. Intern. Med.* 147:1026–1030, 1987) reported results of a study with HCT with or without amiloride, showing that the combination was well tolerated and largely prevented hypokalemia.

Other drugs can be effectively and safely used. Calcium entry blockers may be particularly effective in the elderly and, even though renin levels tend to be low in elderly hypertensives, ACE inhibitors as monotherapy appear to work very well among them (Woo et al.: *Arch. Intern. Med.* 147:1386–1389, 1987).—N.M. Kaplan, M.D.

Secondary Forms of Hypertension

▶ ↓ At all ages, secondary forms of hypertension are relatively infrequent. The next abstract provides excellent data on the frequency of these forms, and the following four abstracts cover some new findings about the two most common secondary causes, renal parenchymal and renal vascular diseases.—N.M. Kaplan, M.D.

Secondary Hypertension in a Blood Pressure Clinic

Anne Marie Sinclair, Christopher G. Isles, Irene Brown, Helen Cameron, Gordon D. Murray, and James W.K. Robertson (Western Infirmary, Glasgow, Scotland)

Arch. Intern. Med. 147:1289–1293, July 1987 6–44

A search for underlying causes of hypertension is justified if the hypertension is cured when the cause is removed. Another reason for searching is to identify patients who may be at risk of the complications of hypertension. To examine the relative importance of these goals, the prevalence, reversibility, and mortality of secondary hypertension were assessed among 3,783 patients, aged 25–84 years, with moderately severe nonmalignant hypertension, who attended the Glasgow (Scotland) Blood Pressure Clinic. Patients were judged to be cured when blood pressure fell to less than 140/90 mm Hg without treatment or improved when a fall of greater than 20/10 mm Hg was achieved with the same treatment or less.

Underlying causes of hypertension were uncommon, being present in only 297 patients (7.9%). A potentially reversible cause of hypertension was evident in 87 patients (2.3%), including the oral contraceptive pill in 38 patients, renovascular disease in 27 patients, and primary hyperaldosteronism in 10 patients. Only 33 patients (0.9%) were cured by specific intervention, mostly those who stopped taking oral contraceptive pills (Fig 6–6). The most common underlying cause of hypertension was renal parenchymal disease, which was present in 210 patients (5.6%). These patients had significantly higher mortality than men and women with other causes of hypertension.

The excess death was attributed to renal failure and vascular causes but not to cancer or other nonvascular diseases, and the most common cause of death was ischemic heart disease followed by stroke. There was no significant risk of death among patients with minor urographic abnormalities, provided renal function was normal.

Investigation of hypertension for an underlying cause will reveal a small number of patients with treatable causes and a moderate number of patients with irreversible renal disease who are at particularly high risk

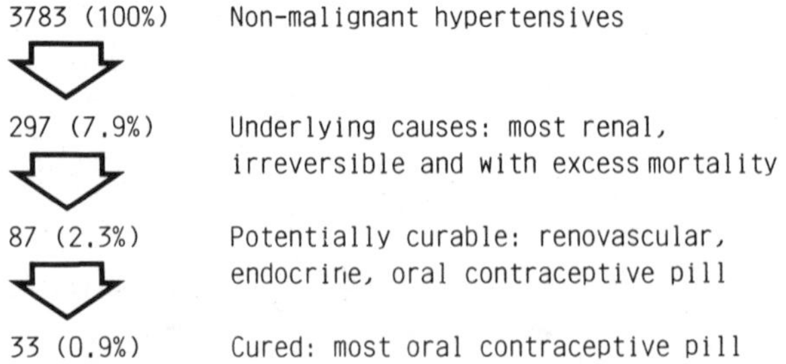

3783 (100%) Non-malignant hypertensives

297 (7.9%) Underlying causes: most renal, irreversible and with excess mortality

87 (2.3%) Potentially curable: renovascular, endocrine, oral contraceptive pill

33 (0.9%) Cured: most oral contraceptive pill

Fig 6–6.—Investigation of hypertension for underlying cause revealed moderate number of patients at high risk with disease that was irreversible, and small number with treatable causes, of whom few were cured by specific intervention. (Courtesy of Sinclair, A.M., et al.: Arch. Intern. Med. 147:1289–1293, July 1987.)

from heart attack and stroke. Attention should therefore be directed toward reducing cardiovascular risk in hypertensive patients with renal disease.

▶ This large group of patients with nonmalignant hypertension is not truly representative of the usual population of patients dealt with by most clinicians. They were referred to a special clinic, likely because many were difficult to treat or because they had suggestive features of a secondary cause. Their blood pressures were fairly high, averaging 183/110 mm Hg at entry.

Nonetheless, even among this population who should have a higher frequency, the findings of a fairly complete evaluation, as shown in Figure 6–7, confirm the relative rarity of secondary forms and the even greater rarity of potentially and actually curable causes. Fortunately, it takes no more than a good history, physical examination, and simple laboratory data to rule out most of these. The only one that is not fairly obvious is renovascular disease, but the search for it may now be much easier.—N.M. Kaplan, M.D.

Renovascular Hypertension Identified by Captopril-Induced Changes in the Renogram

Gijsbert G. Geyskes, Hong Y. Oei, Carl B.A.J. Puylaert, and Evert J. Dorhout Mees (Univ. Hosp., Utrecht, The Netherlands)

Hypertension 9:451–458, May 1987 6–45

Recent studies have shown that a kidney with renal artery stenosis may have impaired excretory function during converting enzyme inhibition (CEI). However, this impairment is detected by physicians only in patients without a normal kidney, because as long as one healthy kidney remains, it maintains the overall glomerular filtration rate and diuresis. A study was done to determine whether a unilateral change in renal function induced by CEI can be detected by radioisotope renography in patients with renovascular hypertension caused by unilateral renal artery stenosis.

Radioisotope renography was performed in 21 hypertensive patients with unilateral renal artery stenosis with and without premedication with 25 mg of captopril. The results were compared with the effect of percutaneous transluminal angioplasty on blood pressure (BP), evaluated 6 weeks after angioplasty. In 15 patients, angioplasty caused a considerable decrease in BP. Of these, captopril induced changes in the time-activity curves of the affected kidney only in 12 patients, suggesting deterioration of the excretory function of that kidney, while the function of the contralateral kidney remained normal.

After angioplasty, the asymmetry in the time-activity curves decreased, despite identical premedication with captopril. Such captopril-induced unilateral impairment of renal function was not observed in the 6 patients whose BP did not change after percutaneous transluminal angioplasty or in 13 hypertensive patients with normal renal arteries. Renal impairment was characterized by a decrease in ^{99m}Tc-diethylenetriamine pentaacetic acid uptake and a delay in ^{131}I-hippurate excretion, while ^{131}I-hippurate uptake was unchanged.

In this study, a positive test result was seen in 12 of 15 patients with renovascular hypertension, as determined by the decline of BP after angioplasty, and a negative result was obtained in 13 patients with normal renal arteries and in all 6 patients with anatomical renal artery stenosis (which apparently was not causing the hypertension, since the BP remained high after adequate angioplasty). Thus, the specificity of this test was 100%.

▶ This article follows up on observations first published by Japanese investigators (Imai et al.: *Jpn. Heart J.* 21:793–802, 1980) and amplified by Muller and coworkers (*Am. J. Med.* 80:633–643, 1986) at John Laragh's unit in New York. Clearly, the ischemic kidney responds to removal of the high levels of angiotensin that are maintaining its blood flow by a further increase in renin release, which presumably reflects a marked decrease in perfusion.

The initial captopril test simply measured peripheral blood plasma renin activity. The addition of radioisotopic renography before and after captopril administration almost certainly adds to the diagnostic accuracy of the procedure. Others have confirmed these results (Fommei et al.: *Hypertension* 10:212–220, 1987), so that I believe when there is a need to rule out renovascular hypertension, a combined captopril test, measuring both peripheral blood PRA and isotopic uptake before and after the drug, is a logical choice.

However, if the diagnosis seems more likely or if there is a strong need to be certain (as with any patient with malignant hypertension), I would still do a renal arteriogram as my first test.

Once the diagnosis is made, therapy must be provided, and there are three choices. For most, surgery is the best.—N.M. Kaplan, M.D.

Surgical Treatment of Renovascular Hypertension Caused by Arteriosclerosis: I. Influence of Preoperative Factors on Blood Pressure Control Early and Late After Reconstructive Surgery

Johan H. van Bockel, Reinout van Schilfgaarde, Willem Felthuis, Jo Hermans, Peter van Bremmelen, and Johan L. Terpstra (Univ. Hosp. Leiden, Leiden, The Netherlands)

Surgery 101:698–705, June 1987 6–46

There is some controversy about the efficacy of surgical treatment for renovascular hypertension caused by arteriosclerosis. Research has yielded conflicting results. A study was done to evaluate the long-term efficacy of such surgery.

Reconstructive surgery was performed in 1959–1983 on 112 patients with renovascular hypertension caused by arteriosclerosis. The patients, with a median age of 49 years, had persistent hypertension despite medical treatment. Their mean blood pressure was 188/113 mm Hg, and the mean duration of objectively documented hypertension was 21 months at the time of surgery. Manifestations of extrarenal arteriosclerosis (ERA) were seen in 57 patients (51%). The results of surgery were assessed at a mean of 8.4 months and a mean of 8.9 years after the operation. Patients were classified as cured, improved, or unsuccessfully treated, as determined by blood pressure response.

At the long-term follow-up, 18% were classified as cured and 61% as improved. At short-term follow-up, 24% were classified as cured and 50% as improved. The results were not affected by patient age or the presence of ERA. The only pertinent clinical feature influencing long-term results was the preoperative duration of hypertension: long-term beneficial responses were observed in 95% of the patients with a duration shorter than the median and in 78% of those with a duration longer than the media.

Surgical therapy for renovascular hypertension caused by arteriosclerosis can effectively reduce blood pressure, and this result can be maintained on a long-term basis. Older age, longer duration of hypertension, and the presence of ERA do not exclude surgical treatment.

▶ Long-term medical therapy is possible for those who cannot or will not have angioplasty or surgery, but there is obviously a danger of progressive loss of function of the ischemic kidney, particularly when the most effective drug, an ACE inhibitor, is used (Wenting et al.: *Kidney Int.* 31(suppl. 20):S180–S183, 1987).

Angioplasty is probably the best choice for older patients, or for any who would have a particularly tough time with surgery. But it is likely not going to provide long-term relief. Surgery is probably the best choice for most patients, even the elderly (Vidt: *Geriatrics* 42:59–70, 1987). But, as this article documents, the diagnosis should be made as early as possible to provide the best chance for relief. That is why more widespread use of the captopril test and renal arteriography *in selected patients* should be encouraged.

The most common form of secondary hypertension, much more common than renovascular disease, is renal parenchymal disease. The diagnosis is easy—a serum creatinine evaluation is all it takes. But the therapy has often come down to the terribly difficult and expensive management of end stage renal disease (ESRD): dialysis and transplantation. There is a rising feeling that we can do better, mainly because of the awareness that hyperperfusion and hypertension in the remaining glomeruli may be the underlying mechanism for progressive loss of renal function, and the hope that ACE inhibitors will provide better reduction of glomerular pressure than other agents.

The largest group of patients vulnerable to progressive nephropathy are diabetics, and it is among them that the most exciting work has been done.—N.M. Kaplan, M.D.

Effect of Antihypertensive Treatment on Kidney Function in Diabetic Nephropathy

Hans-Henrik Parving, Allan R. Andersen, Ulla M. Smidt, Eva Hommel, Elisabeth R. Mathiesen, and Per A. Svendsen (Hvidöre Hosp., Klampenborg, Bispebjerg Hosp., Steno Mem. Hosp., Gentofte, Denmark)

Br. Med. J. 294:1443–1447, June 6, 1987 6–47

About 40% of insulin-dependent diabetic patients develop persistent proteinuria, a decline in glomerular filtration rate. This clinical syndrome is known as diabetic nephropathy. Mortality in insulin-dependent diabetic patients with persistent proteinuria has been shown to be much higher than in diabetic patients without proteinuria. Renal failure is the primary cause of death in insulin-dependent diabetics with nephropathy. A prospective study was done to determine the initial clinical course of diabetic nephropathy and to assess the long-term effect of aggressive treatment of increased blood pressure on glomerular filtration rates and albuminuria in patients with insulin dependent diabetes and diabetic nephropathy.

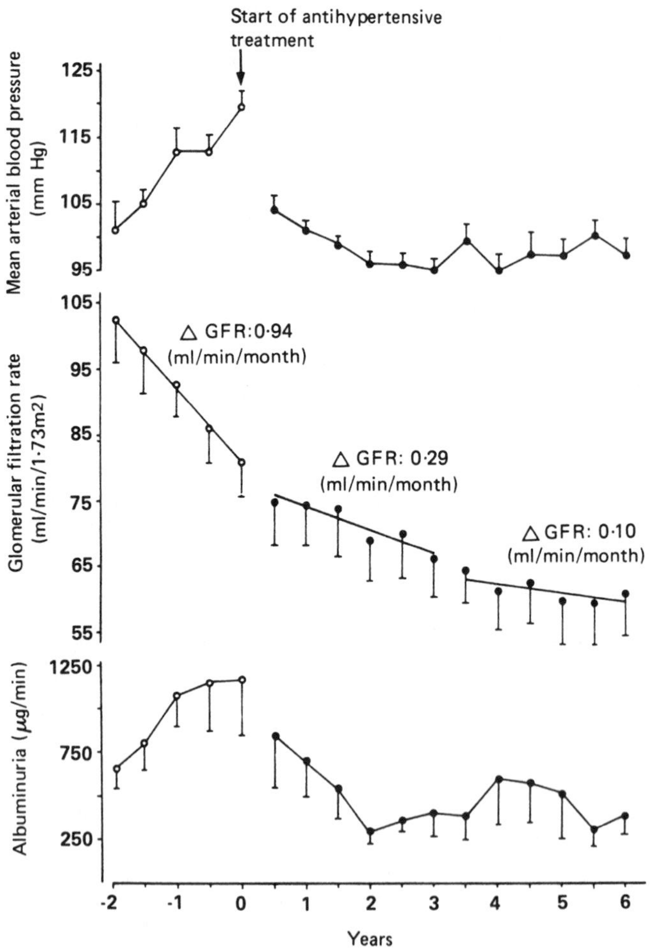

Fig 6–7.—Average course of mean arterial blood pressure, glomerular filtration rate, and albuminuria before *(open circles)* and during *(solid circles)* long-term effective antihypertensive treatment of nine insulin dependent diabetic patients who had nephropathy. (Courtesy of Parving, H.H., et al.: Br. Med. J. 294:1443–1447, June 6, 1987.)

Eleven patients, with a mean age of 30 years, were studied. Antihypertensive treatment was started after a control period of at least 23 months if repeated measurements showed a diastolic blood pressure of 100 mm Hg or more or if the patient had a sustained diastolic blood pressure of 90 mm Hg or greater preceded by an increase in mean arterial blood pressure of 10 mm Hg or more during the past 2 years. Metoprolol, hydralazine, and frusemide or thiazide were given as antihypertensive agents. During the mean pretreatment period of 32 months, the glomerular filtration rate decreased significantly and albuminuria and the arterial blood pressure increased significantly. During the mean 72-month period of antihypertensive treatment, the average arterial blood pressure dropped from 143/96 mm Hg to 129/84 mm Hg (Fig 6–7). Albuminuria decreased from 1,038 μg per minute to 504 μ per minute.

The rate of decline of the glomerular filtration rate dropped from 0.89 ml per minute per month before antihypertensive treatment to 0.22 ml per minute per month during treatment. The rate of decline of the glomerular filtration rate was found to be significantly lower during the second 3 years compared with the first 3 years in patients receiving long-term antihypertensive therapy. One patient, with a glomerular filtration rate of 46 ml per minute per 1.74 sq m, died of an acute myocardial infarction.

Long-term, aggressive antihypertensive therapy induces a progressive reduction in the rate of decline in kidney function and thus postpones renal insufficiency in insulin-dependent diabetic patients with diabetic nephropathy.

▶ Figure 6–7 represents a historic happening: the long-term protection of renal function in patients with diabetic nephropathy. Note that it was obtained with traditional antihypertensive therapy. Whether ACE inhibitors will do better remains to be seen, although equally promising results over shorter intervals with these drugs have been found in both normotensive (Marre et al.: *Br. Med. J.* 294:1448–1452, 1987) and hypertensive (Hommel et al.: *Br. Med. J.* 293:467–470, 1986) patients with diabetic nephropathy.

This is obviously a hot area of clinical research. The promise of stopping what has become the leading cause of death type I diabetes is exciting.

Hypertension occurs with other forms of renal parenchymal disease that may be even easier to treat.—N.M. Kaplan, M.D.

Reversible Hypertension Associated With Unrecognized High Pressure Chronic Retention of Urine

D.A. Jones, N.J.R. George, P.H. O'Reilly, and R.J. Barnard (Univ. Hospital of South Manchester, Stepping Hill Hospital, Stockport, England)

Lancet 1:1052–1054, May 9, 1987 6–48

Patients with high pressure chronic retention of urine are a homogeneous group with clinical features suggesting circulatory overload. The cardiovascular effects of relief of obstruction were studied prospectively in 21 men with high pressure chronic retention and hydroephrosis and hydroureter associated with hypertension, severe peripheral edema, raised jugular venous pressure, or clinical evidence of pulmonary edema.

The 21 patients, aged 34–87 years, had high pressure chronic retention diagnosed by standard clinical and radiologic techniques. All had a tense, painless, palpable bladder. Nineteen underwent intravenous urography, which showed bilateral hydroureter and hydronephrosis. Eleven had hypertension, 8 had peripheral pitting edema, 5 had raised jugular venous pressure, and 5 had clinical evidence of pulmonary edema. Bladder drainage by urethral catheterization resulted in weight loss in 17 patients and blood pressure reduction in all of the hypertensive patients. Postdrainage supine diastolic pressure ranged from 70–100 mm Hg, compared with 95–120 mm Hg before drainage.

All other abnormal cardiovascular signs noted before drainage returned to normal within 3 days after drainage, except for minor residual ankle edema in 2 patients and some pulmonary crepitations in another 2. Cardiovascular responses were associated with a significant increase in urinary volume, 3.112 L/24 hours; absolute sodium excretion, 234 mmole/24 hours; and fractional sodium excretion, 2.8%.

Hypertension related to chronic urinary tract obstruction may be the most common form of surgically correctable renal hypertension. Patients with high pressure chronic retention usually do not have typical prostatic symptoms and will be missed by casual clinical inquiry. Hydronephrosis and painless bladder distension had not previously been suspected in 24% of the patients in this series who were referred for control of cardiovascular symptoms that did not respond to first-line therapy.

▶ I find this, too, exciting: the prospect of relieving hypertension along with urinary tract obstruction. Prostatic hypertrophy is a common problem in older men and its relief may help them in multiple ways.

Interestingly, even unilateral hydronephrosis may occasionally cause hypertension that may be cured after relief of the obstruction (Wanner et al.: *Nephrology* 45:236–241, 1987).—N.M. Kaplan, M.D.

Hypertension With the Pill and Pregnancy

▶ ↓ Among young women, hypertension is not infrequently caused by use of estrogen-containing oral contraceptives, but the number of women whose health is better for using the pill far outweighs the number whose health is made worse. The largest growing group of women who are taking estrogens are the postmenopausal, in whom estrogen replacement therapy clearly protects against osteoporosis and probably coronary disease. Fortunately, estrogen given as replacement therapy will not cause hypertension and may even protect against it.—N.M. Kaplan, M.D.

The Long-Term Effect of Oral and Percutaneous Estradiol on Plasma Renin Substrate and Blood Pressure

C. Hassager, B.J. Riis, V. Strøm, T.T. Guyene, and C. Christiansen (Univ. of Copenhagen, Glostrup Hosp., Glostrup, Denmark, and Hôpital Broussais, Paris)
Circulation 76:753–758, October 1987 6–49

Oral estrogen replacement therapy affects liver metabolism, causing changes in plasma renin substrate and plasma lipoprotein levels, which in turn may increase the risk of hypertension and thromboembolic disease. Although percutaneous estrogen administration avoids the first-pass liver effect, the early results of an ongoing long-term study have demonstrated that after 6 months of percutaneous estrogen therapy, measurable changes in serum lipoproteins do occur. A 2-year placebo-controlled study examined the long-term effect of percutaneous and oral estradiol administration on blood pressure and plasma renin substrate.

The study population comprised 110 early postmenopausal women who were allocated to treatment with either oral cyclical estradiol valerate and cyproterone acetate, oral placebo, percutaneous 17β-estradiol supplemented by oral progesterone during the second year of the study, or percutaneous placebo cream.

Systolic and diastolic blood pressures remained unchanged in both drug-treated groups, but diastolic blood pressure tended to increase in both placebo-treated groups. Plasma renin substrate levels increased during oral estradiol administration, but remained unchanged with percutaneous estradiol treatment. No correlation was observed between blood pressure and plasma renin substrate concentrations. Estrone and estradiol serum levels continued to increase after 3 months of percutaneous estradiol treatment, but reached a plateau at 6 months of treatment. The addition of cyclical oral progesterone to the percutaneous estradiol regimen during the second year did not alter any of the measured variables.

Both oral and percutaneous estradiol therapy may protect women against the age-related increase in diastolic blood pressure observed during the early postmenopausal years. However, the metabolic steady state is not attained until after 3 months of estradiol administration.

▶ This is the best study now available on the effects of estrogen replacement therapy on blood pressure. The news is good: if anything, diastolic pressures fell in those on estrogen compared to those given a placebo. The news is particularly good for percutaneous estrogen, which will likely become the most popular way to give postmenopausal replacement. The addition of progesterone, generally advocated to reduce the likelihood of endometrial cancer, had no adverse effects on either the blood pressure or the renin system.

In younger women who do not take the pill, pregnancy-induced hypertension remains a problem.—N.M. Kaplan, M.D.

Treatment of Cardiovascular Diseases

Kennedy R. Lees and Peter C. Rubin (Stobhill Gen. Hosp., Glasgow, Scotland)
Br. Med. J. 294:358–360, Feb. 7, 1987 6–50

The risks of maternal hypertension during pregnancy are well known, but pharmacologic intervention with antihypertensive or antiarrhythmic agents remains controversial. Some limited studies suggest that treatment of chronic hypertension and pregnancy-induced hypertension is beneficial to the fetus. In one study of the data on 247 women, nine miscarriages or perinatal deaths occurred in the nontreated group, while only one occurred in the treated group. In another group of treated women with pregnancy-induced hypertension, a reduction in maternal blood pressure and neonatal morbidity was observed when compared with a control group. Recommendations on blood pressure levels warranting treatment are controversial; the authors' policy is to treat chronic hypertension at a pressure above 140/90 mm Hg after the first trimester and to treat pregnancy-induced hypertension if systolic or diastolic pressures increase by 30 mm Hg or 15 mm Hg, respectively.

Methyldopa and β-blocking agents are effective antihypertensive medications in pregnancy. Adverse effects such as sedation, depression, and postural hypotension may necessitate discontinuation of methyldopa in 15% of women; however, it has a good safety record. There have been a few reports of fetal abnormalities after β-blocker use, but these must be viewed in the light of the incidence of deformities. Hydralazine should be used as second-line treatment if necessary. The use of loop diuretics as second-line therapy appears to be safe for treatment of cardiac failure in pregnancy. A recent review of thiazide use in pregnancy concluded that there was no evidence of a deleterious effect. However, in preeclampsia, intravascular volume depletion occurs, and further depletion by diuretics may have a critical effect on the comprised uteroplacental blood flow. Therefore, diuretics are generally not used in pregnancy.

Diazoxide has some adverse effects on the fetus and should be reserved for use in intrapartum emergencies. There is little information on the use of sodium nitroprusside in hypertensive emergencies in pregnant women. In small numbers of patients, short-term use has been satisfactory. It is the drug of choice for treating hypertensive emergencies and eclampsia when blood pressure can be accurately and continuously monitored.

▶ This brief review says most everything needed about proper management of pregnancy-induced hypertension (PIH). Obstetricians are appropriately cautious about changing accepted practices, particularly since drug trials are virtually impossible during pregnancy. But the dependency on methyldopa and hydralazine seems to be slowly eroding, with greater use of β-blockers and the combined alpha-beta blocker labetalol (Rasmussen: *Dan. Med. Bull.* 34:170–172, 1987). Calcium entry blockers have attractive features for use in pregnancy (Lawrence and Broughton Pipkin: *Br. J. Clin. Pharmacol.* 23:683–692, 1987).

As for hypertension in general, prevention would be preferable. Interest continues about the apparent deficiency of prostacyclin that may somehow be casual (Soares de Moura: *Br. J. Clin. Pharmacol.* 23:765–768, 1987).

True pregnancy-induced hypertension (preeclampsia) may, in fact, be quite rare. Of 84 women with presumed PIH that appeared before 37 weeks' gestation, renal abnormalities were found in 65% (Ihle et al.: *Br. Med. J.* 294:79–81,

1987). The authors believe that true, self-limited, idiopathic PIH is the diagnosis only in about 10% of primiparas who develop hypertension before week 37 but in more than 75% of cases developing after that time.—N.M. Kaplan, M.D.

Concluding Comments

▶ A lot more has happened during the past year in clinical hypertension than can be covered here, but these are certainly most of the highlights. A few additional points are worth noting:

- A mini-epidemic of misdiagnosed pheochromocytoma is being seen because labetalol gives rise to falsely elevated urinary excretion of both metanephrines and catecholamines (Feldman: *J. Clin. Pharmacol.* 27:288–292, 1987). If you're suspicious of a pheo, either stop the labetalol or measure urinary VMA or plasma catechols.
- Cyclosporine, being widely used with transplants and various autoimmune diseases, frequently causes hypertension as well as renal dysfunction (Bantle et al.: *Am. J. Med.* 83:59–64, 1987). The blood pressure may be difficult to bring down.
- Over-the-counter diet pills and decongestants often contain the sympathomimetic agent, phenylpropanolamine, which may raise the blood pressure considerably, particularly in those with autonomic nervous impairment (Biaggioni et al.: *JAMA* 258:236–239, 1987).—N.M. Kaplan, M.D.

Subject Index

A

D

K

L

M

N

O

P

R

T

W

X

Author Index

A

B

C

D

E

F

M

N